AUTISM SPECTRUM DISORDERS
IN ADOLESCENTS AND ADULTS

Autism Spectrum Disorders in Adolescents and Adults

EVIDENCE-BASED AND PROMISING INTERVENTIONS

Edited by

Matt Tincani
Andy Bondy

THE GUILFORD PRESS
New York   London

© 2014 The Guilford Press
A Division of Guilford Publications, Inc.
370 Seventh Avenue, Suite 1200, New York, NY 10001
www.guilford.com

Paperback edition 2016

Printed in the United States of America

This book is printed on acid-free paper.

Last digit is print number: 9 8 7 6 5 4

The authors have checked with sources believed to be reliable in their efforts to provide information that is complete and generally in accord with the standards of practice that are accepted at the time of publication. However, in view of the possibility of human error or changes in behavioral, mental health, or medical sciences, neither the authors, nor the editors and publisher, nor any other party who has been involved in the preparation or publication of this work warrants that the information contained herein is in every respect accurate or complete, and they are not responsible for any errors or omissions or the results obtained from the use of such information. Readers are encouraged to confirm the information contained in this book with other sources.

Library of Congress Cataloging-in-Publication Data

Autism spectrum disorders in adolescents and adults : evidence-based and promising interventions / edited by Matt Tincani, Andy Bondy.

    pages cm
    Includes bibliographical references and index.
    ISBN 978-1-4625-1717-6 (hardback)
    ISBN 978-1-4625-2615-4 (paperback)
    1. Autism spectrum disorders in children—Treatment. 2. Autism spectrum disorders—Treatment. I. Tincani, Matt. II. Bondy, Andy.
    RJ506.A9A92392 2014
    618.92′85882—dc23

                                                                2014006718

For Lisa, Colin, and Cash
—M. T.

To Lori, my wife and partner in so many ways
—A. B.

About the Editors

Matt Tincani, PhD, is Associate Professor of Special Education and Applied Behavior Analysis at Temple University, where he chairs the Department of Psychological, Organizational, and Leadership Studies in the College of Education. He has worked in the field of autism spectrum disorders (ASD) for over 20 years as a therapist, program supervisor, university teacher, and researcher. A Board Certified Behavior Analyst, he has developed several university-based programs to prepare professionals who support people with ASD and has held a variety of state and national leadership positions. Dr. Tincani is author or coauthor of dozens of articles, book chapters, and books featuring research and strategies to teach communication, socialization, academic, and self-help skills to people with ASD and other disabilities.

Andy Bondy, PhD, has over 40 years of experience working with children and adults with ASD and related developmental disabilities. For more than a dozen years he served as the director of a statewide public school program for students with autism. He and his wife, Lori Frost, pioneered the development of the Picture Exchange Communication System (PECS). Dr. Bondy designed the Pyramid Approach to Education as a comprehensive combination of broad-spectrum behavior analysis and functional communication strategies. Dr. Bondy is a cofounder of Pyramid Educational Consultants, Inc., in Newark, Delaware, and serves as Vice-Chair of the Board of Directors of the Cambridge Center for Behavioral Studies.

Contributors

Angelica Aguirre, MA, BCBA, Rehabilitation Institute, Southern Illinois University, Carbondale, Illinois

Ruth Aspy, PhD, The Ziggurat Group, Plano, Texas

Andy Bondy, PhD, Pyramid Educational Consultants, Inc., Newark, Delaware

Valerie Boyer, PhD, CCC-SLP, Rehabilitation Institute, Southern Illinois University, Carbondale, Illinois

Amarie Carnett, MEd, BCBA, Department of Educational Psychology and Pedagogy, Victoria University of Wellington, Wellington, New Zealand

Staci Carr, EdM, MS, VCU Autism Center for Excellence, Virginia Commonwealth University, Richmond, Virginia

Amy Bixler Coffin, MS, Ohio Center for Autism and Low Incidence, Westerville, Ohio

Phyllis Coyne, MS, private practice, Portland, Oregon

Shannon Crozier, PhD, Center for Autism Spectrum Disorders and Department of Educational and Clinical Studies, College of Education, University of Nevada, Las Vegas, Las Vegas, Nevada

Anthony Foglia, MA, The McCarton School, New York, New York

Beverly L. Frantz, PhD, Institute on Disabilities, Temple University, Philadelphia, Pennsylvania

Ann Fullerton, PhD, Department of Special Education, Graduate School of Education, Portland State University, Portland, Oregon

Maria Fernanda Garcia, BA, Teachers College, Columbia University, New York, New York

Peter F. Gerhardt, EdD, JPG Consultation Group, Montclair, New Jersey

Vanessa A. Green, PhD, School of Educational Psychology and Pedagogy, Victoria University of Wellington, Wellington, New Zealand

Barry G. Grossman, PhD, The Ziggurat Group, Plano, Texas

Sandra L. Harris, PhD, Douglass Developmental Disabilities Center, Rutgers, The State University of New Jersey, New Brunswick, New Jersey

Shawn A. Henry, MS, Ohio Center for Autism and Low Incidence, Columbus, Ohio

Giulio E. Lancioni, PhD, Department of Neuroscience and Sense Organs, University of Bari, Bari, Italy

Russell Lang, PhD, Department of Curriculum and Instruction, College of Education, Texas State University, San Marcos, Texas

Carol Markowitz, MA, MEd, Eden Autism Services, Princeton, New Jersey

Brenda Smith Myles, PhD, Ohio Center for Autism and Low Incidence, Westerville, Ohio; The Ziggurat Group, Plano, Texas

John O'Neill, MA, BCBA, Rehabilitation Institute, Southern Illinois University, Carbondale, Illinois

Mark F. O'Reilly, PhD, Department of Special Education, College of Education, University of Texas at Austin, Austin, Texas

Donna J. Owens, MA, Ohio Center for Autism and Low Incidence, Westerville, Ohio

Lauren Pepa, MS, Douglass Developmental Disabilities Center and Department of Clinical Psychology, Rutgers, The State University of New Jersey, New Brunswick, New Jersey

Cathy Pratt, PhD, BCBA-D, Indiana Resource Center on Autism, University of Indiana, Bloomington, Indiana

Ruth Anne Rehfeldt, PhD, BCBA-D, Rehabilitation Institute, Southern Illinois University, Carbondale, Illinois

Carol Schall, PhD, VCU Autism Center for Excellence, Virginia Commonwealth University, Richmond, Virginia

Jeff Sigafoos, PhD, School of Educational Psychology and Pedagogy, Victoria University of Wellington, Wellington, New Zealand

Daniel Steere, PhD, Department of Special Education and Rehabilitation, East Stroudsburg University, East Stroudsburg, Pennsylvania

Pamela Sherron Targett, MEd, Rehabilitation Research and Training Center, Virginia Commonwealth University, Richmond, Virginia

Jane Thierfeld Brown, EdD, University of Connecticut School of Law, Hartford, Connecticut

Matt Tincani, PhD, BCBA-D, Department of Psychological, Organizational, and Leadership Studies, College of Education, Temple University, Philadelphia, Pennsylvania

Jason C. Travers, PhD, BCBA-D, Department of Special Education, College of Education, University of Kansas, Lawrence, Kansas

Larah van der Meer, PhD, School of Educational Psychology and Pedagogy, Victoria University of Wellington, Wellington, New Zealand

Paul Wehman, PhD, VCU Autism Center for Excellence and Division of Research, Department of Physical Medicine and Rehabilitation, Virginia Commonwealth University, Richmond, Virginia

Michael L. Wehmeyer, PhD, Bureau of Child Research and Department of Special Education, School of Education, University of Kansas, Lawrence, Kansas

Christine Wenzel, MA, Center for Students with Disabilities, University of Connecticut, Storrs, Connecticut

Peggy Schaefer Whitby, PhD, BCBA-D, Department of Curriculum and Instruction, College of Education and Health Professions, University of Arkansas, Fayetteville, Arkansas

Lorraine E. Wolf, PhD, Office of Disability Services, Boston University, Boston, Massachusetts

Courtney Yantes, MBA, Ohio Center for Autism and Low Incidence, Columbus, Ohio

Dianne Zager, PhD, Division of Communication Sciences and Disorders, Dyson College of Arts and Sciences, Pace University, New York, New York

David W. Zellis, JD, Zellis Law, LLC, Langhorne, Pennsylvania

Preface

We have edited this collection of chapters on evidence-based and promising practices for adolescents and adults with autism spectrum disorders (ASD) for several key reasons. The recent tremendous explosion in cases of children with ASD is well known and documented throughout the world (Baron-Cohen et al., 2009; Baio, 2012; Gal, Abiri, Reichenberg, Gabis, & Gross, 2012; Kim et al., 2011). During the past 25 years or so there has been a concomitant increase in research and publications regarding the identification, assessment, and education of these children. This heavy focus on children is understandable given the promise of early identification and intervention. However, there remains a paucity of research and guidelines that focus on the issues that face adults with ASD.

One of us (Andy Bondy) served as a statewide director of a public school for students with ASD. Our primary challenge was to design a program that would confer an educational advantage to all students. In seeking to accomplish this goal, we asked ourselves a crucial question: What is the long-term goal of sending children with ASD to school? To answer this question, we engaged in many discussions with parents and professionals. We noted a common theme. Education in society at large aims to provide skills that lead to successful employment in the real world, living independently away from one's parents, and being reasonably happy. We concluded that the goal of educating a student with ASD is exactly the same: to help him or her to get a good job in the community, to live away from home (even if support is still warranted), and to be reasonably happy. Thus all of our educational efforts had to conform to achieving these functional life goals in adulthood.

However, teaching communication, job skills, living skills, leisure skills, and so forth, would all be for naught if the posteducation community could not maintain and sustain these skills in the long term. For example, if a young woman learned to communicate about various wants and needs; acquired skills associated with shopping for food, preparing and cooking meals, and cleaning up; and then moved into a home in which all of these tasks were performed for her, it should not surprise us if these skills faded away over time. Conversely, if she had not acquired these skills in school, would adult service providers or parents teach these skills? These are some of the daunting challenges facing adults with ASD and their families. Yes, we need to identify and diagnose ASD early and provide an excellent education, but learning and growth do not stop at a particular age. This book is designed to offer hope and research-based guidelines about available strategies to help adults with ASD lead productive and happy lives.

We asked a number of leading researchers to write chapters on critical issues related to the well-being of adolescents and adults with ASD. Each set of authors was asked to review the current literature associated with a wide array of topics. In addition to reviewing key research, each chapter provides some examples of how specific features and strategies may influence a hypothetical case in terms of practical decision making. Some of the case studies provide detailed accounts of how real adults with ASD benefited from application of particular strategies; other case studies are hypothetical examples based on real-world experiences as detailed by the chapter authors.

Chapter 1, by Myles, Coffin, Owens, and Yantes, provides a lucid description of many of the characteristics and challenges faced by adults with ASD. The chapter begins with a review of many issues associated with communication and social interaction, including issues related to sexuality. The authors then describe some of the key factors related to the often unique sensory and motor issues among this group of individuals. Next, they present a review of various cognitive factors, including a discussion of executive function, central coherence, and emotional vulnerability. Chapter 2, by Pepa and Harris, focuses on ASD in the context of the family, especially the transition from the teenage years into adulthood. The authors review factors relating to the central role that families play in supporting their children with ASD in terms of service coordination, educational transitioning, employment, and potential residential transitioning. The chapter also provides guidance for finding social support on an ongoing basis. The last section of the chapter reviews research on a variety of family coping strategies and factors that may best help families through different types of transitions.

Chapter 3, by Wehmeyer and Zager, deals specifically with the transitional issues associated with leaving secondary school. The chapter begins with a review of the federal requirements for transitional services, as well as college and career readiness issues. The authors provide clear guidelines for the elements considered essential to preparing an adequate transitional plan. These include clear suggestions for elements that should be included in a student's individualized education program (IEP). The chapter also reviews issues that may promote self-determination among adults with ASD. Finally, the authors provide guidance connected with transitioning into community living. Chapter 4, by Thierfeld Brown, Wolf, and Wenzel, addresses similar issues in postsecondary education. The chapter offers a comprehensive review of strategies that help those with higher functioning ASD cope with the academic and social demands that college may bring. The authors then discuss the supported education service model and how it can provide aid, often via coaching, for many adults with ASD. Another model that provides help with university issues is described in a model identified as Beyond Access. Finally, the authors provide examples of various uses of technology on campus that may help adults with ASD successfully navigate the requirements of a college education.

Chapter 5, by Aguirre, O'Neill, Rehfeldt, and Boyer, switches gears by looking at behavioral interventions that promote complex communication and social skills. The authors begin by reviewing components and research regarding behavioral skills training. They next review evidence of several specific strategies, including modeling, prompting, and reinforcement, with regard to specific skill acquisition for adults with ASD. A comprehensive review of the literature regarding script fading and peer-mediated instruction is offered, along with case examples. Finally, there is a fascinating discussion on the role of and strategies for promoting response variability, as well as the use of virtual environments, with this population. Chapter 6, by Lang and colleagues, also addresses issues related to communication, but from an augmentative and alternative communications (AAC) perspective. The chapter opens with a review of the term *communication* from both traditional and behavioral perspectives, including the importance of an analysis of the functional units of language. There ensues a description of AAC and a variety of modalities that may prove helpful in promoting functional communication, including manual signs, picture-exchange systems (e.g., the PECS), and speech-generating devices (SGDs). The authors provide a clear review of tactics and evidence on various modalities and strategies, including an overview of teaching strategies to promote acquisition and maintenance.

Chapter 7, by Tincani and Crozier, provides details of a broad approach to behavior intervention and life enhancement called positive behavior support (PBS). The chapter opens with a review of the historical context in which PBS was developed and how it is distinct from other approaches and orientations (including applied behavior analysis), including its emphasis on prevention. Among the key factors associated with successful implementation of PBS are service delivery systems, autonomy and choice, and medical and health issues. The chapter concludes with a thorough review of primary, secondary, and tertiary support factors that must be addressed for comprehensive changes to occur and last.

Applied behavior analysis (ABA) is widely recognized as a strongly research-validated practice for young children with ASD, but for many years researchers and practitioners have successfully applied the principles and strategies of ABA to adults. Chapter 8, by Gerhardt, Garcia, and Foglia, gives an overview of ABA-based strategies for teaching a variety of skills to adolescents and adults with ASD, with an emphasis on adaptive and vocational skill domains. They review important considerations in arranging for stimulus control to teach skills to adults, as well as strategies for promoting generalization of skills in the community.

Chapter 9, by Travers and Whitby, looks specifically at the broad issue of sexuality and relationships. The opening section notes the rationale for sexuality education for people with ASD, and well as a review of their rights with regard to relationships, marriage, and parenthood. This discussion is complemented by noting the responsibility of society to report and prevent sexual abuse. The discussion continues by addressing sexual health and hygiene, self-determination, and specialized instruction. The core components of a wide-ranging sexuality education package are elucidated, including how cultural factors may influence training issues. The authors then review the extant literature on evidence-based practices regarding general and specific issues (including menstrual care and masturbation) and follow with case examples. In Chapter 10, Coyne and Fullerton provide information on the related topic of recreation and leisure. They review many studies regarding the overall importance of adults with ASD having fulfilling recreational and leisure skills and opportunities. The chapter includes a review of how factors associated with ASD may have an impact on the development and maintenance of recreational and leisure activities. This section is followed by a discussion of how incorporating an individual's strengths may inform the proper selection of leisure activities. The chapter ends with a detailed description of how to assess and plan the expansion of leisure activities.

Chapter 11, by Wehman, Targett, Schall, and Carr, focuses on the crucial issue of meaningful employment. The authors open with a frank discussion about the notoriously poor rate of community-based employment participation for adults with ASD. They review the general and research-based literature on this topic. From that review, the authors provide a number of promising practices that should help improve the likelihood of employability in this population, including supported and customized employment strategies. The chapter also provides information on planning a career beyond a successful single job. The authors next provide strategies that may help businesses in hiring and supporting the employment of adults with ASD. A second major issue—independent living—is addressed in Chapter 12, by Myles and colleagues. They focus specifically on strategies that may help those identified with ASD described as high functioning. For successful independent living, many strategies have been shown to be effective, including modification of technology to promote aspects of such a life (e.g., financial and domestic issues). To help achieve these broad goals, the authors describe the Ziggurat Model as well as the Comprehensive Autism Planning System.

Chapter 13, by Markowitz, deals with an aspect of life that many families are reluctant to face: aging and its associated issues of estate planning and funding. The growth in the number of individuals with ASD has had a great impact on the number of adults needing services and lifelong oversight. The author reviews several life-sustaining factors, including appropriate medical care, the role of parents and guardians as advocates, and the transition from work to retirement. Markowitz provides a careful review of residential alternatives and what factors may influence their selection. Finally, there is a review of issues related to funding for services and support. The last chapter, Chapter 14, by Frantz and Zellis, provides invaluable information regarding the legal rights and challenges associated with adults with ASD. They review cultural misrepresentations of individuals with ASD and how these may influence opportunities and reactions, including by police personnel. They review several cases of adults with ASD whose behaviors led to involvement with our judicial system. The chapter ends with suggestions on what a family may consider when seeking legal advice and representation.

We hope the reader will find these chapters both informative and provocative. There are some clear suggestions and guidance based on research. However, the reality is that solid research on the well-being of adults with ASD is in its infancy. We hope that each chapter will provoke discussion, debate, and thoughtful discourse about how to best help those with ASD lead productive and satisfying lives. We also hope that these discussions will lead to a new area of research dedicated to providing professionals and caregivers with more evidence-based guidance to help make crucial choices regarding strategies and goals for adolescents and adults with ASD.

REFERENCES

Baio, J. (2012). Prevalence of autism spectrum disorders—autism and development disabilities monitoring network, 14 sites, United States, 2008. *MMWR Surveillance Summaries, 61*(SS03), 1–19.

Baron-Cohen, S., Scott, F. J., Allison, C., Williams, J., Bolton, P., Matthews, F. E., et al. (2009). Prevalence of autism-spectrum conditions: UK school-based population studies. *British Journal of Psychiatry, 194*(6), 500–509.

Gal, G., Abiri, L., Reichenberg, A., Gabis, L., & Gross, R. (2012). Time trends in reported autism spectrum disorders in Israel, 1986–2005. *Journal of Autism and Developmental Disorders, 42*(3), 428–431.

Kim, Y., Leventhal, B. L., Koh, Y., Fombonne, E., Laska, E., Lim, E., et al. (2011). Prevalence of autism spectrum disorders in a total population sample. *American Journal of Psychiatry, 168*(9), 904–912.

Contents

PART I

Introduction

CHAPTER 1

• • • • • •

Characteristics of Adults with High-Functioning Autism Spectrum Disorders

- **Brenda Smith Myles, Amy Bixler Coffin, Donna J. Owens, and Courtney Yantes**

You definitely don't want to get rid of all of the autism genetics because if you did that, there'd be no scientists. After all, who do you think made the first stone spear back in the caves? It wasn't the really social people.
—TEMPLE GRANDIN (Plank, 2013)

This chapter presents an overview of the characteristics of adults with high-functioning autism spectrum disorders (HFASD), with a special focus on social/communication, sensory–motor, and cognitive skills, including special interests, as well as emotional vulnerability. It is important to emphasize from the outset that although individuals with HFASD may experience challenges in these areas, they are not necessarily limited by them. That is, when there is a match between characteristics and the environment and when instruction is relevant, the potential of adults on the spectrum is unlimited.

Social/Communication Skills

"One of my closest friends has autism. She is caring and loyal, and listens with interest to what I say. I know that she will always tell me the truth—even when others cannot. Her unique way of interpreting a situation helps me realize that there are multiple perspectives and that . . . her social and communication errors largely have to do with not having the information she needs to interact with others. My friend wants to learn new ways of interacting with others—and her interest in doing this is far greater than mine. She tolerates my social errors with a kindness that many others do not exhibit."

Social interactions are unpredictable and often require participants to understand the perspective as well as the verbal and nonverbal communication of others, many of whom are unfamiliar to them. In addition, social mores, including the hidden curriculum (Endow, 2012), add a subtle and ever-changing layer of complexity to social interactions. This unpredictability adds complexity, uncertainty, and anxiety to interactions because adults on the spectrum do not have access to the information they need to be successful (Levy & Perry, 2011).

Social challenges experienced by those with HFASD are pervasive and long-lasting, unlike other ASD-related traits that may lessen over time (see the later section on emotional vulnerability; cf. Frith, 2004; Levy & Perry, 2011; Stokes, Newton, & Kaur, 2007). Such demands can cause great distress, thereby contributing to social anxiety, stress, and even depression, depending on the specific social context (Hintzen, Delespaul, Van Os, & Myin-Germeys, 2010).

Many of these challenges may be attributed to weak theory of mind (ToM) skills—the cognitive ability to attribute beliefs, thoughts, desires, feelings, and intentions to oneself and others in order to understand and predict behaviors (Baron-Cohen, 1995). Thus interference in the development of ToM results in what is referred to as "mind-blindness," that is, the inability to recognize the thoughts and feelings of others. Not surprisingly, therefore, individuals with HFASD tend to be less proficient "mind readers" than persons with neurotypical development.

Because many individuals with HFASD struggle to understand others' emotions, they often miss nuances such as eye contact, body language, proximity, or facial expressions. In addition, they may have difficulty with pragmatic language, misinterpret others' communicative intent, and struggle with responding appropriately, either verbally or nonverbally. As a result, they may appear to lack tact in their social communications, to be literal, and to seem egocentric, selfish, and apathetic; they may even come across as too honest or domineering, inadvertently turning others off. In turn, this social skill deficit may contribute to significant difficulty in forming long-term personal relationships (Barnhill, 2007). The following brief conversation occurred between Barbara, a recently divorced neurotypical woman, and Joan, a woman on the spectrum.

JOAN: My brother has finally started to date after being divorced for five years. His first date came from *Match.com*.

BARBARA: I was thinking about doing the same thing, but I am a bit concerned about no one contacting me.

JOAN: You should be just fine. You are fat, but so are most people. And even though you aren't beautiful or even pretty, some people might think that you are cute. I think that you will be fine on *Match.com*.

BARBARA: Okay. I will try to remember only the best parts of your description of me.

Examples of pragmatic skills that are challenging for adults with HFASD include:

- Engaging in reciprocal conversation
- Making relevant contributions to a topic
- Asking relevant or clarifying questions
- Using appropriate strategies to gain attention or to interrupt
- Understanding language with multiple meanings, humor, sarcasm
- Turn-taking
- Adjusting language based on the context of a situation (Vermeulen, 2012).

The following telephone conversation between Bridget, who is neurotypical, and her friend, Jeanne, who has autism, illustrates a minor and somewhat humorous misunderstanding.

BRIDGET: I just rescued a dog. He is very sweet and his name is Schumann. He's 3 or 4 years old. Schumann was in rescue for over a year; no one wanted him.

JEANNE: Why not?

BRIDGET: Probably because he has three legs.

JEANNE: All dogs have three legs.

BRIDGET: What I meant to say was that he doesn't have four legs. He only has three legs.

JEANNE: I must be following you with a literal interpretation. You know that it happens more when I am tired.

Many adults with HFA recognize that they have social challenges and are able to report them either verbally or in written format. Montgomery and colleagues (2008) and Montgomery, Stoesz, and McCrimmon (2013), in their study of the resilience of young adults with HFASD, attempted to quantify their emotional intelligence. Even though the adults in their study demonstrated a relative strength in understanding complex emotions and transitions from one emotion to another, they experienced difficulty in applying this information to everyday situations. That is, they demonstrated "a disconnect between 'knowing' and 'doing'" (Montgomery et al., 2008, p. 86). Similar findings were reported by Samson, Huber, and Gross (2012). Common social challenges identified by adults with HFASD themselves appear in Table 1.1.

The majority of adults with HFASD want to engage in personal and professional relationships. They desire involvement in social opportunities and want to be considered as valued members of society, yet stigma, isolation, and exclusion are major concerns. Indeed, many individuals with HFASD report that they feel an almost overwhelming sense of isolation and social frustration (Jobe & White, 2007) that increases as they grow older and become more aware of being "different" from others (Muller, Schuler, & Yates, 2008). As a result, it is not uncommon for adults on the spectrum to have few "real" social contacts. Often, their contacts include family members—they generally live with their parents, often not as their first choice (Balfe & Tantam, 2010)—or individuals they meet using social media (Levy & Perry, 2011).

Recent research has focused on endeavors by adults on the spectrum to develop romantic relationships. However, the characteristics involved—communication and social interactions—often cause heightened challenges in this area. Even though adults with HFASD targeted the same types of potential partners as their peers without HFASD (e.g., colleagues, acquaintances, friends, ex-partners), adults on the spectrum

TABLE 1.1. Social Challenges Identified by Adults with HFASD

- Reading other people's feelings: 91%
- Being bullied: 95%
- Responding to people's feelings: 86%
- Feeling left out of things: 77%
- Feeling misunderstood: 63%
- Feeling put down by others: 62%
- Feeling sexually frustrated: 56%
- Being sexually or financially exploited: 40%
- Having trouble showing own feelings: 42%
- Having distressing family problems: 31%

Note. Based on Balfe and Tantam (2010).

were more likely to attempt to develop romantic attachments with strangers and celebrities, using inappropriate courtship behaviors that include (1) touching inappropriately, (2) showing obsessional interest, (3) making inappropriate comments, (4) monitoring activities, (5) following, (6) pursuing in a threatening manner, and (7) making threats toward themselves or others. In addition, attempts to develop relationships generally lasted longer than those of neurotypical peers when faced with lack of interest or downright refusal by the targeted partner. Adults on the spectrum reported having little or no instruction in developing and maintaining romantic relationships (Gougeon, 2010; Stokes et al., 2007).

Similar results were found by Mehzabin and Stokes (2011). That is, these authors noted that, compared with typical peers, adults with HFASD had received less sex education, had fewer sexual experiences, and had more concerns about their sexual and romantic futures. Nevertheless, Mehzabin and Stokes (2011) also found that the adults they surveyed shared similar levels of knowledge about sexual behavior as adults without HFASD. Because these results were contrary to findings by Stokes and colleagues (2007) and other anecdotal reports (Davies & Dubie, 2012; Henault, 2005), Mehzabin and Stokes (2011) attributed their findings to a lack of insight or ToM challenges experienced by adults with ASD.

Difficulties in understanding sexuality and romantic relationships can lead to problems in many environments, including on the job.

> Khan ended up with serious problems because he didn't understand that his daily compliments to a female coworker were considered sexual harassment. Each day, he gave this coworker what he considered very nice compliments, such as "You have very pretty legs" or "You look hot when your shirts are tight." Eventually, the coworker reported the situation to her boss. When questioned afterward, Khan not only admitted that he had made these (and similar) comments but defended himself by saying that because his comments were truthful, there wasn't anything wrong with them. After all, he had often been told that telling the truth would not get you into trouble. Khan was told to stop making these types of comments. He did, but unwittingly he substituted comments that were even worse. Once again, he thought he was following the rules, because he did stop saying the comments his boss specifically told him to stop saying, but he substituted new truths. Ultimately, he was fired for telling the female coworker, "I wish I was your boyfriend so I could have sex with you." (Myles, Endow, & Mayfield, 2013, p. 5)

Farley and colleagues (2009) found more positive social outcomes for a group of adults with HFASD who were members of a strongly church-influenced community. Of these adults, 85% engaged in myriad organized social group activities, almost one-half had dated in both group and couple formats, and 7% were married. These positive outcomes were attributed to participation in the faith-based community.

Challenges in social interaction and communication are a key component of HFASD and are often the single most disabling factor in the everyday life of adults on the spectrum. Many individuals with HFASD experience a range of significant social and communication challenges. Such challenges are often related to understanding the subtleties of communication, establishing, negotiating, and maintaining relationships, and managing levels of social anxiety. Although the social competence of individuals with HFASD in these areas improves with age (Levy & Perry, 2011; Orsmond, Krauss, & Seltzer, 2004), challenges still exist.

Sensory–Motor Skills

"The world is replete with overwhelming sensory demands. It appears that sensory information comes into the life of an adult with autism with great intensity—some of which is problematic and some of which can be enjoyable. I once attended an art exhibit with a friend who is on the spectrum. It was an amazing experience. I always enjoy this type of activity, but my friend guided me to experience the art in a more in-depth manner. We considered the impact of light, shading, depth, and even the reactions of others to the artwork. She put considerable effort into tolerating the sensory elements in the exhibit. After the exhibit, my friend needed some downtime because she was overwhelmed by the many sensory aspects in the museum."

Historically, despite overwhelming anecdotal reports, sensory sensitivities have not been considered a diagnostic criterion of ASD due to a lack of empirical evidence. However, that has now changed given a growing body of research. Thus, the fifth edition of the *Diagnostic and Statistical Manual of Mental Disorders* (American Psychiatric Association, 2013) includes hyper- or hyporeactivity to sensory input as an aspect of the core autism component of restricted patterns of behavior. In recent years, it has been widely acknowledged that sensory challenges affect the vast majority of children on the spectrum (cf. Harrison & Hare, 2004; Klintwall et al., 2011) to the extent that it affects family routines at home and limits participation in activities outside the home environment (Schaaf, Toth-Cohen, Johnson, Outten, & Benevides, 2011).

A similar profile is emerging for adults. Billstedt, Gillberg, and Gillberg (2005, 2007) found that sensory issues in children with autism continue into adulthood. Crane, Goddard, and Pring (2009) found that 94% of the adults with HFASD reported significant sensory challenges in one of four quadrants identified by Brown and Dunn (2002; see Table 1.2). They further found that sensory differences persisted across adulthood. This is contrary to the findings of Kern and colleagues (2007) and of Leekam, Nieto, Libby, Wing, and Gould (2007), who reported that sensory challenges in some areas tend to dissipate with age.

Because there appears to be no one profile of sensory challenges experienced by adults on the spectrum (Crane et al., 2009; Kern et al., 2007), first-person accounts are valuable in understanding the diverse impact of sensory input. Based on interviews with nine adults with HFASD, Smith and Sharp (2013) contextualized their sensory challenges using the following categories:

1. *Heightened senses.* Sensory experiences are generally more extreme than those experienced by neurotypical individuals. Heighted senses may be fascinating, pleasurable, calming, or distracting. Some heightened senses, such as attention to visual detail, can have practical applicability to jobs or hobbies. Table 1.3 highlights job experiences that match a heightened visual sense. Others, such as sensitivities to specific sounds, may be stressful or painful, resulting in isolation.

2. *Moderating factors.* Single inputs (e.g., one sound) are generally less stressful than multiple inputs. A similar profile was found for low- versus high-intensity input and sensory impact in ordered versus chaotic environments. Stress level is a moderating factor. That is, sensory issues have

TABLE 1.2. Sensory Profile Quadrants

Quadrant name	Quadrant descriptor
Low registration	Responds more slowly than others to or is unaware of sensory stimuli. For example, the person may not notice a scent that is apparent to others.
Sensory sensitivity	Is distracted or uncomfortable in the presence of sensory stimuli. For example, the person may be sensitive to specific textures or may not be able to concentrate in the presence of noise.
Sensation seeking	Prefers sensory stimulation and seeks it out. For example, the person may need high levels of movement or bright lights.
Sensation avoiding	Engages in behaviors to reduce exposure to sensory stimuli and prefers environments in which such stimuli can be controlled. For example, sensation-avoiding individuals may prefer to work alone and stay away from sensory-laden environments, such as lunchrooms or shopping malls.

Note. Based on Brown and Dunn (2002).

TABLE 1.3. Job Matches for Visual Learners Who Have a High Need for Structure and Predictability

• Draft technician	• Web designer
• Photographer	• Veterinary technician
• Animal trainer	• Auto mechanic
• Graphic artist	• Lighting technician
• Jewelry maker	• Landscape designer

Note. Based on Myles et al. (2013).

a more marked impact on an already stressed person than on a calm person. The term *sensory avalanche* was used to describe a situation whereby stress causes the adult with autism "to become more sensitive to adverse sensory events, causing them subsequently to become more stressed and therefore more sensitive, creating a vicious cycle" (Smith & Sharp, 2013, p. 896). Other people are described as sometimes being a source of stress either by their personal characteristics (e.g., voice volume) or environments in which they wish to interact (e.g., noisy lunch or break room), often resulting in individuals with HFASD isolating themselves from others. Still other people may be seen as supportive and understanding of sensory challenges, resulting in greater self-acceptance.

3. *Coping strategies.* Adults on the spectrum have identified or developed coping strategies to address the moderating factors described above; however, there appears to be no link between coping strategies and sensory events. Adults reported that they identified some coping strategies purely by serendipity. Coping strategies consisted of dampeners, such as earplugs or sunglasses, to make input less intense; blocking out input by closing eyes when listening to someone or avoiding eye contact; creating order by having a schedule or priming for an event; and calming strategies that included deep pressure or carrying a weighted bag.

What is most characteristic about sensory differences is their variability across individuals, across senses, across time, and across circumstances. Unusual sensory reactions can include hypersensitivity to stimuli, as in a reaction to noises, light, smells, or certain tactile input, such as the feel of some foods in the mouth or certain fabrics against the skin. Conversely, hyposensitivity to sensory input, even to pain, can cause some individuals to ignore otherwise irritating stimuli such as a fire alarm or a doorbell buzzing (Standifer, 2009). Those who are hyposensitive may seek intense sensory input, such as bear hugs or tight-fitting clothes, as a way to regulate their sensory systems.

Fatigue and anxiety can exacerbate the intensity of reactions to sensory stimuli, making reactions variable over time. Furthermore, the same individual can experience hypersensitivity in some circumstances and require increased sensory input in others. For example, Temple Grandin (1992) built her "squeeze machine" to provide deep pressure across her body, an experience she found to be calming.

Cognitive Skills

"The people with HFASD that I have the pleasure to know often amaze me. They are bright and see things in a unique way. They speak with great passion and knowledge, sharing information unabashedly. They are efficient and goal-directed—and this is enhanced by the presence of routines. Flexibility can be a challenge for some of my adult friends on the spectrum—a characteristic I share; however, as a neurotypical, I do not put forth as much effort as they do in trying to be accommodating to changes."

Although intelligence quotient (IQ) has been reported as the best predictor of outcome in individuals with autism (cf. Levy & Perry, 2011), it provides limited insight into the adult with HFASD. An examination of cognition, including executive function (EF) and central coherence characteristics, provides a more comprehensive picture of adults on the spectrum. EF and central coherence may also contribute to some extent to the cognitive differences often observed in adults with HFASD. However, further studies are needed to identify the exact roles these cognitive areas play in the lives of adults with HFASD (Happé & Charlton, 2012). We discuss, in addition to the cognitive challenges, a cognitive strength—special interests.

Executive Function

EF describes the cognitive processes that regulate, control, and manage other cognitive processes, such as information acquisition and management, working memory, attention, problem solving, inhibition, mental flexibility, shift, and initiation and monitoring of actions (cf. Brown, Reichel, & Quinlan, 2009; Chan, Shum, & Toulopoulou, 2008). EF also includes the ability to manage frustration and modulate emotions (Brown et al., 2009; Chan et al., 2008), discussed in the later section on emotional vulnerability.

Regardless of IQ, adults with autism often have difficulties learning and organizing information if it is complex and/or contains multiple components (Cederlund, Hagberg, & Gillberg, 2010; Sumiyoshi, Kawakubo, Suga, Sumiyoshi, & Kasai, 2011). Working memory, the ability to actively hold multiple items in mind so that they can be manipulated, is also problematic for adults with HFASD. When coupled with challenges with distractibility and attention, these can affect life success (Kenworthy et al., 2005).

Even though individuals with ASD have good rote skills and are able to interpret discrete or small units of information (Bowler, Gardiner, & Grice, 2000), difficulties ensue when they are asked to integrate and organize multiple variables or more complex information (Sachse et al., 2013; Tsatsanis, Noens, Illmann, Pauls, & Volkmar, 2011). For example, Bowler and colleagues (2000) found that when asked to recall and organize information, adults on the spectrum do not rely on *remembering* but focus instead on *knowing*. Remembering occurs when a person "brings back to mind contextual details of previous events and experiences that include an awareness of one's self, usually at a particular time, and a particular place" (2000, p. 295). Knowing, on the other hand, includes general information about previous events.

Time management is another area that is often challenging for a number of reasons, including difficulty with time perception and working memory, which affects the ability to monitor elapsed time; planning the steps necessary to complete a project or task to meet timelines; and shifting or maintaining attention from one thing to another to complete tasks to meet time requirements (Kenworthy et al., 2005; Sumiyoshi et al., 2011; Wallace & Happé, 2008). Concomitant challenges are seen in planning, flexibility, and integrating and evaluating multiple variables, particularly when tasks become more difficult (Sachse et al., 2013).

Individuals with HFASD often recognize that they experience these challenges. For example, in a survey of adults with HFASD with IQs greater than 70, Balfe and Tantam (2010) found that they experienced difficulties that included managing time and planning (64%), coping with unexpected changes and being flexible (84%), and changing tasks (85%). These challenges were linked with managing time spent on special interests (84%), managing money (67%), cooking (60%), tidying and cleaning (52%), and bathing (31%).

In addition, many individuals with autism demonstrate a gap between knowledge and the ability to act. That is, although some adults on the spectrum recognize that they need materials for a task at work, they have difficulty acting on this information (Gilotty, Kenworthy, Sirian, Black, & Wagner, 2002). Thus they often become "stuck" on the idea that they need materials; they do not know how to move to the next stage—obtaining them.

Central Coherence

Related to EF, central coherence is loosely defined as the ability to integrate information to understand context or "the big picture." Many persons with HFASD are described as having poor or weak central coherence (cf. Frith, 2003). Those who struggle with identifying general ideas by integrating details have difficulty interpreting incoming information in order to understand the larger context. "Those who are affected tend to a detail oriented, selective perception and have great difficulties in capturing the overall context—their central coherence is deficient" (Roy, Dillo, Emrich, & Ohlmeier, 2009, p. 59).

Although the research on central coherence in individuals with HFASD is equivocal and some studies demonstrate that these individuals show skills similar to or better than those of same-age typical peers (cf. Mottron, Peretz, & Menard, 2000; Plaisted, O'Riordan, & Baron-Cohen, 1998), it is generally believed that weak central coherence is present under specific conditions. These include circumstances in which individuals on the spectrum must (1) process multiple items simultaneously (Lopez & Leekam, 2003); (2) rely on inference or self-monitoring rather than direct instruction (Joliffe & Baron-Cohen, 2001); and (3) process information in an open format rather than a forced-choice format (Beaumont & Newcombe, 2006).

Social interactions and employment situations, for example, present constant challenges for central coherence skills, requiring effective information processing in order to concentrate on the whole social situation or the purpose of a task rather than discrete details. Illustrations of this difficulty might be a person with HFASD who focuses only on what is being said in a social interaction and not on the speaker's tone of voice or body language or the adult who is concerned with her section of a task with little concern for how it will be integrated into the work of others (Ambery, Russell, Perry, Morris, & Murphy, 2006; Jarrold, Butler, Cottington, & Jimenez, 2000).

Furthermore, many individuals with HFASD struggle in areas such as organization, problem solving, attention, figurative concepts, generalization, and abstract reasoning—skills that are imperative for obtaining and maintaining employment and for basic everyday functioning and social interactions.

Special Interests

Many adults on the spectrum display skills, strengths, and talents associated with special interests and often display extensive knowledge in a particular interest area. Special interests "may seem unusual because of their subject matter or the intensity with which" they are pursued (Roy et al., 2009, p. 59).

Larry Moody, a retired registered engineer, highlighted the importance of special interests:

> My first engineering-related job was as a draftsman. I had taken a half-year of drafting in high school and found it interesting, detailed and mostly solitary work. I took the State Civil Service exam for drafting, passed it and was hired. Later my supervisor told me he chose me because I had scored higher on the drafting exam than anyone he had met in the more than 10 years he had been a supervisor. I realize now that it was one of my special interests. (Grandin & Duffy, 2008, p. 163)

Although these special interests may be helpful in targeting employment opportunities, they have not been fully utilized. Table 1.4 provides a brief example of special interests and potential job matches.

Emotional Vulnerability

> Even though Lilia enjoys her job as a tax accountant, she is continually challenged by stress. In order to understand her stress, Lilia has learned to identify stress by her behavior. As her stress level increases, her visual sense becomes overwhelmed. While Lilia initially could not track this in real time, once she identified the behaviors she engaged in, she had no difficulty knowing which level of stress she was experiencing at any given time and was able to take precautions accordingly. When her stress level is low, Lilia takes off her glasses. She knows her stress level is medium when she rubs her eyes, and when she needs to use tissues to wipe her watering eyes her stress level is high. Using concrete, easily observable behavior indicators matched to stress levels enables Lilia to track her stress level accurately, which in turn allows her to employ regulation strategies known to be most effective at each level of stress. Lilia uses this plan periodically throughout the day, employing the self-regulation techniques she knows will be most helpful to her according to her stress level at the time. Besides using her stress level to manage her regulation needs, Lilia has matched each of her stress levels with a personal reminder of how she will react to various situations. For example, like most with ASD, as Lilia's stress level increases, she becomes less flexible at dealing with perceived change or interruption in her routine/plan. Lilia finds that it is easier to outsmart this aspect of her ASD by being ready to implement a personal reminder. (Myles et al., 2013, p. 53)

Individuals with HFASD have difficulty navigating the world of emotions, causing significant challenges in their capacity for emotional

TABLE 1.4. Special Interests and Potential Job Matches

Special interest	Sample job match
Bridges	Construction laborer
	Crane driver
	Architect
Insects	Entomologist
	Gardener
Autism	Advocate
	Mentor
	Educator
Dinosaurs	Paleontologist
	Paleontologist assistant
History	Historical librarian
	Genealogical society researcher
	History professor
	Historical researcher
Drawing and/or artistry	Graphic designer
	Illustrator
	Architect
Airplanes	Pilot
	Navigator
	Air traffic controller
	Aeronautical engineer

regulation. This problem is often evidenced by the presence of depression, anxiety, anger, and self-esteem differences.

According to Roy and colleagues (2009), depression is linked to impairments in the personal and professional domains. For example, college students with HFASD reported intense feelings of loneliness, with fewer and shorter-term friendships and romantic relationships than their typical peers (Jobe & White, 2007). Furthermore, Jobe and White (2007) reported that young adults with HFASD "do not necessarily prefer aloneness, as once assumed, but rather experience increased levels of loneliness related to lack of social skill and understanding" (p. 1479), which may lead to depression—a major debilitating mental health issue in HFASD. Indeed, Cederlund and colleagues (2010) reported a prevalence rate of 12%, whereas Balfe and Tantam (2010) stated that 40% of adults with ASD experienced this mental health condition. Furthermore, in their study of adults with HFASD, Lugnegard, Hallerback, and Gillberg (2011) found that 70% of their sample suffered from least one episode of major depression and that 50% experienced recurrent depression.

Related to depression are suicidal ideations and suicide attempts. Researchers suspect that suicidal behavior among those with HFASD occurs more often than is recognized (Barnhill, 2007; Ghaziuddin, 2005; Ghaziuddin, Ghaziuddin, & Greden, 2002; Tantam & Prestwood, 1999). More specifically, Balfe and Tantum (2010) reported that 40% of their sample had contemplated suicide and 15% had attempted to kill themselves.

Anxiety, another common condition experienced by adults with HFASD, also affects all areas of life, from independent living to employment. For example, after interviewing six adults with Asperger syndrome about their job experiences, Hurlbutt and Chalmers (2004) concluded, "the stress of not understanding the social rules of the environment, not knowing which topics are appropriate to talk about and which are not, having difficulty asking for help, and being exhausted from concentrating so hard all day to understand the world of neurotypicals can become overwhelming" (p. 219). Similarly, Lugnegard and colleagues (2011) found that more than one-half of the adults in their study had experienced at least one anxiety disorder, with others having a diagnosis of two or more, including social anxiety disorder, generalized anxiety disorder, and obsessive–compulsive disorder.

Social isolation plays a significant role in the anxiety of individuals with HFASD as adults. As children they were often the objects of bullying and teasing by their peers, setting the stage for a state of social isolation that persists in adulthood (Balfe & Tantam, 2010). Furthermore, their social and communication challenges complicate their ability to interact comfortably with others, especially those who are unfamiliar to them, despite a desire for social relationships.

Adults with HFASD also report experiencing more negative than positive emotions, including anger, than their neurotypical counterparts. According to Quek, Sofronoff, Sheffield, White, and Kelly (2012), 17% of adults on the spectrum experience clinically significant levels of anger. In their study, anxiety and depression were positively associated with anger, with depression explaining 25% of the variance in anger. Similar results were found by Matson and Nebel-Schwalm (2007) and Tantam (2000).

Aggression—actions that often follow anger and include threatening, rough play, provoked lashing out, hitting, biting, or violent behavior—is a challenge experienced by approximately 50% of children through the age of 14; however, it declines significantly after age 15 (Kanne & Mazurek, 2011). Langstrom, Grann, Richkin, Sjostedt, and Fazel (2009) and Murphy (2003) reported that these behaviors are evidenced in only a small percentage of adults on the spectrum. In fact, researchers investigating violent behavior in adults on the spectrum found that they were less likely to engage in violence than the general population, but that these behaviors were associated with substance abuse, personality disorder, or psychotic behavior (Langstrom et al., 2009). However, Balfe and Tantam (2010) noted quite different results. Thus their study, a self-report by adults with HFASD, indicated that anger and aggression may be more pervasive than otherwise thought, with 84% indicating that they anger easily and 31% stating that they often hit others.

Research into challenges in emotional regulation has attributed the cause to deficits in theory of mind (ToM) and perspective taking. Specifically, in addition to the difficulty individuals with HFASD have in identifying the mental states of others, ToM deficits are linked to their inability to identify and differentiate their own mental states (Aspy & Grossman, 2011). Kanne and Mazurek (2011) ascribed emotional regulation challenges to inflexibility, whereas Barrett, Gross, Conner, and Benvenuto (2001) and Samson and colleagues (2012) reported that adults with HFASD typically use less effective methods for emotional regulation than do neurotypical adults. That is, they tend to rely on emotional suppression, a less effective coping strategy, rather than employing emotional reappraisal to shift their perspective in troubling circumstances.

Not surprisingly, the difficulties experienced in these areas can lead to self-esteem challenges (Barnhill, 2007; Hurlbutt & Chalmers, 2004). This outcome is significant because self-esteem is positively correlated with quality of life (Burgess & Gutstein, 2007). For example, Montgomery and colleagues (2013) and others (Palmer, Donaldson, & Stough, 2002; Saklofske, Austin, & Minski, 2003), in their investigation of self-esteem and related characteristics (e.g., optimism, self-awareness, and self-actualization), found that these traits predict life satisfaction, social network quality, loneliness, and depression. Eugene, an adult with Asperger syndrome, reported, "I have to struggle so hard to achieve what NTs [neurotypicals] take for granted, and I was a little envious of their ease in socializing. It would be good to understand socialization completely, but, with the developing autistic society, these feelings of envy are beginning to go away in my mind" (Hurlbutt & Chalmers, 2004, p. 219).

Summary
• • • • • •

Ongoing research indicates that although progress has been made in recent years regarding services and supports for individuals with ASD, the overall system leaves much to be desired, especially as these individuals transition to postsecondary education and adulthood. Increasing ASD prevalence rates mean not only significant stress on families and services today but also increased stress on families and services tomorrow, simply because the system is not equipped to handle what will eventually be an influx of adults with ASD. Elevating the success of those with HFASD hinges on collaborative efforts to bridge the gaps between high school, competitive employment, and postsecondary education, as well as independent living and community involvement (Myles et al., 2013; Shattuck et al., 2012).

As individuals with ASD attempt to make the transition from high school to postschool outcomes, they find themselves facing an often broken structure of support and assistance. Those who wish to obtain employment generally not only are the victims of poor transition services that inhibit their ability to find jobs but also encounter a public that perceives them as unemployable (Gerhardt, 2009). Failure to collaborate on the part of educational entities, employers, and community services leaves these individuals and their families with limited means and opportunities to pursue meaningful and competitive employment (Chiang, Cheung, Li, & Tsai, 2013), resulting in tremendous loss of potential for the individual on the spectrum, as well as a loss to society.

Those who choose not to seek employment directly upon leaving high school but instead pursue postsecondary education face an equal share of barriers in the postsecondary education setting. Institutions of higher education are ill equipped to assist students with disabilities in ways that are relevant to their learning abilities and styles and are, in fact, just beginning to explore ways in which to support this growing student population (Camarena & Sarigiani, 2009). Nevertheless, multiple predictors indicate that students with HFASD can be successful in postsecondary educational settings (Chiang et al., 2013; Taylor & Seltzer, 2011).

Beyond academics and employment, efforts to enhance and support lifelong success and satisfaction in the lives of individuals with ASD include assessing their family lives and community participation. There is much to be done in this regard. According to Gerhardt (2009):

> An entire generation of our nation's most vulnerable citizens is about to leave the entitlement-based world of special education and enter the already overwhelmed and under-funded world of non-entitlement adult services. While exceptional adult programs and services exist in every state, they tend to be more the exception than the rule; leaving many individuals and their families to fend for themselves. (p. 40)

There is reason for hope, however, as young children today are reaping the benefits of intensive early intervention, which may diffuse long-term complications as they enter adulthood (Henninger & Taylor, 2013). In addition, society as a whole is beginning to realize that individuals with HFASD, and indeed anyone across the spectrum, can make meaningful contributions to their communities (Gerhardt, 2009) and live happy and satisfying lives.

REFERENCES

Ambery, F. Z., Russell, A. J., Perry, K., Morris, R., & Murphy, D. G. M. (2006). Neuropsychological functioning in adults with Asperger syndrome. *Autism, 10,* 551–564.

American Psychiatric Association. (2013). *Diagnostic and statistical manual of mental disorders* (5th ed.). Arlington, VA: Author.

Aspy, R., & Grossman, B. (2011). *Designing comprehensive interventions for high-functioning individuals with autism spectrum disorders: The Ziggurat model* (2nd ed.). Shawnee Mission, KS: AAPC.

Balfe, M., & Tantam, D. (2010). A descriptive social and health profile of a community sample of adults and adolescents with Asperger syndrome. *BMC Research Notes, 3,* 300–307.

Barnhill, G. P. (2007). Outcomes in adults with Asperger syndrome. *Focus on Autism and Other Developmental Disabilities, 22,* 116–126.

Baron-Cohen, S. (1995). *Mindblindness: An essay on autism and theory of mind.* Cambridge, MA: MIT Press.

Barrett, L. F., Gross, J., Conner, T., & Benvenuto, M. (2001). Emotion differentiation and regulation. *Cognition and Emotion, 15,* 713–724.

Beaumont, R., & Newcombe, P. (2006). Theory of mind and central coherence in adults with high-functioning autism or Asperger syndrome. *Autism, 10,* 365–382.

Billstedt, E., Gillberg, I. C., & Gillberg, C. (2005). Autism after adolescence: Population-based 13- to 22-year follow-up study of 120 individuals with autism diagnosed in childhood. *Journal of Autism and Developmental Disorders, 35,* 351–360.

Billstedt, E., Gillberg, I. C., & Gillberg, C. (2007). Autism in adults: Symptom patterns and early childhood predictors. Use of the DISCO in a community sample followed from childhood. *Journal of Child Psychology and Psychiatry, 48,* 1102–1110.

Bowler, D. M., Gardiner, J. M., & Grice, S. J. (2000). Episodic memory and remembering in adults with Asperger syndrome. *Journal of Autism and Developmental Disorders, 30,* 533–542.

Brown, C., & Dunn, W. (2002) *Adolescent Adult Sensory Profile: User's manual.* San Antonio, TX: Psychological Corporation.

Brown, T. E., Reichel, P. C., & Quinlan, D. M. (2009). Executive function impairments in high IQ adults with ADHD. *Journal of Attention Disorders, 31,* 161–167.

Burgess, A. F., & Gutstein, S. E. (2007). Quality of life for people with autism:

Raising the standard for evaluating successful outcomes. *Child and Adolescent Mental Health, 12,* 80–86.

Camarena, P. M., & Sarigiani, P. A. (2009). Postsecondary educational aspirations of high-functioning adolescents with autism spectrum disorders and their parents. *Focus on Autism and Other Developmental Disabilities, 24,* 115–128.

Cederlund, M., Hagberg, B., & Gillberg, C. (2010). Asperger syndrome in adolescent and young adult males: Interview and self- and parent assessment of social, emotional, and cognitive problems. *Research in Developmental Disabilities, 31,* 287–298.

Chan, R. C. K., Shum, D., & Touloupoulou, T. (2008). Assessment of executive functions: Review of instruments and identification of critical issues. *Archives of Clinical Neuropsychology, 23,* 201–216.

Chiang, H., Cheung, Y. K., Li, H., & Tsai, L. Y. (2013). Factors associated with participation in employment for high school leavers with autism. *Journal of Autism and Developmental Disorders, 43,* 1832–1842.

Crane, L., Goddard, L., & Pring, L. (2009). Sensory processing in adults with autism spectrum disorders. *Autism, 13,* 215–228.

Davies, C., & Dubie, M. (2012). *Intimate relationships and sexual health: A curriculum for teaching adolescents/adults with high-functioning autism spectrum disorders and other social challenges.* Shawnee Mission, KS: AAPC.

Endow, J. (2012). *Learning the hidden curriculum: The odyssey of one autistic adult.* Shawnee Mission, KS: AAPC Publishing.

Farley, M. A., McMahon, W. M., Fombonne, E., Jenson, W. R., Miller, J., Gardner, M., et al. (2009). Twenty-year outcome for individuals with autism and average or near-average cognitive abilities. *Autism Research, 2,* 109–118.

Frith, U. (2003). *Explaining the enigma* (2nd ed.). London: Wiley-Blackwell.

Frith, U. (2004). Emanuel Miller lecture: Confusion and controversies about Asperger syndrome. *Journal of Child Psychology and Psychiatry, 45,* 672–686.

Gerhardt, P. (2009). *The current state of services for adults with autism.* New York: New York Center for Autism.

Ghaziuddin, M. (2005). A family history study of Asperger syndrome. *Journal of Autism and Developmental Disorders, 35,* 177–182.

Ghaziuddin, M., Ghaziuddin, M., & Greden, J. (2002). Depression in persons with autism: Implications for research and clinical care. *Journal of Autism and Developmental Disorders, 32,* 299–305.

Gilotty, L., Kenworthy, L., Sirian, L., Black, D. O., & Wagner, A. E. (2002). Adaptive skills and executive function in autism spectrum disorders. *Child Neuropsychology, 8,* 241–248.

Gougeon, N. A. (2010). Sexuality and autism: A critical review of selected literature using a social-relationship model of disability. *American Journal of Sexuality Education, 5,* 328–361.

Grandin, T. (1992). Calming effects of deep touch pressure in patients with autistic disorder, college students, and animals. *Journal of Child and Adolescent Psychopharmacology, 2,* 63–70.

Grandin, T., & Duffy, K. (2008). *Developing talents: Careers for individuals with Asperger syndrome and high-functioning autism* (2nd ed.). Shawnee Mission, KS: AAPC.

Happe, F., & Charlton, R. A. (2012). Aging in autism spectrum disorders: A mini-review. *Gerontology, 58*, 70–78.

Harrison, J., & Hare, D. J. (2004). Brief report: Assessment of sensory abnormalities in people with autism spectrum disorders. *Journal of Autism and Developmental Disorders, 34*, 727–730.

Henault, I. (2005). *Asperger's syndrome and sexuality: From adolescence through adulthood.* London, UK: Jessica Kingsley.

Henninger, M., & Taylor, J. L. (2013). Outcomes in adults with autism spectrum disorder: A historical perspective. *Autism, 17*, 103–116.

Hintzen, A., Delespaul, P., van Os, J., & Myin-Germeys, I. (2010). Social needs in daily life in adults with pervasive developmental disorders. *Psychiatry Research, 179*, 75–80.

Hurlbutt, K., & Chalmers, L. (2004). Employment and adults with Asperger syndrome. *Focus on Autism and Developmental Disabilities, 19*, 215–222.

Jarrold, C., Butler, D. W., Cottington, E. M., & Jimenez, F. (2000). Linking theory of mind and central coherence bias in autism and in the general population. *Developmental Psychology, 36*, 126–138.

Jobe, L. E., & White, S. W. (2007). Loneliness, social relationships, and a broader autism phenotype in college students. *Personality and Individual Differences, 42*, 1479–1489.

Joliffe, T., & Baron-Cohen, S. (2001). A test of central coherence theory: Can adults with high-functioning autism or Asperger syndrome integrate fragments of an object? *Cognitive Neuropsychiatry, 6*, 193–216.

Kanne, S. M., & Mazurek, M. O. (2011). Aggression in children and adolescents with ASD: Prevalence and risk factors. *Journal of Autism and Developmental Disorders, 41*, 926–937.

Kenworthy, L. E., Black, D. O., Wallace, G. L., Ahluvalia, T., Wagner, A. E., & Sirian, L. M. (2005). Disorganization: The forgotten dysfunction in the high-functioning autism spectrum disorders. *Developmental Neuropsychology, 28*, 809–827.

Kern, J. K., Garver, C. R., Grannemann, B. D., Trivedi, M. H., Carmody, R., Andrews, A. A., et al. (2007). Response to vestibular sensory events in autism. *Research in Autism Disorders, 1*, 67–74.

Klintwall, L., Holm, A., Eriksson, M., Carlsson, L. H., Olsson, M. B., Hedvall, A., et al. (2011). Sensory abnormalities in autism: A brief report. *Research in Developmental Disabilities, 32*, 795–800.

Langstrom, N., Grann, M., Richkin, V., Sjostedt, G., & Fazel, S. (2009). Risk factors for violent offending in autism spectrum disorder: A national study of hospitalized individuals. *Journal of Interpersonal Violence, 24*, 1358–1370.

Leekam, S. R., Nieto, C., Libby, S. J., Wing, L., & Gould, J. (2007). Describing the sensory abnormalities of children and adults with autism. *Journal of Autism and Developmental Disorders, 37*, 894–910.

Levy, A., & Perry, A. (2011). Outcomes in adolescents and adults with autism: A review of the literature. *Research in Autism Spectrum Disorders, 5*, 1271–1282.

Lopez, B., & Leekam, S. R. (2003). Do children with autism fail to process information in context? *Journal of Child Psychology and Psychiatry, 44*, 285–300.

Lugnegard, T., Hallerback, M. U., & Gillberg, C. (2011). Psychiatric comorbidity in young adults with a clinical diagnosis of Asperger syndrome. *Research in Developmental Disabilities, 32,* 1910–1917.

Matson, J. L., & Nebel-Schwalm, M. S. (2007). Comorbid psychopathology with autism spectrum disorder in children: An overview. *Research in Developmental Disabilities, 28,* 341–352.

Mehzabin, P., & Stokes, M. A. (2011). Self-assessed sexuality in young adults with high-functioning autism. *Research in Autism Spectrum Disorders, 5,* 614–621.

Montgomery, J. M., Schwean, V., L., Burt, J. G., Dyke, D. I., Thorne, K. J., Hindes, Y. L., et al. (2008). Emotional intelligence and resiliency in young adults with Asperger's disorder: Challenges and opportunities. *Canadian Journal of School Psychology, 23,* 70–93.

Montgomery, J. M., Stoesz, B. M., & McCrimmon, A. W. (2013). Emotional intelligence, theory of mind, and executive functions as predictors of social outcomes in young adults with Asperger syndrome. *Focus on Autism and Other Developmental Disabilities, 28,* 4–13.

Mottron, L., Peretz, I., & Menard, E. (2000). Local and global processing of music in high-functioning persons with autism: Beyond central coherence? *Journal of Child Psychiatry and Psychology, 41,* 1057–1065.

Muller, E., Schuler, A., & Yates, G. B. (2008). Social challenges and supports from the perspective of individuals with Asperger syndrome and other autism spectrum disabilities. *Autism, 12,* 173–190.

Murphy, D. (2003). Admission and cognitive details of male patients diagnosed with Asperger's syndrome detained in a special hospital: Comparison with a schizophrenia and personality disorder sample. *Journal of Forensic Psychiatry and Psychology, 14,* 506–524.

Myles, B. S., Endow, J., & Mayfield, M. (2013). *The hidden curriculum and getting and keeping a job: Navigating the social landscape of employment.* Shawnee Mission, KS: AAPC.

Orsmond, G. L., Krauss, M. W., & Seltzer, M. M. (2004). Peer relationships and social and recreational activities among adolescents and adults with autism. *Journal of Autism and Developmental Disorders, 34,* 245–256.

Palmer, B., Donaldson, C., & Stough, C. (2002). Emotional intelligence and life satisfaction. *Personality and Individual Differences, 33,* 1091–1100.

Plaisted, K. C., O'Riordan, M. A. F., & Baron-Cohen, S. (1998). Enhanced discrimination of novel highly similar stimuli by adults with autism during a perceptual learning task. *Journal of Child Psychology and Psychiatry, 39,* 765–775.

Plank, A. (2013, January 2). Interview with Temple Grandin. Retrieved from *www.wrongplanet.net/article295.html.*

Quek, L., Sofronoff, K., Sheffield, J., White, A., & Kelly, A. (2012). Co-occurring anger in young people with Asperger's syndrome. *Journal of Clinical Psychology, 68,* 1142–1148.

Roy, M., Dillo, W., Emrich, H. M., & Ohlmeier, M. D. (2009). Asperger's syndrome in adulthood. *Deutsches Artzeblatt International, 105,* 59–64.

Sachse, M., Schlitt, S., Hainz, D., Ciaramidaro, A., Schirman, S., Walter H., et al. (2013). Executive and visuo-motor function in adolescents and adults with autism spectrum disorder. *Journal of Autism and Developmental Disorders, 43,* 1222–1235.

Saklofske, D. H., Austin, E. J., & Minski, P. S. (2003). Self-reported emotional intelligence: Factor structure and evidence for construct validity. *Personality and Individual Differences, 34,* 1091–1100.

Samson, A. C., Huber, O., & Gross, J. J. (2012). Emotion regulation in Asperger's syndrome and high-functioning autism. *Emotion, 12,* 659–665.

Schaaf, R. C., Toth-Cohen, S., Johnson, S. L., Outten, G., & Benevides, T. W. (2011). The everyday routines of families of children with autism: Examining the impact of sensory processing difficulties on the family. *Autism, 15,* 373–389.

Shattuck, P. T., Narendorf, S. C., Cooper, B., Sterzing, P. R., Wagner, M., & Taylor, J. L. (2012). Postsecondary education and employment among youth with an autism spectrum disorder. *Pediatrics, 129,* 1042–1049.

Smith, R. S., & Sharp, J. (2013). Fascination and isolation: A grounded theory exploration of unusual sensory experiences in adults with Asperger syndrome. *Journal of Autism and Developmental Disorders, 43,* 891–910.

Standifer, S. A. (2009). *Adult autism and employment: A guide for vocational rehabilitation professionals.* Columbia: University of Missouri, School of Health Professions.

Stokes, M., Newton, N., & Kaur, A. (2007). Stalking, and social and romantic functioning among adolescents and adults with autism spectrum disorder. *Journal of Autism and Developmental Disorders, 37,* 1969–1986.

Sumiyoshi, C., Kawakubo, Y., Suga, M., Sumiyoshi, T., & Kasai, K. (2011). Impaired ability to organize information in individuals with autism spectrum disorders and their siblings. *Neuroscience Research, 69,* 252–257.

Tantam, D. (2000). Psychological disorder in adolescents and adults with Asperger syndrome. *Autism, 4,* 47–62.

Tantam, D., & Prestwood, S. (1999). *A mind of one's own.* London: National Autistic Society.

Taylor, J. L., & Seltzer, M. (2011). Employment and post-secondary educational activities for young adults with autism spectrum disorders during the transition to adulthood. *Journal of Autism and Developmental Disabilities, 41,* 566–574.

Tsatsanis, K. D., Noens, I. L., Illmann, C. L., Pauls, D. L., & Volkmar, F. R. (2011). Managing complexity: Impact of organization and processing style on nonverbal memory in autism spectrum disorders. *Journal of Autism and Developmental Disorders, 41,* 135–147.

Vermeulen, P. (2012). *Autism as context blindness.* Shawnee Mission, KS: AAPC.

Wallace, G. L., & Happe, F. (2008). Time perception in autism spectrum disorders. *Research in Autism Spectrum Disorders, 2,* 447–455.

CHAPTER 2

• • • • • • •

Autism Spectrum Disorders and the Family

• **Lauren Pepa and Sandra L. Harris**

Living our lives is a process of continual evolution. We go from infancy to kindergarten to high school to adult employment to retirement. We move from a family of babies to a family of school-age children to a family of adolescents to a family of adults and to the deaths of the family elders. If we are lucky and resilient, we grow in wisdom and judgment along with growing older. This process of growth can be stressful, exciting, alarming, fascinating, and very challenging for typically developing children and their parents. As parents we suffer all of the normative losses of life, including the deaths of our own parents, sometimes a divorce, sometimes a child who gets into trouble with drugs or crashes the family car, and sometimes our own health problems. In spite of these common losses and challenges, most of us rebound from the events, and life regains its usual equilibrium.

Parents of children with autism spectrum disorders (ASD) face some very special problems as their children mature from toddler to teen to adult and, within adulthood, pass from young adult to middle-aged adult. Although parents rarely live long enough to see their own children become elderly, they must still plan for the future welfare of their adult children with ASD. The fact of the diagnosis remains with the family members in an enduring way and affects their daily lives.

In this chapter we summarize the research on adults with ASD and their families. That includes the role of families in supporting adults on the autism spectrum and the shift in responsibility that occurs as the individual transitions from adolescence to adulthood. We describe the family's role in several domains of an individual's life, including service coordination, educational planning, employment, residential placement, and social support. We also discuss the impact of the transition from adolescence to adulthood on mothers, fathers, and siblings. We examine the changes in coping methods that occur as the children and parents grow older. We also consider how intellectual functioning level, behavioral problems, and medical issues of the person with ASD influence living arrangements and affect the family unit. Finally, we illustrate how parental age influences the plans they make for the adult with ASD.

Brief Review of the Literature

Although many families report significant challenges in managing the transition from adolescence to adulthood for their family member with ASD, the literature, unfortunately, yields very little empirical examination or support in documenting these concerns. Even though the impact of ASD on the family unit has been well researched, the emphasis has largely been placed on first diagnosis and childhood (Taylor & Warren, 2012). For families, this includes the coordination of a diagnostic evaluation, emotional response to the diagnosis of ASD, and then the process of acquiring appropriate services for their children. However, it is clear that the transition from adolescence to adulthood brings specific challenges to both individuals with ASD and their families. Some research even suggests that the parental stress increases as the family member with ASD ages (Scorgie, Wilgosh, & McDonald, 1998). For families of typically developing children, the transition to adulthood usually involves a decrease in direct parental responsibility as children transition to college, live away from home, form romantic relationships, and develop families of their own. However, for families of individuals with ASD, their caretaking responsibilities are often lifelong (Baker, Smith, Greenberg, & Seltzer, 2011). Although this involvement will certainly vary depending on the intellectual ability and behavioral disposition of the individual with ASD, family concern and support are nonetheless sustained and can often encompass new challenges. Furthermore, just as the level of parent involvement has a direct impact on family stress, the role of parents is also extremely important for the well-being of the child. As with typically developing children, research suggests that positive parent–child relationship quality is related to better behavioral and psychological outcomes for individuals with ASD as they transition from adolescence to adulthood (Smith, Greenberg, Seltzer, & Hong, 2008). Given the importance of family for individuals with ASD, it becomes crucial to outline the roles that family members play in the lives of their adolescent and adult children, as well as the impact of these roles on the family members themselves.

The Role of Families in Supporting Adults

Service Coordination

Once an ASD diagnosis has been made, the acquisition and coordination of appropriate services typically follows. This initial step involves significant stress for the family because parents are required to quickly become fluent in the services needed, to identify pathways for securing these services, and to endure the hardships that are often part of the journey (Taylor & Warren, 2012). Fortunately, as children become situated in an academic placement, the parents' role in the coordination of service delivery is often supplemented by school personnel, including caseworkers, child study teams, and the children's teachers. Although parents are considered primary caregivers, they are not required to navigate the waters of service coordination independently.

As families prepare for the transition to adulthood, they may receive less assistance and perhaps even a reduction in the services themselves (Howlin, Alcock, & Burkin, 2005). This may include a reduction in direct therapy services, such as applied behavior analysis, speech, or occupational therapy. The experience will be different between higher and lower functioning individuals with ASD. Higher functioning individuals typically have greater cognitive abilities, are in more mainstream academic settings, and have a greater repertoire of functional skills than their lower functioning counterparts. As they approach adulthood, higher functioning individuals on the autism spectrum are preparing for a transition away from the support of a high school setting and toward a more challenging college or occupational setting (Taylor & Seltzer, 2011). For families, this transition often involves taking primary responsibility for the coordination of their children's services. This increase in parental responsibility begins in adolescence and lasts as long as they assume the role. It should be noted that this increase in responsibility requires many resources on the part of the family unit, including time and money. These practical requirements can often be stressful for parents and may result in some hardship.

Additionally, this increased accountability has been shown to directly affect familial relationships. Research suggests that families of higher functioning individuals on the autism spectrum experience significant strain following the child's exit from college (Taylor & Seltzer, 2011). Additionally, studies reveal that the mother–child relationship can be negatively affected during this time due in part to the parents' difficulties with acquiring appropriate services and activities for their children (Taylor & Seltzer, 2011). Additionally, for higher functioning individuals with ASD, there are several avenues that the child may take following the transition from secondary school. Families of high-functioning individuals on the autism spectrum often have to support their children in obtaining postsecondary education, finding jobs, and, in some cases, living independently. We explore these issues more fully in later sections. Although the role of parents of individuals with ASD mimics the typical parenting experience, they often maintain a more active and sustained involvement with their children.

For families of young adults with more limited functional skills, especially individuals with significant behavior problems, coordination of services can be significantly more cumbersome. Research suggests that individuals on the more impaired end of the autism spectrum continue to require support into adulthood and that these individuals will often transition out of their secondary school settings into supportive day programs or will remain at home (Esbensen et al., 2010). Because appropriate placements are extremely limited and often have extensive wait lists, it often falls to parents to independently initiate coordination of these services many years prior to the children's reaching adulthood. This requires the family to find appropriate day programs, align themselves with support organizations (e.g., the Department of Human Services' Division of Developmental Disabilities), and follow up with these placement requests year after year until a spot is secured. Parents therefore struggle to maintain appropriate services for their children if placements do not become readily available, and they may require leaves of absence from work or need to hire respite workers to supervise their children at home. The families of lower functioning individuals with ASD also experience a transition in service coordination between adolescence and adulthood, often requiring them to play a significantly more active role during this sensitive time (Kring, Greenberg, & Seltzer, 2008).

Educational Transition

In terms of educational services, the transition from adolescence into adulthood involves leaving high school and finding a new placement. The research in this area is limited, but Taylor and Seltzer (2011) investigated the vocational and day activities of individuals with ASD following their exit from secondary school. The authors sampled 66 young adults with ASD who were recruited from an ongoing research project. Individuals of all functioning levels were included in the sample. Results suggested that almost 50% of the sample moved on to postsecondary education with some support. For families with children who pursued higher education, the parents' experience paralleled a typical transitional experience. These families helped their children find appropriate educational settings, filled out application materials, and helped with the transition to placement once admitted. However, unlike families of typically developing individuals, familial involvement was more demanding. Families helped their children secure appropriate academic accommodations after admission and provided consistent support throughout their children's enrollment.

For lower functioning individuals with ASD, the family role in the educational transition also holds challenges. As these adults do not move on to postsecondary education, families must coordinate other opportunities, including employment settings or skills-based adult day programs. In either scenario, due to the limited independence of their children with ASD, families will play a more active role in decision making and setting up these opportunities.

Employment Opportunities

As with their typically developing peers, the transition from adolescence to adulthood for individuals with ASD often involves entry into the workforce. For many individuals on the autism spectrum, families and school districts anticipate the child's needs after graduation and offer work-training opportunities in high school. However, as individuals with ASD age out of their public education, families are required to take an active role in pursuing these employment opportunities for their children. Research suggests that approximately one-third of individuals with ASD obtain some employment; however, very few are in competitive employment settings (Taylor & Seltzer, 2011). Research on the predictors of independent employment for people with ASD is minimal, but there is some research to suggest that functioning level, or intelligence more specifically, has the most direct correlation with obtaining occupational placements. Specifically, those individuals with lower intellectual functioning are less successful than those with higher intelligence scores (Taylor & Seltzer, 2011).

Whereas individuals with ASD who have cognitive impairment or behavioral challenges are largely unemployed or underemployed, employment opportunities for higher functioning individuals are more available, and in some cases these individuals work in relatively independent settings through competitive employment. These individuals can often find placements within job sites that are created for individuals with special needs, or they may even function adaptively in a typical job setting. For these individuals, family involvement in finding job opportunities may be modest and can be done independently by the adolescent after high school. Although families may have to facilitate transportation or other resources, employment itself can often be completed autonomously. This modest involvement is often a relief for families and may alleviate some stress for families who are experiencing financial difficulties (Taylor & Seltzer, 2011).

For individuals with lower intellectual functioning or significant behavioral issues, securing employment opportunities may be more difficult. Overall, the research suggests that individuals with ASD are at a disadvantage when it comes to functional independence, for example, when compared with individuals with Down syndrome (Esbensen et al., 2010). However, the two groups were found to be comparable with regard to vocational independence, with the majority of both groups in supportive employment or sheltered workshops (Esbensen et al., 2010). Although these results would suggest comparable outcomes, the research suggests that individuals with ASD require more highly supported settings than do people with Down syndrome (Ballaban-Gil, Rapin, Tuchman, & Shinnar, 1996). For families of children with ASD, finding appropriate employment for their children can be quite challenging and labor intensive.

Residential Transition

For typical adolescents, the transition to adulthood often involves a change in residency status. They may move out of their parents' houses, into dorm rooms or their own apartments, and then move into a home to start a family of their own. For individuals with ASD entering adulthood, families also have to consider the long-term residential status of their children. Esbensen and colleagues (2010) compared individuals with ASD and Down syndrome on several measures of independence typically found in adult populations: residential independence, social interaction, and vocational independence. Results suggested that individuals with ASD showed less overall functional independence in adulthood than those with Down syndrome. While not differing on vocational status, individuals with ASD were found to have less social contact with friends and were more likely to live in community residences than were the adults with Down syndrome (Esbensen et al., 2010).

For families of individuals with ASD, the transition from adolescence to adulthood involves many difficult decisions. The parents of higher functioning individuals may often discuss with their sons or daughters the wisdom of staying at home or moving out and living on their own. As with their typically developing peers, the family and the adolescent evaluate whether the child is "ready" to live independently. This evaluation involves close consideration of their adaptive skills, employment status, and social network. For those individuals who are better suited to continue living at home, the families will adjust to this decision and plan for the future. For those who are ready to live on their own, the families can prepare their children for this change. For many, this decision requires considerable thought and planning on the part of the entire family unit. It is important to recognize that this decision may change over time, requiring families to incorporate new information about their children's abilities and maturity.

Families of lower functioning individuals undergo a similar process in the transition to adulthood. For these individuals, they are often deciding whether their children will remain in the home or move to a supportive residential placement (e.g., supported residence, group home). To keep an adult child in the home involves a continuation of the direct care responsibilities of the parents, which may place stress on the family unit (Smith et al., 2010). Furthermore, families of individuals with behavior problems often have to adapt behavior plans to meet the needs of their adult children. Research suggests that this responsibility can be further exacerbated by health problems, which are common in adolescents and adults with ASD (Kring, Greenberg, & Seltzer, 2010). The combination of these factors leads to increased maternal burden and to stress on the family as a whole (Kring et al., 2010). Although there are significant family considerations over keeping an adult child in the home, families also experience great difficulty in making the decision to place their children in residential or group settings. Families prefer to find a facility with which they feel comfortable. The limited availability of these placements requires the family to prepare for this transition many years in advance. Additionally, despite the hardship and stress that families often experience, parents and siblings alike often have difficulty separating from the individual with ASD (Glasberg, Martins, & Harris, 2006). This transition can therefore be very emotionally stressful for the whole family.

Finally, for families of children at any functioning level on the autism spectrum, it is crucial to recognize the importance of the entire family in making decisions regarding residency and caregiving. For most families, parents take primary caregiving and guardianship responsibilities for their children with ASD until late adolescence or adulthood. However, research on siblings of these individuals suggests that many begin to consider their own caregiving responsibilities as they reach adolescence (Glasberg, 2000). During this time, typically developing siblings may think about the role they want to have in their sibling's life, and parents may initiate discussions about the role they envision. While siblings frequently have some caregiving responsibilities throughout childhood, this time of transition makes future responsibilities extremely salient (Glasberg, 2000).

Finding Social Support

Families are also involved in the acquisition of social support and social networks. One of the core symptoms of ASD is impairment in social interaction, and this deficit is no different for adolescents and adults. A study by Shattuck and colleagues (2007) suggests that limited social relationships was the most commonly reported autism symptom in their sample of adolescents and adults. Furthermore, a study by Hofvander and colleagues (2009) sampled 122 individuals of normal intelligence with autism spectrum diagnoses. Results of their analysis revealed that 56% of participants had been bullied by peers and only 16% had lived in a long-term relationship. In considering how to provide services to address these deficits, one might keep in mind that research suggests that social contact helps to increase independence and broaden social support (Esbensen et al., 2010).

Given the importance of social networks and the impairments in social functioning experienced by individuals with ASD, families play a crucial role in acquiring services. Their involvement may include facilitating participation in social skills groups or creating socialization opportunities. As in other areas, parents of lower functioning individuals may take a more active role in the coordination of these services. Families of higher functioning individuals may see more independence and initiative on the part of the adolescents.

Supporting Families

Given the significant role that parents play in the lives of adolescents and adults with ASD, it becomes increasingly important to address not only the well-being of the affected children but also that of the family members providing support. This section addresses the research on family coping strategies, factors that affect individual coping, and ways to best support families during this transitional time.

Changes in Coping Methods across Time

The concept of coping refers to how parents address the many stressful problems they face over the years, from the time they first learn of the young child's ASD diagnosis to the demands of the adult years (Glasberg et al., 2006). Raising a child on the spectrum is inherently stressful because of the specialized care the child requires and the need to find appropriate educational services, to manage disruptive behaviors, and to balance the multiple needs of the child with ASD with the needs of the rest of the nuclear family, including spouse, siblings, and aging parents.

One example of how family life is influenced as the person with an ASD grows up is found in how the strategies for parental coping may change as their child with ASD becomes an adult. A longitudinal study by Gray (2006) looked at parental coping over 10 years, using in-depth interviews with 19 mothers and 9 fathers to explore how they coped with the needs of their children with ASD. At the 10-year follow-up, the children had a mean age of 18 years. Gray found at follow-up that parents relied less on problem-focused strategies—such as utilizing service providers, seeking family support, withdrawing from outside relationships to focus on the child with ASD, and relying on individualism—as their coping methods. These problem-focused strategies aim to directly address and reduce the source of a stressor. Instead, parents employed more emotion-focused strategies, such as religious faith and valuing their child's strengths. These strategies are not focused on reducing the source of stress but rather on adapting one's emotional reaction to a life stressor.

Although parents of children of any age may draw upon their spiritual values or religious faith (e.g., Ekas, Whitman, & Shivers. 2009), as people get older they are more likely to put greater emphasis on these and other emotion-based values. This shift in coping methods is not unique to parents of children with ASD but is related to one's stage of maturity. The research suggests that as people grow older they depend less on problem-focused and more on emotion-focused strategies (e.g., Carstensen et al., 2011; Scheibe, 2012). In the case of parents of children with ASD, the shift may be heightened by the relative lack of public resources for adults on the spectrum and by the deaths of grandparents who might have played a key support role for the family (Glasberg et al., 2006). Gray (2006) also notes that the children as a group exhibited fewer problem behaviors at the 10-year follow-up and that this reduction enabled most parents to use fewer problem-focused strategies.

Maternal Well-Being

In terms of maternal adjustment, a longitudinal study by Lounds, Seltzer, Greenberg, and Shattuck (2007) found that mothers of 140 adolescents and young adults with ASD reported fewer behavior problems over time. The mother–child relationship also improved during this interval. The mothers appeared to have made an adaptation to their children's behavior during the transition period between adolescence and young adulthood. They were less anxious. Nonetheless, almost 25% reported an increase in depression, and 16% had an increase in anxiety, so this period is not one of universal improvement. Consistent with other studies, Lounds and colleagues (2007) found that the young people as a group had a decline in overall symptoms of ASD and problem behaviors. The decline in problem behaviors may be linked to the improvement in maternal well-being. The reduction in ASD symptoms per se was not related to maternal outcome.

One important subgroup of young people who appear to be quite challenged after high school are young adults on the high-functioning end of the spectrum. A 2010 report by Taylor and Seltzer notes that after these young people leave high school, they experience a decline in the warmth of the mother–child relationship. This change may reflect in part the frustration mothers feel when their intelligent children with ASD do not complete college or find jobs and begin to engage in more maladaptive behavior. These young people, although bright in many skill areas, often have few resources available to them in the community and may sit at home for months, perhaps engaging in ritualized behaviors.

As part of a longitudinal study of the families of people with ASD, Barker and her colleagues (2011) studied the emotional well-being of mothers of 379 adolescents and adults with ASD over a decade. They measured depressive symptoms and anxiety in midlife and in old age of the mothers of these teenagers and adults with ASD. When they controlled for maternal age, they found that anxiety declined over 10 years for the entire sample and that older women were less anxious than younger women at the start of the study. Symptoms of depression were stable over this same decade. They also found that when the adolescent or adult with ASD moved out of the home, there was a drop in maternal anxiety, although maternal depression remained stable. Mothers also described greater anxiety when their social support networks were diminished or when they faced other difficult family events.

Adult Siblings

Our brothers and sisters offer us an enduring relationship. If we are fortunate, long after the deaths of our parents, our siblings will still be part of our lives. Having a brother or sister with ASD creates challenges for siblings that most people with typically developing siblings do not encounter. Fortunately, most children who have a brother or sister on the spectrum learn to manage their feelings of frustration, disappointment, and anger and are as psychologically healthy as their peers who have typically developing brothers or sisters (Harris & Glasberg, 2012). Almost all of the sibling research has focused on childhood relationships, and there are relatively few data on the relationships of typically developing adults and their siblings with ASD. Because the problem behaviors of the person with ASD often become less intense over time and the typically developing adult sibling has grown in perspective, there may be changes in the sibling-to-sibling relationship as each matures.

Seltzer, Orsmond, and Esbensen (2009) used a cross-sectional design to compare the relationship between persons with ASD and their typically developing siblings during both the adolescence and the adulthood of the siblings. They write that although the adult siblings had less contact with their siblings with ASD than did the adolescents, their ratings of the positive affect in the sibling relationship did not differ. Seltzer and colleagues note that interactions between typically developing siblings tend to diminish in adolescence and early adulthood and then increase later in life. Like their same-age peers, the typically developing adolescent siblings of persons with ASD reported more emotion-focused coping methods and fewer problem-focused methods than did the adults. Interestingly, the adolescents said they had more social support from their friends and from their parents than did the adults. However, Seltzer and colleagues note that among those adults who did report support from their parents, there was a relationship between that parental support and the adult's positive evaluation of the relationship with the sibling with ASD. They also found gender differences for the adult siblings, with men who had sisters with ASD showing the least involvement with their sisters and those women who had sisters with ASD showing the most engagement.

Case Examples of Families Supporting Adults

We have had the privilege of working with families of adults on the autism spectrum. In some instances, we knew the adults from childhood, and in other cases they came to our program when they aged out of the school system. To protect their identities, we have altered names and other minor details that could potentially compromise the identities of the families involved.

Independent Work Setting

The Martin Family

Jessica and Mark Martin have four children, and their youngest son, Christopher, has ASD. Christopher was first diagnosed at the age of 4, after his parents became concerned about his lack of interest in other children and repetitive play with toys. At this time, Christopher received therapeutic services that included speech therapy and occupational therapy. When Christopher turned school age, he was enrolled at the mainstream elementary school in a special education classroom with other children who had special learning concerns. During these first few years, Christopher's language ability flourished, but he experienced more significant impairments in social functioning and academic demands.

Christopher's parents enrolled him in social skills groups in the community and received educational accommodations at school that allotted him extra help and time to complete tests and assignments. During this time, Christopher was mainstreamed in several academic subjects, and he began to interact more readily with peers. When Christopher entered high school, he was enrolled in the local vocational school and attended classes there as part of his school day. At this program, he learned important job skills training that included exposure to different job opportunities. During this time, Christopher and his parents had conversations about the skills he was learning and what he might want to do in the future. Christopher also expressed interest in going to college, but was unsure about what academic area he wanted to pursue.

When Christopher graduated from high school, his parents helped to find him a job at a local accounting office doing clerical work. The individuals who owned the office were affiliated with the vocational school and had previously hired individuals with ASD with great success. They provided Christopher with extensive work training, a structured schedule, and many opportunities to ask questions when needed. Both Christopher and his parents agreed that working at the office would provide him with the opportunity to work and build his job skills, while also allowing him the opportunity to explore future endeavors more fully. Christopher is continuing to live at home and is currently planning to apply to local colleges for the next academic year.

Discussion

Christopher is an example of a very high-functioning individual with ASD who was able to succeed in a mainstream school with appropriate educational and social supports. Christopher's family obtained services from the time of first diagnosis that extended all the way through his high school career. Christopher knew that he wanted to attend college one day, and Christopher's parents and his support team at school knew that it was important for him to learn vocational skills in addition to academic skills. During this time, Christopher learned crucial skills for working in a professional setting, including organizational skills, time management, and social skills necessary for working with others. Christopher also tried different areas of employment, including clerical work, veterinary assistance, and food preparation. Allowing Christopher to try all of these areas allowed him to better identify areas of interest that may translate into a future career.

Although Christopher and his parents all want him to attend college, they also recognized that Christopher was not ready to make this transition upon graduation and would benefit from work experience prior to that commitment. The family was disappointed that he could not attend college along with many students in his class, but they were also relieved to find a work setting in which Christopher could work independently and gain valuable experience.

Supported Work Setting

The Walker Family

Francine and Randall Walker have one child, Belle, who was diagnosed with ASD at 2 years old. Francine and Randall began to suspect a developmental delay when Belle reached 18 months of age without saying her first word. Following an evaluation, Belle received early intervention services in the home, including applied behavior analysis (ABA), speech therapy, and occupational therapy. In addition to Belle's language delay, she also had intellectual impairments and engaged in significant maladaptive behaviors, including repetitive flapping of her hands and aggression directed at others when access to preferred items was denied. When Belle came of school age, she briefly attended a public elementary school in a self-contained classroom. Unfortunately, after a year, the school district decided that they could not accommodate Belle's educational and behavioral needs. Belle was then sent to an out-of-district placement that specialized in ABA services.

In this setting, school personnel sufficiently addressed Belle's educational needs, and she began to acquire important academic and adaptive skills. In the beginning, adaptive activities focused on skills for daily living, including basic hygiene, setting the table, and selecting her own clothing. Once these skills were acquired and Belle got older, the school stressed the importance of vocational skills to Belle's parents. They noted that it would be unlikely that Belle would work completely independently at a job site in the future; however, it was important for her to learn job skills in order to achieve some functional independence. Belle's parents agreed, and she began training with school personnel at a local grocery store stocking shelves and at a local restaurant setting tables.

When Belle transitioned out of her school placement, her parents were concerned that she would not find comparable opportunities in the community. Her parents had placed themselves on wait lists for adult day programs, and they had to wait almost 2 years before Belle was accepted into a program. This delay was stressful for Belle and her parents. Her parents were required to hire respite workers to be with Belle during the day, and they practiced vocational skills with Belle in the home when they returned from work. Fortunately, after 2 years Francine and Randall were offered a placement with an applied behavior analysis–based adult day program. In addition to providing skills training, they found Belle a supported position at a restaurant where she could use the skills she had learned in high school. Although this transition was somewhat difficult for Belle, she adapted and functioned at the restaurant with the help of day program staff. Belle's family was very relieved at her opportunity to attend the program and her continued access to employment opportunities.

Discussion

Belle's situation is a difficult one that involves significant family stress and adaptation. Belle's parents were called into action while Belle was at a young age to coordinate appropriate educational and therapeutic services. The decision by parents to enroll their child in a specialized placement can be difficult. Parents will grieve the realities of their child's abilities and the support that is required to maintain his or her skills and prosocial behaviors. Belle's family also experienced significant challenges during the transition out of high school and into her adult life. Whereas she had received skills training in a very supportive setting in school and was exposed to several different vocational placements, the high demand for adult programs left her without a placement upon graduation. During this time, Belle's parents assumed the responsibility of coordinating her daily activities and maintaining vocational skills when possible. This obligation was extremely stressful for Francine and Randall. Fortunately, they connected with a local parent support group where they met other parents of disabled adults and shared their experiences. Then, after 2 years, Belle was placed in an adult day program, and her vocational placements could be continued.

Case Examples of Strategies for Coping

The Diaz Family

Sophia and Santiago Diaz had a daughter, Pilar, who was diagnosed with ASD at the age of 3 years. They enrolled her in a specialized preschool for children with ASD within a few months of receiving that diagnosis. Pilar made good progress in the preschool, and when she turned 5 she was enrolled in a regular kindergarten with some extra classroom support. Sophia and Santiago were pleased to see Pilar making good academic progress but were concerned about her difficulties with establishing friendships in school. Many of the other children were kind to her, and in the lower grades they invited her to birthday parties, but Pilar was baffled by how to connect with her peers and actually had little interest in doing so.

When she graduated from high school Pilar had done well academically, but she remained naive about how to navigate the world outside of school. She knew she wanted to go to college and become an engineer. The school guidance counselor suggested that she first take some courses at the local community college and then, if she did well, transfer to a 4-year college. Fortunately for Pilar and her family, the community college had a support program for students with ASD. Support program staff helped students get oriented to the campus, organized social activities for the students with ASD, and coached them in how to interact with faculty members and peers. Pilar was assigned a peer buddy who kept an eye on her and included her in some activities on campus. Once again, Pilar did well academically, and thanks to the support program she learned to be a little more "savvy" about how to interact with people. After 2 years at the community college, Pilar transferred to a 4-year college, where there was also a support program for people on the spectrum.

Although Pilar lived at home while she attended the community college, her parents discussed with her the possibility of living in a dormitory when she started the new college. They talked to the residence counselors about how to arrange for Pilar to live on campus. Based on the residence staff's experience with other students on the spectrum, they recommended that Pilar have her own room and be assigned a "big sister" who would help Pilar adapt to living in the dorm and on campus.

Discussion

Pilar, who was very bright, did well in high school and in the community college. One of her primary challenges was learning how to understand and relate to other people, including her peers and teachers. It was her very good fortune to be born to parents who quickly realized that she needed a great deal of specialized help if she were to maximize her potential. They enrolled her in a preschool program within a short time after they got the diagnosis and collaborated fully with the teaching staff in the preschool. They were also very responsive to suggestions of her teachers throughout her public school years, and most of the teachers, in turn, looked to Sophia and Santiago for suggestions about how best to support Pilar in school. By the time she enrolled in the community college, Pilar had learned some basic self- advocacy skills, and with her parents and the staff of the support program coaching her behind the scenes, she made requests of her professors and asked for the accommodations she some-times needed. In addition, her peer buddy helped Pilar begin to interact with other students at the community college. These skills transferred when Pilar made the very major move from the small community college to a much larger 4-year college and to living in a dormitory on campus. When last we heard, Pilar had found an entry-level job as an engineer and was living at home with her parents. Sophia and Santiago told us they hoped she would eventually move into a supervised apartment where she would have someone who would check on her periodically and teach her how to do things such as pay bills.

The Sullivan Family

Dan and Emily Sullivan had married relatively late in life and were both in their mid-50s when Bobby, who had ASD, turned 18. At that point Bobby was taller and stronger than his father, and when he did not get the things he wanted, he would sometimes have tantrums and lash out at his parents. Dan had been diagnosed with high blood pressure and cardiac problems and realized he could no longer safely control his son. There was a serious risk that Dan or Emily might be seriously injured by Bobby, even though he had no deliberate intent to harm them. Although they had been caring and devoted parents, they knew they could no longer meet Bobby's needs and remain safe at home.

The Sullivans struggled with their decision to request a group home placement, but they could find no other reasonable option and some-what reluctantly accepted a placement. They toured several different group homes and were impressed by the one in which they placed Bobby because of the warmth they felt there and the ability of the men and women on the staff to protect Bobby and keep him safe as well as happy. Moving day for Bobby was difficult for his parents and confusing for him, but over the course of the next few months Dan and Emily realized that their son had made a good adjustment to the residence and in fact went into the community far more often than they had taken him.

Discussion

The decision to move an adult child from the family home to a group home is difficult for almost every family who makes that choice. Some-times, as was the case with Bobby, the child's challenging behavior, per-haps combined with parental health issues, makes keeping the adult with ASD in the family home against the best interest of both the parents and the adult child. Even a compliant adult child at some point is probably best served by making the move from family home to group home. If this move is delayed too long, the parents may die, leaving no one to help their adult child make the transition from family home to community.

Some families make advance arrangements for a sibling to assume the care of the adult with ASD. That provision can vary from asking the sibling to keep a loving watch over a brother or sister who resides in a group home to having the adult with ASD live with the sibling. In every case in which a sibling plays an active role, parents and the adult sibling (and his or her partner, if there is one) need to have discussed this option and made a joint decision about how things will be handled. Learning after one's parents have died that one is supposed to assume a direct care role for the adult with ASD may work out very poorly and ultimately result in a group home placement.

A Checklist for Parents

Between the two of us, we have 50 years of experience working with people who have ASD and their families. That experience, in various settings, has given us a wonderful opportunity to know parents and siblings and the challenges they face when there is someone with ASD in the family. These family members have been among our best teachers. Between what we have learned from families and what we have learned from evidence-based research, we have some suggestions for parents and supporting professionals who are facing the challenges and opportunities of the transition from high school to postsecondary life for a child with ASD.

1. The transition from early adolescence into adulthood is often accompanied by a reduction in some of the troubling behaviors of a teen with ASD (e.g., Lounds et al., 2007). Under these conditions, parental distress may diminish. But other young adults continue to pose serious management problems that may intensify parental worry and sadness. It makes sense under those conditions to seek support from a therapist or religious advisor. Support groups are another valuable resource, and friendships are to be treasured as a place to seek comfort.

2. When children with ASD are in the public schools, much of the coordination of their services is done by the professionals who work in that setting in consultation with parents. Services for adults with ASD are often more limited, and it becomes the role of parents to do much of the coordination. Learn as much as you can about the resources that are potentially available to your adult child and begin making plans to access appropriate resources while he or she is still in middle school and high

school. Don't wait until your child has completed high school to begin that planning. Make sure your child is on all appropriate waiting lists for resources, including adult day programs, vocational training programs, and group homes or supervised apartments.

3. Make realistic plans. If your child has ASD and intellectual disability, look for resources that are appropriate to her or his skills and abilities. If your child is of average or higher intelligence and has developed a number of potentially marketable skills, find the educational or vocational resources that will support that level of ability. That could be a community college, a 4-year university, or a vocational program that focuses on your child's special skills and interests, such as the area of information technology.

4. If you are hoping your typically developing children will assume some responsibility for your child with ASD when you can no longer fill that role, you need to discuss those plans with your children and, if they are married, with their partners, as well.

5. If your child is not capable of managing his or her own affairs, be sure you have established guardianship so that you oversee his or her needs. Also make plans for the transfer of guardianship when you are no longer able to manage that responsibility.

6. Consult an attorney who specializes in creating trusts for people with disabilities so that you can ensure that your adult child's resources will be protected.

Conclusion
• • • • • • •

The research findings provided in this chapter, in conjunction with the case studies, help to illustrate the essential role that families play in the lives of adults with ASD. This involvement is particularly salient during the sensitive transition from adolescence to adulthood, when several important changes and decisions are being made. Research suggests that parents are significantly involved in several aspects of the child's life and often feel significant emotional ramifications from this involvement. However, as clear and salient as these feelings and behaviors are, the research evidence to support these claims is lagging behind the experience of families. In our clinical work, every day we encounter parents and families who are going through this transitional period and who echo the sentiments that the small literature conveys. While it is unfortunate that the research has not yet captured this experience in full, this area is fertile for future research and investigation.

REFERENCES

Baker, J. K., Smith, L. E., Greenberg, J. S., & Seltzer, M. M. (2011). Change in maternal criticism and behavior problems in adolescents and adults with autism across a seven-year period. *Journal of Abnormal Psychology, 120*(2), 465–475.

Ballaban-Gil, K., Rapin, L., Tuchman, T., & Shinnar, S. (1996). Longitudinal examination of the behavioral, language, and social changes in a population of adolescent and young adults with autistic disorder. *Pediatric Neurology, 15,* 217–223.

Barker, E. T., Hartley, S. L., Seltzer, M. M., Floyd, F. J., Greenberg, J. S., & Orsmond, G. I. (2011). Trajectories of emotional well-being in mothers of adolescents and adults with autism. *Developmental Psychology, 47,* 551–561.

Carstensen, L. L., Turan, B., Scheibe, S., Ram, N., Ersner-Hershfield, H., Samanez-Larkin, G. R., et al. (2011). Emotional experience improves with age: Evidence based on over 10 years of experience sampling. *Psychology and Aging, 26,* 21–33

Ekas, N. V., Whitman, T. L., & Shivers, C. (2009). Religiosity, spirituality, and socioemotional functioning in mothers of children with autism spectrum disorder. *Journal of Autism and Developmental Disorders, 39,* 706–719.

Esbensen, A. J., Bishop, S. L., Seltzer, M. M., Greenberg, J. S., & Taylor, J. L. (2010). Comparisons between individuals with autism spectrum disorders and individuals with Down syndrome in adulthood. *American Journal of Intellectual and Developmental Disabilities, 115*(4), 277–290.

Glasberg, B., Martins, M., & Harris, S. L. (2006). Stress and coping among family members of individuals with autism. In M. G. Baron, J. Groden, G. Groden, & L. P. Lipsett (Eds.), *Stress and coping in autism* (pp. 277–301). New York: Oxford University Press.

Glasberg, B. A. (2000). The development of siblings' understanding of autism spectrum disorders. *Journal of Autism and Developmental Disorders, 30*(2), 143–156.

Gray, D. E. (2006). Coping over time: The parents of children with autism. *Journal of Intellectual Disability Research, 50,* 970–976.

Harris, S. L., & Glasberg, B. (2012). *Siblings of children with autism* (3rd ed.). Bethesda, MD: Woodbine House.

Hofvander, B., Delorme, R., Chaste, P., Nyden, A., Wentz, E., Stahlberg, O., et al. (2009). Psychiatric and psychosocial problems in adults with normal-intelligence autism spectrum disorders. *BMC Psychiatry, 9,* 35.

Howlin, P., Alcock, J., & Burkin, C. (2005). An 8-year follow-up of a specialist-supported employment service for high-ability adults with autism or Asperger syndrome. *Autism, 9,* 533–549.

Kring, S. R., Greenberg, J. S., & Seltzer, M. M. (2008). Adolescents and adults with autism with and without co-morbid psychiatric disorders: Differences in maternal well-being. *Journal of Mental Health Research in Intellectual Disabilities, 1*(2), 53–74.

Kring, S. R., Greenberg, J. S., & Seltzer, M. M. (2010). The impact of health problems on behavior problems in adolescents and adults with autism spectrum disorders: Implications for maternal burden. *Social Work Mental Health, 8*(1), 54–71.

Lounds, J., Seltzer, M. M., Greenberg, J. S., & Shattuck, P. T. (2007). Transition and change in adolescents and young adults with autism: Longitudinal effects on maternal well-being. *American Journal of Mental Retardation, 112,* 401–417.

Scheibe, S. (2012). The golden years of emotion. *Association for Psychological Science Observer, 25,* 19–21.

Scorgie, K., Wilgosh, L., & McDonald, L. (1998) Stress and coping in families of children with disabilities: An examination of recent literature. *Developmental Disabilities Bulletin, 26*(1), 22–42.

Seltzer, M. M., Orsmond, G. I., & Esbensen, A. J. (2009). Siblings of individuals with autism spectrum disorder: Sibling relationships and well-being in adolescence and adulthood. *Autism, 13,* 59–80.

Shattuck, P. T., Seltzer, M. M., Greenberg, J. S., Orsmond, G. I., Bolt, D., Kring, S., et al. (2007). Change in autism symptoms and maladaptive behaviors in adolescents and adults with an autism spectrum disorder. *Journal of Autism and Developmental Disorders, 37*(9), 1735–1747.

Smith, L. E., Greenberg, J. S., Seltzer, M. M., & Hong, J. (2008). Symptoms and behavior problems of adolescents and adults with autism: Effects of mother–child relationship quality, warmth, and praise. *American Journal of Mental Retardation, 113*(5), 387–402.

Smith, L. E., Hong, J., Seltzer, M. M., Greenberg, J. S., Almeida, D. M., & Bishop, S. L. (2010). Daily experiences among mothers of adolescents and adults with autism spectrum disorder. *Journal of Autism and Developmental Disorders, 40*(2), 167–178.

Taylor, J. L., & Seltzer, M. M. (2010). Changes in the mother–child relationship during the transition to adulthood for youth with autism spectrum disorders. *Journal of Autism and Developmental Disorders, 41,* 1397–1410.

Taylor, J. L., & Seltzer, M. M. (2011). Employment and post-secondary activities for young adults with autism spectrum disorders during the transition to adulthood. *Journal of Autism and Developmental Disorders, 41*(5), 566–574.

Taylor, J. L., & Warren, Z. E. (2012). Maternal depressive symptoms following autism spectrum diagnosis. *Journal of Autism and Developmental Disorders, 42,* 1411–1418.

PART II
• • • • •
Transitioning from Adolescence to Adulthood

CHAPTER 3

● ● ● ● ● ●

Effective Secondary Education and Transition for Adolescents with Autism Spectrum Disorders

● **Michael L. Wehmeyer and Dianne Zager**

The purpose of this book is to provide a comprehensive overview of evidence-based and promising practices for adults with autism spectrum disorders (ASD). Adulthood begins with the process of individuation and the transition from adolescence to young adulthood. Making the transition from high school to adulthood represents a period during which all adolescents face multiple responsibilities and changing roles that include establishing independence, attending postsecondary education or training, developing social networks, choosing careers, participating in their communities, and managing health care and financial affairs (Wehmeyer & Webb, 2012). Transition to postsecondary education, employment, independent living, and community integration is especially challenging for people with autism because transitions require skills and abilities that, by nature, are difficult for these people to acquire due to characteristics related to this disability (Zager & Wehmeyer, in press). This chapter examines effective secondary education practices for youth and young adults with ASD that lead to successful adulthood.

Secondary Education and Transition Services for Adolescents with ASD

Access to the General Education Curriculum

As per federal requirements, the educational programs of all students receiving special education services must ensure that students are involved with and progress in the general education curriculum and are provided instruction in *other educational needs* not addressed in the general education curriculum. A comprehensive discussion of the former with regard to academic instruction for high school students with ASD is beyond the scope of this chapter; but, of course, success in adulthood is predicated on acquiring the literacy, math, science, and other content knowledge and skills associated with the general education curriculum. Ensuring that students receiving special education services have access to the general education curriculum was a key feature of the 1997 and 2004 amendments to the Individuals with Disabilities Education Act (IDEA; the federal law requiring a free appropriate education for all students with disabilities), and these requirements were intended to ensure that students with disabilities were held to high expectations and had access to a high-quality, challenging curriculum.

We highlight these federal requirements to emphasize that, although our chapter focuses principally on transition services and college and career readiness issues pertaining to the secondary education of students with ASD, it is important to remember that, like all students, students with ASD must receive high-quality instruction in core academic content and also the supplementary aids and services, specially designed instruction, and related services that they need in order to progress in core content courses with their peers without disabilities. Furthermore, with the advent of a focus on college and career readiness for all students (discussed subsequently), it is clear that transition-related services are increasingly becoming more aligned with content in the general education curriculum for all students (Morningstar, Bassett, Cashman, Kochhar-Bryant, & Wehmeyer, 2012).

Transition Services

The federal focus on transition services for youth receiving special education services has its roots in the work study programs of the 1960s and the career education movement of the 1970s (Halpern, 1994). The 1990 amendments to IDEA mandated that transition services be provided to students 16 and older or students 14 and older, if appropriate. The 2004 reauthorization of IDEA required that transition services be considered for all students ages 16 and over receiving special education services, though many state plans kept the age at 14, and defined "transition services" as a coordinated set of activities for a child with a disability that:

- Is designed to be within a results-oriented process, that is, focused on improving the academic and functional achievement of the child with a disability to facilitate the child's movement from school to postschool activities, including postsecondary education, vocational education, integrated employment (including supported employment), continuing and adult education, adult services, independent living, or community participation;
- Is based on the individual child's needs, taking into account the child's strengths, preferences, and interests; and
- Includes instruction, related services, community experiences, the development of employment and other postschool adult living objectives, and, if appropriate, acquisition of daily living skills and functional vocational evaluation [34 CFR 300.43 (a)] [20 U.S.C. 1401(34)].

IDEA also requires that when transition services are discussed at an individualized education program (IEP) meeting, students must be invited and, as noted above, that needed transition services must take into account student strengths, preferences, and interests. These so-called *student-involvement* requirements have, in part, led to an emphasis on promoting the self-determination of students with disabilities in transition supports and services, an emphasis that is discussed in some detail subsequently.

Wehmeyer and Patton (2012) identified a number of guiding principles essential to the transition process for all youth, including youth with ASD. These principles follow.

- Transition efforts should start early.
- Planning must be comprehensive.
- Planning processes must consider a student's preferences and interests.
- The transition planning process should be considered a capacity-building activity (i.e., considering a student's strengths).
- Student participation throughout the process is essential.
- Family involvement is desired, needed, and crucial.
- The transition planning process must be sensitive to diversity.
- Supports and services are useful, and we all use them.

- Community-based activities provide extremely beneficial experiences.
- Interagency commitment and coordination is essential.
- Timing is crucial if certain linkages are to be made and a seamless transition to life after high school is to be achieved.

The federally funded National Secondary Transition Technical Assistance Center (NSTTAC) has established a taxonomy for transition programming (Kohler, 1996) that embodies the above-referenced principles and that provides a guide for educators focusing on the transition of youth with ASD. Kohler's (1996) taxonomy conceptualizes high-quality transition programming as addressing five overarching areas: (1) student-focused planning activities (IEP development, student involvement, planning strategies); (2) student development activities (life skills instruction, career and vocational curricula, structured work experiences, assessment support services); (3) family involvement (family training, family involvement, family empowerment); (4) program structure (program philosophy, program policy, strategic planning, program evaluation, resource allocation, human resource development); and (5) interagency collaboration (collaborative framework, collaborative service delivery).

The NSTTAC (2010) has identified evidence-based practices in secondary transition for students with disabilities linked to Kohler's primary areas, provided in Table 3.1. In addition, NSTTAC has identified 16 evidence-based predictors of postschool employment, education, and independent living success, listed in Table 3.2. These evidence-based transition practices and predictors of successful adult outcomes should form the basis for high-quality instructional supports to promote transition for all students, including students with ASD. It is not feasible to discuss each of these in any depth in the context of this chapter, and readers are referred to other sources for more detailed information (Wehmeyer & Webb, 2012), but because several of these instructional areas (social skills, self-determination, student involvement, family involvement) are particularly important for students with ASD, we discuss them in greater depth in subsequent sections.

College and Career Readiness

One of the outcomes of efforts by the Council of Chief State School Officers (CCSSO) and the National Governors Association to promulgate academic content standards in reading and mathematics (e.g., the Common Core State Standards) has been an emphasis on "college and career readiness" for all students. The discussion pertaining to standards that

TABLE 3.1. Evidence-Based Practices in Secondary Transition

Kohler's taxonomy category	Evidence-based practices	
Student-focused planning	• Involving students in the IEP process • Using the Whose Future Is It Anyway? process • Using the self-advocacy strategy • Using the self-directed IEP	
Student development	• Teaching functional life skills:	
	o banking o restaurant purchasing o employment skills using computer-assisted instruction (CAI) o grocery shopping o home maintenance o leisure o personal health o job-specific employment o purchasing using the "one more than" strategy o life skills using CAI o life skills using computer-based instruction (CBI) o goal setting and attainment using the self-determined learning model of instruction	o safety o self-care o self-determination o self-management for life o self-management for employment o self-advocacy o purchasing o functional reading o functional math o social o purchasing o completing a job application o job-related social communication o cooking and food preparation o employment skills using CBI
Family involvement	• Training parents about transition services	
Program structure	• Providing community-based instruction • Extending services beyond secondary school • Using *check and connect*	
Interagency coordination	• None	

Note. From National Secondary Transition Technical Assistance Center (2010).

lead to college and career readiness harkens back to our earlier point that transition-related knowledge and skills are important for all students and are increasingly becoming a part of the general education curriculum. Although discussions of college and career readiness standards have focused principally on core content areas (math, reading), there is an emerging discussion pertaining to career and college readiness for students with disabilities, including students with significant cognitive

TABLE 3.2. Evidence-Based Predictors of Postschool Employment, Education, and Independent Living Success

Predictors/outcomes	Education	Employment	Independent living
Career awareness	×	×	
Community experiences		×	
Exit exam requirements/high school diploma status		×	
Inclusion in general education	×	×	×
Interagency collaboration	×	×	
Occupational courses	×	×	
Paid employment/work experience	×	×	×
Parental involvement		×	
Program of study		×	
Self-advocacy/self-determination	×	×	
Self-care/independent living	×	×	×
Social skills	×	×	
Student support	×	×	×
Transition program	×	×	
Vocational education	×	×	
Work study		×	

Note. From National Secondary Transition Technical Assistance Center (2010).

disabilities (Kearns et al., 2010). The conversation pertaining to college and career readiness for youth with ASD tends to focus on college preparation; the issue of postsecondary education and students with ASD is a topic covered more in depth in a subsequent section. One should not, however, ignore the importance of transition services leading to employment and meaningful community inclusion. The following sections examine what is known about transition outcomes and transition services for youth and young adults with ASD.

Transition and Students with ASD

Few studies have focused on transition-related services and outcomes for youth with ASD as a group (Seltzer, Greenberg, Floyd, & Hong, 2004). That is not to say, however, that there isn't a need to do so. Data from the most recent federal longitudinal study of transition-related outcomes (National Longitudinal Transition Study 2 [NLTS2]) certainly suggest otherwise. Newman (2007) reported on data from the NLTS2 for 1,000 students with ASD. Findings were of the glass-half-full nature. On the positive side, 77% of these youth had at least one vocational education course during high school, and 71% of students had taken at least one life skills course. On the other hand, just over three-quarters of the students who had a vocationally related course received their instruction in a separate, special education setting. The insufficiency of this is seen in the few studies of transition-related outcomes for this population, which show that most young people with ASD continue to live at home with their parents after graduation from high school (Hendricks & Wehman, 2009), are unemployed (Standifer, 2009), and are socially isolated (Wehmeyer & Patton, 2012).

Social skills and transition outcomes are closely linked in the lives of young people with ASD. Findings that young adults with ASD are socially isolated are self-evidently tied to issues of social competence and skills. Even outcomes such as employment tie directly to these issues of social competence. Research shows that social skill limitations are a major reason that people with ASD have difficulty finding or retaining jobs (Schall & Wehman, 2009). Other common issues that impinge on success in post–high school settings include communication difficulties and behavioral issues (Schall & Wehman, 2009) as well as, importantly, the lack of adequate supports within the system to mitigate the effects of these barriers (Targett & Wehman, 2009).

Educational and Transition Planning and IEP Development

Like other educational endeavors, instruction in transition and in college and career readiness begins with planning and assessment. For students receiving special education services, the IEP meeting is often the focal point for such activities as curriculum design, program development, assessment of needed instruction, instructional goal setting, and the identification of needed supports and accommodations.

There are a limited number of transition assessment tools, and fewer still that are particularly targeted only for students with ASD. Again, the NSTTAC provides a useful starting point for consideration of assessment in transition. The Age-Appropriate Transition Assessment Toolkit (NSTTAC, 2013) summarizes important aspects of assessment in transition, among which are that such assessment is an ongoing, and not a static, process; that assessment must begin with information about student needs, preferences, interests, and strengths; and that assessment will, necessarily, use a wide array of techniques, from questionnaires and surveys to observation and interviews. The NSTTAC toolkit identified several informal and formal assessment methods, including:

- Interviews and questionnaires developed to determine a youth's needs, preferences, and interests relative to planning for postsecondary outcomes;
- Direct observation of student performance in vocational, employment, or community living domains;
- Environmental or situational analyses to determine the specific skills needed in environments in which students might live, learn, work, or play and the types of accommodations and supports or context modifications necessary to ensure success;
- Curriculum-based assessments linked to vocational or transition programs or materials;
- Aptitude tests and interest inventories;
- Career development measures;
- Transition planning inventories that provide a scan of student strengths and needs across a wide array of settings.

Three illustrations of the latter (planning inventories) show the process when planning transitions for students with ASD. The first, the Transition Planning Inventory—Updated Version (TPI; Clark & Patton, 2009), is a testing system designed to identify and plan for the comprehensive transition needs of students, with data gathered from the students, parents, and school personnel, across all major transition domains. Rehfeldt, Clark, and Lee (2012) examined whether IEP teams that used the TPI generated significantly more transition-related IEP goals and determined that, among IEP teams for 56 students, including some students with ASD, those IEP teams that used the TPI did develop significantly more transition-related goals.

One autism-specific planning system is the Comprehensive Autism Planning System—Transition (CAPS-TR; Henry & Myles, 2007; Myles, Smith, Aspy, Grossman, & Henry, 2012). The CAPS-TR is "a system that ties the type and intensities of supports that individuals require to their daily schedule of activities" (Myles et al., 2012, p. 138) and is organized around 10 elements, from the time of day and time of activity and associated tasks to the training needed to be an effective employee to social skills in transition areas and to the types of supports needed for the student to succeed. For example, the CAPS-TR assists planning teams in the consideration of transition-related factors, such as employee training needed; social skills and communication supports necessary to daily living and transition-related domains; environmental supports, modifications, and accommodations needed to ensure greater independence; natural supports provided by coworkers, community members, neighbors, and others; and the types of data that can be collected to document progress in transition-related domains.

The third planning inventory is the Treatment and Education of Autistic and Related Communications Handicapped Children (TEACCH) Transition Assessment Profile (TTAP)—Second Edition (Mesibov, Thomas, Chapman, & Schopler, 2007). The TTAP was developed for adolescents with ASD and provides information on six transition-related domains: vocational skills, vocational behavior, independent functioning, leisure skills, functional communication, and interpersonal behavior.

Student Involvement in Educational and Transition Planning

In large part because of the student involvement requirements in IDEA mentioned previously, active student engagement in transition planning has become an important component of the transition IEP development process. Research documents the positive impact of efforts to promote student involvement in educational and transition planning on more positive transition outcomes (Martin, Van Dycke, Christensen, Greene, Gardner, & Lovett, 2006; Mason, Field, & Sawilowsky, 2004; Test, Mason, Hughes, Konrad, Neale, & Wood, 2004). A number of interventions designed to promote student involvement in educational and transition planning have some evidence of efficacy, including the *Self-Directed IEP* (Martin, Marshall, Maxson, & Jerman, 1993), the *Self-Advocacy Strategy* (Van Reusen, Bos, Schumaker, & Deshler, 2002), *Whose Future Is It Anyway?* (Wehmeyer, Palmer, Lee, Williams-Diehm, & Shogren, 2011), *TAKE CHARGE for the Future* (Powers, Turner, Westwood, Matuszewski, Wilson, & Phillips (2001) and the *NEXT S.T.E.P.* curriculum (Halpern et al., 1997). Research using these interventions has shown that involvement in the planning process significantly increased the percentage of time students talked in and started or led their IEP meetings, that students involved with the process showed more positive perceptions about their capacity to self-direct planning and held more positive expectations for the success of such self-directed planning, and that students receiving such interventions gained knowledge about transition planning and had significantly more positive perceptions of self-efficacy about transition planning and more positive outcome expectations.

One of the frequently cited benefits of student involvement in educational planning and decision making has been that such efforts and experiences lead to the enhanced self-determination of adolescents with disabilities. Williams-Diehm, Wehmeyer, Palmer, Soukup, and Garner (2008) studied the differences in levels of self-determination among 276 students with disabilities divided into groups that differed by level of student involvement in the IEP meeting. Multivariate analysis showed significant differences among self-determination scores using two different measures for students in a high-involvement group versus students in a low-involvement group, indicating that students who were more involved in their meetings were more self-determined. A second multivariate analysis found, though, that students who were more self-determined (two groups, high or low self-determination) were more likely to be involved in their IEP meetings, suggesting a reciprocal relationship between being self-determined and being involved with one's own transition planning.

Promoting Self-Determination

Promoting self-determination is best practice in transition and college and career readiness for several reasons, including that research has established that young people who leave school as more self-determined achieve more positive postsecondary outcomes (Shogren, Wehmeyer, Palmer, Rifenbark, & Little, in press). Self-determined behavior refers to "volitional actions that enable one to act as the primary causal agent in one's life and to maintain or improve one's quality of life" (Wehmeyer, 2005, p. 117). An act or event is self-determined if the person's action reflects four essential characteristics: (1) the individual acted autonomously, (2) the behaviors were self-regulated, (3) the person initiated and responded to event(s) in a "psychologically empowered" manner, and (4) the person acted in a self-realizing manner. Self-determination refers to self- (vs. other-) caused action, to people acting volitionally based on their own will. Volitional refers to the act or instance of making a *conscious* choice or decision, so volitional behavior implies that one acts with intent. Self-determined behavior is volitional and intentional, not simply random and nonpurposeful.

The concept of causal agency is central to this perspective. Broadly defined, *causal agency* implies that it is the person who makes or causes things to happen in his or her life. Self-determination emerges across the lifespan as children and adolescents learn skills and develop attitudes and beliefs that enable them to be causal agents in their lives. These skills and attitudes are referred to in this model as *component elements* of self-determined behavior and include choice making, problem solving, decision making, goal setting and attainment, self-advocacy, and self-management skills.

As noted previously, promoting self-determination is important for several reasons. First, student self-determination status has been linked to the attainment of more positive transition outcomes, including more positive employment and independent living (Shogren et al., in press; Wehmeyer & Palmer, 2003; Wehmeyer & Schwartz, 1997), as well as more positive quality of life and life satisfaction (Lachapelle et al., 2005; Shogren, López, Wehmeyer, Little, & Pressgrove, 2006; Wehmeyer & Schwartz, 1998). Next, research with students from multiple disability categories has established the need for intervention to promote self-determination, documenting that students with intellectual disability (Wehmeyer & Metzler, 1995), learning disabilities (Field, Sarver, & Shaw, 2003; Pierson, Carter, Lane, & Glaeser, 2008), emotional and behavioral disorders (Carter, Lane, Pierson, & Glaeser, 2006; Pierson et al., 2008), and ASD (Ward & Meyer, 1999; Wehmeyer, Shogren, Zager, Smith, & Simpson, 2010) are less self-determined than their nondisabled peers.

Though such research is only now emerging pertaining to the relative self-determination of students with ASD, those findings support the need for such instruction. Chou, Skorupski, Wehmeyer, and Palmer (2013) compared the self-determination of 222 middle and high school students with ASD, intellectual disability, or learning disabilities and found that, in the autonomous functioning domain, students with ASD scored lower than did students with learning disabilities or students with intellectual disability and lower than did students with learning disabilities in all domains.

Space does not allow a comprehensive treatment of interventions to promote the self-determination of youth with ASD, and readers are referred to Wehmeyer and colleagues (2010) or Wehmeyer and Patton (2012) for more detail. As noted previously, there is a reciprocal relationship between promoting student involvement in transition planning and self-determination, so efforts to promote self-determination need to include activities to engage students with ASD in educational and transition planning. Furthermore, research has established that students across disability categories can acquire knowledge and skills pertaining to important component elements of self-determined behavior, including goal setting and attainment, problem solving, decision making, self-regulation and self-management, and self-advocacy if provided adequate instruction (Algozzine, Browder, Karvonen, Test, & Wood, 2001; Cobb, Lehmann, Newman-Gonchar, & Alwell, 2009). There are multiple intervention methods, materials, and strategies that have proven efficacy. Wehmeyer, Palmer, Shogren, Williams-Diehm, and Soukup (2013) conducted a randomized-trial, placebo control group study that showed that providing students across disability categories, including ASD, with instruction to promote student involvement and using interventions that included the Self-Determined Learning Model of Instruction (SDLMI; Shogren, Palmer, Wehmeyer, Williams-Diehm, & Little, 2012; Wehmeyer et al., 2012) resulted in enhanced self-determination and more positive employment and independent living outcomes. Given the characteristics of young people with ASD, Wehmeyer and colleagues (2010) suggested that special attention may need to be paid to instruction to promote goal setting and problem solving and that all instruction should take into account issues pertaining to social interactions and social skills, discussed next.

Considerations in Transition Programming for Students with ASD

The transition from secondary school to adult environments is especially challenging for students on the spectrum. Transitions require skill in social interaction, interpersonal communication, and executive functioning, all areas of known difficulty for persons with autism. These qualities are central to the diagnostic criteria related to ASD (Zager & Wehmeyer, in press). Understanding the nature and culture of autism and how these core characteristics of ASD affect performance and interpersonal interaction can result in improved learning and transition outcomes (Zager, Alpern, McKeon, Maxam, & Mulvey, 2013). In planning for transition for students on the spectrum, it is crucial to consider: (1) how to build on strengths and interests in employment preparation and intervention; (2) how to present opportunities to learn in varied ways to accommodate challenges associated with autism, such as sensory issues (e.g., hypersensitivity to noise, smell, or touch; distractibility; restricted interests; repetitive behaviors); and (3) how to redirect behaviors that could be perceived negatively into work-related assets (e.g., overattention to detail, persistent attraction to specific activities, rigidity).

Enhancing Social Communication, Social Skills, and Social Inclusion

Obviously, strategies to develop social skills, promote positive social interactions, and enhance social inclusion are important to emphasize in preparing students for transition to college and careers. Social skills are essential throughout a person's life; however, during the developmental years their importance can be critical, with school success being minimized if the student has poor social skills (Smith & Gilles, 2003). Social skills affect all areas during secondary school, including popularity (Boutot, 2007), and are important for success in community living and work, as well. At the secondary level, friendships and other social activities may be more important than parental relationships and approval (Polloway, Miller, & Smith, 2011). Students with ASD experience difficulties in the social domain for a variety of reasons, one of which is theory of mind. They may be unaware of the feelings and thoughts of others and may seem to be unaware or unconcerned with how their comments or actions may be perceived. Problems in understanding behaviors and feelings of others (Baron-Cohen, Tager-Flusberg, & Cohen, 2000) can be frustrating and can lead to inappropriate responses and feelings of isolation.

Because interpersonal communication is so challenging for people with autism, social behavior and preferences should be considered in preparing for transition. Although they may wish to have friendships, individuals with autism tend to have difficulty initiating and engaging in social behaviors. Scripted social stories, video modeling, and role playing in actual situations can help build understanding of others' feelings and reactions and teach socially expected behaviors, reducing problems that may arise from misunderstandings.

Accommodating Information-Processing Differences

The ability to take in, register, decode, and comprehend unfamiliar abstract concepts is often difficult for persons with ASD. Individuals with ASD may struggle at various stages of comprehension building, including (1) input of new information, (2) organization of information, (3) encoding information for storage and later retrieval, and (4) expressing new concepts (Zager & Wehmeyer, in press). Difficulty in understanding abstract language and concepts affects learning and interaction. Understanding the core language and communication differences associated with autism helps to foster engagement (Zager et al., 2013). Relating concepts to actual experiences can enhance meaning when acquiring new knowledge.

The Role of Executive Functioning

Executive functioning refers to the process of managing oneself and one's activities in order to accomplish goals. Executive dysfunction can affect self-regulation and the ability to control attention to task, language, social behavior, and functional skills. These neurologically based skills are necessary to perform day-to-day tasks. They are required for planning and organizing thoughts and activities. Time management, organization of tasks, punctuality, pacing oneself, and maintaining focus enable satisfactory performance in school and in work. Assistive technology supports, such as alarm buzzers to remind students to be on time for appointments, can prove helpful in accommodating students.

Accommodating Sensory Needs

Stimuli such as noise, lighting, and smells may cause sensory discomfort in individuals with ASD. Ben-Sasson and colleagues (2009) noted that hyper- or hyposensitivity to environmental stimuli may affect individuals' sense of well-being and behavior. By taking into account these considerations, agitation and maladaptive behaviors may be reduced, thereby increasing the likelihood of learning and skill mastery. Ecological inventories of potential worksites, in which environmental factors are assessed, can illuminate physical features of work settings and facilitate productive job matches.

In summary, the core characteristics of autism as they affect behavior and learning should be considered at each stage of development, particularly in transition to employment. Individual talents, interests, and preferences are key factors in designing programs for students with autism. Personal interests, as well as challenges and educational needs, change over time as individuals progress though different stages of development. By understanding and addressing the underlying characteristics of autism and building on student strengths while accommodating cognitive, sensory and social challenges, practitioners involved in transition programs can increase their students' success (Zager & Wehmeyer, in press).

Promoting the Transition to Community Living

Teaching Independent Living Skills

During the transition years, beginning by age 14, educators should provide person-centered planning and instruction in home and community living skills. While benefits of access to the general education curriculum are clear and all students have the right to receive their education among their chronological peers, it is also critical that students with ASD have IEPs that address independent community living goals, including personal grooming and hygiene, home living skills (food preparation, housekeeping and laundry, safety, money management), community navigation, social and leisure activities, and use of community resources (post office, restaurants, community events). Cameto, Levine, and Wagner (2004) reported that goals pertaining to living skills were found on 58% of the IEPs, though only 28% focused on independent living.

Life skills instruction that is based on students' individual preferences and needs can be provided concomitantly in school and home by collaborating with parents or caregivers to share responsibility for teaching home and community living skills, thereby maximizing teaching effectiveness and enhancing generalization of learned skills. Universal Design for Transition (UDT; Thoma, Bartholomew, & Scott, 2009), originally developed for use with secondary school students with intellectual disabilities, offers instruction that is designed to meet individual learning preferences and prepare young adults for transition, taking into account individual learning characteristics; it has been used with success with students with autism (Thoma et al., 2009). Through use of evidence-based practices, such as UDT and task analysis, along with systematic prompting and reinforcement in the actual environment in which skills will be used, educators can facilitate successful transition to community living.

Community-Based Instruction

Community-based instruction should be a priority that is balanced with general education inclusion (Spooner, Browder, & Uphold, 2011). With a limited number of hours in the school day and with students with disabilities spending a significant part of their school time in general education classes, special educators may find it challenging to provide life skills instruction in appropriate instructional settings. To achieve a balance of community-based instruction and inclusion in general education, it is helpful to consider the chronological age of the student, increasing the amount of time spent in community-based, out-of-school instructional environments as students enter late adolescence.

Many of the requisite skills in the community living domain, as well as supports and services, overlap and interact with skills needed for successful postsecondary education and employment. Unfortunately, these supports (e.g., positive behavior supports) are not readily accessible in community settings. To build skills needed for adulthood and to increase the likelihood of community engagement, instruction in this domain should be provided both in the school and in the natural environments in which they will be required. When instruction is provided in the community, naturally occurring reinforcers are more likely to help build and sustain new behaviors. Of great importance in developing adult living skills is the area of self-determination. Recognizing and respecting students' choices and encouraging self-advocacy and self-management can enhance person-centered programming and empower individuals to take their place in the community.

Promoting the Transition to Postsecondary Education

Nearly four decades after the Education for All Act (Public Law 94-142) was passed in 1975, colleges and universities across the United States are experiencing an influx of students with autism and other significant disabilities. These students, who have benefited from inclusive education from elementary school through secondary school, may now desire to continue their education at the postsecondary level, rather than remaining in secondary schools till age 21, 3 years after their peers without disabilities graduate. In response to the need for increased access to postsecondary programs, in 2009 the U.S. Department of Education brought together stakeholders and experts to discuss issues related to postsecondary education for students with disabilities (Zager et al., 2013). The purpose of the meeting was to bring together participants from government agencies and universities to increase access to high-quality postsecondary education.

Studies have shown that postsecondary education leads to improved employment and adult living opportunities (Migliore & Butterworth, 2009). As the demand for increased access to postsecondary education has grown, college offices for disabilities have been required to meet the needs of this population of students for appropriate services. Colleges must provide supports and accommodations to ensure equal education opportunities (Eisenman & Mancini, 2010).

Case Example: Collaboration and Outcomes-Based Practices for Transition to College

Chester is 21 years old and in his final year of secondary school. Beginning in the fall, he will be attending the local community college. In planning for the transition to postsecondary education, an interdisciplinary team of school personnel, family members, and Chester himself have joined together to build a cohesive plan to enable and empower Chester to succeed in the next phase of his education. An essential program component has been to involve Chester in all decisions about his transition to college.

Chester's transition counselor has been preparing him to engage actively in college life by building self-determination, self-advocacy competence, and independent living skills. The transition counselor has worked with Chester and his family to ensure that he independently manages his morning routine, including setting the alarm, completing personal hygiene tasks, and leaving for school with the necessary supplies. The counselor has coached Chester on how to access the campus disabilities office and helped him to gather all necessary documents to advocate for accommodations for himself.

The speech–language pathologist (SLP) has been working on improving cooperative group participation and responsive conversational skills to help Chester participate in his classes. The SLP has been especially focused on helping Chester learn to recognize when others are no longer interested in a topic on which he may be perseverating.

Chester's English teacher has been addressing time management and organization of written assignments. She has been assigning lengthy projects that have 2- and 3-week time frames so that Chester can learn to adhere to a work plan and schedule. The English teacher has shown Chester how to use technology, such as his iPhone alarm, to alert himself when he needs to leave for class. She has helped him make weekly schedules so that he paces himself in his assignments.

The SLP has been working with a small group of students, in which Chester has the opportunity to participate in interactive group conversations. Sessions are sometimes videotaped and critiqued by the group, with attention to active listening and conversational behaviors. The SLP has also attended Chester's English class to facilitate group discussions.

Each member of the team has participated in each domain so that time management and organization skills learned at home have been reinforced in school. Several trips to the community college have helped to familiarize Chester with the campus, and social communication skills have been incorporated into all aspects of the transition plan.

When Chester enters college in the fall, he'll be familiar with the campus, know where his classes and important offices are located, and will have a routine in place. Even with the multi-tiered preparation that he has received, college will be an enormously new and challenging experience. But he will be prepared to meet new challenges, make choices, and engage in his new community.

Promoting the Transition to Employment

Wehman, Targett, Schall, and Carr (Chapter 11, this volume) provide a comprehensive look at supporting adults with ASD to achieve meaningful employment, and therefore we do not cover this topic in any depth in this chapter other than to emphasize the importance of a focus on employment as an outcome of the transition process for youth with ASD. As discussed previously, the IEPs of students with ASD must include transition goals and transition services to achieve those goals from the age of 16 on (and earlier in some states). Part of the problem with regard to successful transition to employment involves the low expectations held for students with ASD with regard to employment. Cameto and colleagues (2004) analyzed data from the NLTS2 study and found that among secondary-age students with ASD, 22% of IEPs had a goal for competitive employment and 39% had goals for supported employment (e.g., supported work in a competitive, inclusive workplace), but that the same amount (39%) had a goal for sheltered employment. The latter is, of course, almost always subminimum wage or piece-rate payment.

Conclusion

• • • • • • •

Effective transition for adolescents with ASD begins with student-focused inclusive secondary school education that fosters development of academic skills, independence, and social engagement. Ensuring that students with ASD have access to the general education curriculum and that they are actively engaged in their school community prepares them for participation in their adult community. Individual talents, interests, and preferences are key factors in designing programs for students with autism. Active involvement of the student, family, and team members in the transition process is critical to the success of the transition process. In student-focused planning, individual strengths, interests, and preferences should form the basis of the transition plan. Finally, interdisciplinary collaboration helps students learn to generalize skills learned to new environments and increases the likelihood that necessary skills and behaviors will be maintained in postsecondary settings.

REFERENCES

• • • • • • • •

Algozzine, B., Browder, D., Karvonen, M., Test, D. W., & Wood, W. M. (2001). Effects of interventions to promote self-determination for individuals with disabilities, *Review of Educational Research, 71,* 219–277.

Baron-Cohen, S., Jager-Flusberg, A., & Cohen, D. J. (2000). *Understanding other minds.* Oxford, UK: Oxford University Press.

Ben-Sasson, A., Hen, L., Fluss, R., Cermak, S. A., Engel-Yeger, B., & Gal, E. (2009). A meta-analysis of sensory modulation symptoms in indiviuals with autism dspectrum disorder. *Journal of Autism and Developmental Disorders, 39*(1), 1–11.

Boutot, E. A. (2007). Fitting in: Tips for promoting acceptance and friendships for students with autism spectrum disorders in inclusive classrooms. *Intervention in School and Clinic, 42,* 156–161.

Cameto, R., Levine, P., & Wagner, M. (2004). *Transition planning for students with disabilities: A special topic report from the National Longitudinal Transition Study-2 (NLTS2).* Menlo Park, CA: SRI International.

Carter, E. W., Lane, K. L., Pierson, M. R., & Glaeser, B. (2006). Self-determination skills and opportunities of transition-age youth with emotional disturbance and learning disabilities. *Exceptional Children, 72*(3), 333–346.

Chou, Y. C., Skorupski, W., Wehmeyer, M. L., & Palmer, S. (2013). *Comparisons of self-determined behaviors among students with autism, intellectual disability, and learning disabilities: A multivariate analysis.* Manuscript submitted for publication.

Clark, G., & Patton, J. (2009). *Transition Planning Inventory-Updated Version.* Austin, TX: Pro-Ed.

Cobb, B., Lehmann, J., Newman-Gonchar, R., & Alwell, M. (2009). Self-determination for students with disabilities: A narrative metasynthesis. *Career Development for Exceptional Individuals, 32*(2), 108–114.

Eisenman, L., & Mancini, K. (2010). College perspectives and issues. In M. Grigal & D. Hart (Eds.), *Think college: Postsecondary education options for students with intellectual disabilities* (pp. 161–188). Baltimore: Brookes.

Field, S., Sarver, M. D., & Shaw, S. F. (2003). Self-determination: A key to success in postsecondary education for students with learning disabilities. *Remedial and Special Education, 24*(6), 339–349.

Halpern, A. S. (1994). The transition of youth with disabilities to adult life: A position statement of the Division on Career Development and Transition. *Career Development for Exceptional Individuals, 17*(2), 115–124.

Halpern, A. S., Herr, C. M., Wolf, N. K., Doren, B., Johnson, M. D., & Lawson, J. D. (1997). *NEXT S.T.E.P.: Student transition and educational planning.* Austin, TX: Pro-Ed.

Hendricks, D. R., & Wehman, P. (2009). Transition from school to adulthood for youth with autism spectrum disorders: Review and recommendations. *Focus on Autism and Other Developmental Disabilities, 24,* 77–88.

Henry, S. A., & Myles, B. S. (2007). *The Comprehensive Autism Planning Systems (CAPS) for individuals with Asperger syndrome, autism and related disabilities: Integrating best practices throughout the student's day.* Shawnee Mission, KS: AAPC.

Kearns, J., Kleinert, H., Harrison, B., Sheppard-Jones, K., Hall, M., & Jones, M. (2010). *What does "college and career ready" mean for students with significant cognitive disabilities?* Lexington: University of Kentucky.

Kohler, P. (1996). *Taxonomy for transition programming.* Champaign: University of Illinois.

Lachapelle, Y., Wehmeyer, M. L., Haelewyck, M. C., Courbois, Y., Keith, K. D., Schalock, R., et al. (2005). The relationship between quality of life and self-determination: An international study. *Journal of Intellectual Disability Research, 49,* 740–744.

Martin, J. E., Marshall, L., Maxson, L. L., & Jerman, P. (1993). *Self-directed IEP.* Longmont, CO: Sopris West.

Martin, J. E., Van Dycke, J., Christensen, W. R., Greene, B. A., Gardner, J. E., & Lovett, D. L. (2006). Increasing student participation in IEP meetings: Establishing the self-directed IEP as an evidence-based practice. *Exceptional Children, 72,* 299–316.

Mason, C., Field, S., & Sawilowsky, S. (2004). Implementation of self-determination activities and student participation in IEPs. *Exceptional Children, 70,* 441–451.

Mesibov, G. B., Thomas, J. B., Chapman, S. M., & Schopler, E. (2007). *TEACCH Transition Assessment Profile, Second Edition (TTAAP).* Austin, TX: Pro-Ed.

Migliore, A., & Butterworth, J. (2009). *Postsecondary education and employment outcomes for youth with intellectual disabilities.* Boston: Institute for Community Inclusion. Available at *www.communityinclusion.org/article-php?article_ id-267.*

Morningstar, M., Bassett, D. S., Cashman, J., Kochhar-Bryant, C., & Wehmeyer,

M. L. (2012). Aligning transition services with secondary education reform. *Career Development and Transition for Exceptional Individuals, 35*(3), 132–142.

Myles, B. S., Smith, S. M., Aspy, R., Grossman, B. G., & Henry, S. A. (2012). The Ziggurat Model and a comprehensive autism planning system. In D. Zagar, M. L. Wehmeyer, & R. Simpson (Eds.), *Educating students with autism spectrum disorders: Research-based principles and practices* (pp. 126–148). New York: Taylor & Francis.

National Secondary Transition Technical Assistance Center. (2010). *Evidence-based practices and predictors in secondary transition: What we know and what we still need to know.* Charlotte, NC: Author.

National Secondary Transition Technical Assistance Center. (2013). *Age-Appropriate Transition Assessment Toolkit–Third Edition.* Charlotte, NC: Author.

Newman, L. (2007). *Facts from NLTS2: Secondary school experiences of students with autism.* Menlo Park, CA: SRI International. Retrieved from *www.nlts2.org/fact_sheets/nlts2_fact_sheet_2007_04.pdf.*

Pierson, M. R., Carter, E. W., Lane, K. L., & Glaeser, B. C. (2008). Factors influencing the self-determination of transition-age youth with high-incidence disabilities. *Career Development for Exceptional Individuals, 31*(2), 115–125.

Polloway, E. A., Miller, L., & Smith, T. E. C. (2011). *Language instruction for students with disabilities* (4th ed). Denver, CO: Love.

Powers, L. E., Turner, A., Westwood, D., Matuszewski, J., Wilson, R., & Phillips, A. (2001). TAKE CHARGE for the Future: A controlled field test of a model to promote student involvement in transition planning. *Career Development for Exceptional Individuals, 24*(1), 89–103.

Rehfeldt, J. D., Clark, G. M., & Lee, S. W. (2012). The effects of using the Transition Planning Inventory and a structured IEP process as a transition planning intervention on IEP meeting outcomes. *Remedial and Special Education, 33*(1), 48–58.

Schall, C., & Wehman, P. (2009). Understanding the transition from school to adulthood for students with autism. In P. Wehman, M. D. Smith, & C. Schall (Eds.), *Autism and the transition to adulthood: Success beyond the classroom* (pp. 1–14). Baltimore: Brookes.

Seltzer, M. M., Greenberg, J. S., Floyd, F. J., & Hong, J. (2004). The trajectory of development in adolescents and adults with autism. *Mental Retardation and Developmental Disabilities Research Reviews, 10*, 234–247.

Shogren, K., Palmer, S., Wehmeyer, M. L., Williams-Diehm, K., & Little, T. (2012). Effect of intervention with the Self-Determined Learning Model of Instruction on access and goal attainment. *Remedial and Special Education, 33*(5), 320–330.

Shogren, K. A., Lopez, S. J., Wehmeyer, M. L., Little, T. D., & Pressgrove, C. L. (2006). The role of positive psychology constructs in predicting life satisfaction in adolescents with and without cognitive disabilities: An exploratory study. *Journal of Positive Psychology, 1*, 37–52.

Shogren, K. A., Wehmeyer, M. L., Palmer, S. B., Rifenbark, G., & Little, T. (in press). Relationships between self-determination and postschool outcomes for youth with disabilities. *Journal of Special Education.*

Smith, S. W., & Gilles, D. O. L. (2003). Using key instructional elements to systematically promote social skills generalization for students with challenging behavior. *Intervention in School and Clinic, 39*, 30–37.

Spooner, F., Browder, D. M., & Uphold, N. (2011). Transition to adult living. In D. M. Browder & F. Spooner (Eds.), *Teaching students with moderate and severe disabilities* (pp. 364–382). New York: Guilford Press.

Standifer, S. (2009). *Adult autism and employment; A guide for vocational rehabilitation professionals.* Columbia: University of Missouri.

Targett, P. S., & Wehman, P. (2009). Integrated employment. In P. Wehman, M. D. Smith, & C. Schall (Eds.), *Autism and the transition to adulthood: Success beyond the classroom* (pp. 163–188). Baltimore: Brookes.

Test, D. W., Mason, C., Hughes, C., Konrad, M., Neale, M., & Wood, W. M. (2004). Student involvement in individualized education program meetings. *Exceptional Children, 70*, 391–412.

Thoma, C. A., Bartholomew, C. C., & Scott, L. A. (2009). *Universal design for transition: A roadmap for planning and instruction.* Baltimore: Brookes.

Van Reusen, A. K., Bos, C. S., Schumaker, J. B., & Deshler, D. D. (2002). *The self-advocacy strategy for enhancing student motivation and self-determination.* Lawrence, KS: Edge Enterprises.

Ward, M. J., & Meyer, R. N. (1999). Self-determination for people with developmental disabilities and autism. *Focus on Autism and Other Developmental Disabilities, 14*(3), 133–139.

Wehmeyer, M. L. (2005). Self-determination and individuals with severe disabilities: Reexamining meanings and misinterpretations. *Research and Practice for Persons with Severe Disabilities, 30*, 113–120.

Wehmeyer, M. L., & Metzler, C. (1995). How self-determined are people with mental retardation?: The National Consumer Survey. *Mental Retardation, 33*, 111–119.

Wehmeyer, M. L., & Palmer, S. B. (2003). Adult outcomes from students with cognitive disabilities three years after high school: The impact of self-determination. *Education and Training in Developmental Disabilities, 38*, 131–144.

Wehmeyer, M. L., Palmer, S. B., Lee, Y., Williams-Diehm, K., & Shogren, K. A. (2011). A randomized-trial evaluation of the effect of Whose Future Is It Anyway? on self-determination. *Career Development for Exceptional Individuals, 34*(1), 45–56.

Wehmeyer, M. L., Palmer, S., Shogren, K., Williams-Diehm, K., & Soukup, J. (2013). Establishing a causal relationship between interventions to promote self-determination and enhanced student self-determination. *Journal of Special Education, 46*(4), 195–210.

Wehmeyer, M. L., & Patton, J. R. (2012). Transition to postsecondary education, employment, and adult living. In D. Zagar, M. L. Wehmeyer, & R. Simpson (Eds.), *Educating students with autism spectrum disorders: Research-based principles and practices* (pp. 247–261). New York: Taylor & Francis.

Wehmeyer, M. L. & Schwartz, M. (1997). Self-determination and positive adult outcomes: A follow-up study of youth with mental retardation or learning disabilities. *Exceptional Children, 63*, 245–255.

Wehmeyer, M. L. & Schwartz, M. (1998). The relationship between self-determination, quality of life, and life satisfaction for adults with mental retardation. *Education and Training in Mental Retardation and Developmental Disabilities, 33*, 3–12.

Wehmeyer, M. L., Shogren, K., Palmer, S., Williams-Diehm, K., Little, T., & Boulton, A. (2012). The impact of the Self-Determined Learning Model of Instruction on student self-determination. *Exceptional Children, 78*(2), 135–153.

Wehmeyer, M. L., Shogren, K. A., Zager, D., Smith, T. E. C., & Simpson, R. (2010). Research-based principles and practices for educating students with autism spectrum disorders: Self-determination and social interactions. *Education and Training in Autism and Developmental Disabilities, 45*(4), 475–486.

Wehmeyer, M. L., & Webb, K. W. (Eds.). (2012). *Handbook of adolescent transition and disability.* New York: Taylor & Francis.

Williams-Diehm, K., Wehmeyer, M. L., Palmer, S., Soukup, J. H., & Garner, N. (2008). Self-determination and student involvement in transition planning: A multivariate analysis. *Journal on Developmental Disabilities, 14*, 25–36.

Zager, D., Alpern, C., McKeon, B., Maxam, S., & Mulvey, J. (2013). *Educating college students with autism spectrum disorders.* New York: Routledge/Taylor & Francis.

Zager, D., & Wehmeyer, M. L. (in press). Transition to postsecondary environments for students with autism spectrum disorders. In E. A. Boutot (Ed.), *Autism spectrum disorders: Foundations, characteristics, and effective strategies* (2nd ed.). Boston: Pearson.

CHAPTER 4

● ● ● ● ● ●

Postsecondary Education for Students with Autism Spectrum Disorders

● **Jane Thierfeld Brown, Lorraine E. Wolf, and Christine Wenzel**

Autism spectrum disorders (ASD) are neurodevelopmental. For many, especially those at the mildest end of the autism spectrum, there is a favorable prognosis for independent functioning in adulthood. Many individuals complete high school and college and go on to successful careers. Accordingly, colleges and universities are now reporting a marked increase[1] in the numbers of students who carry this diagnosis and often are at a loss as to how best to accommodate their disability (Wolf & Thierfeld Brown, 2005a).

Students with ASD often have a varied range of IQ and academic ability. Yet these students often struggle in both the academic and social environments. In our experience, traditional accommodations designed to mitigate the academic effects of other disabilities are typically not helpful in this population. Part of the difficulty lies in the fact that many persons with ASD display deficits in executive functioning (Happé, Booth,

---

[1]In 2001, when we began to present to the disability service community (Wolf, Thierfeld Brown, & Bork, 2001), the diagnosis of ASD was largely unfamiliar to disability providers. A 2006 informal survey by one of us (Thierfeld Brown) of 42 colleges found an average of 4.28 students with ASD at 4-year institutions and 8.9 students at community and technical colleges. The recent prevalence estimate of 1:68 by the Centers for Disease Control and Prevention (CDC, 2014) predicts that this increase will continue.

Charlton, & Hughes, 2006; Hill, 2004; Russell, 1997). Deficits in the central tasks of organizing and shifting among concepts, behaviors, ideas, and goals may be especially problematic in college students, as so much of academic life requires good planning (Wolf, 2001; Wolf & Kaplan, 2007). Students with ASD who also have executive dysfunction thus require interventions specifically targeted to those deficit areas.

Asperger Syndrome

Although only recently codified in the diagnostic schema in the United States, Asperger syndrome (AS) has been recognized for a long time. Traditional views in child psychiatry held that autism was a rare and severe condition. Original incidence rates for autism hovered around 4–5 per 10,000 births (Lotter, 1966; also see a review in Yeargin-Allsopp et al., 2003). As familiarity with the diagnosis has spread, a concomitant increase in the number of index cases has been reported worldwide. Indeed, widely popular press reports have predicted rates rising to what some fear may be an "epidemic."

Although the reasons for the reported increase remain controversial, it is clear that the diagnosis of autistic disorders is becoming more common (Gillberg & Wing, 1999). The diagnoses of AS and consequent requests for services are increasing exponentially. A recent study reported that the increase in autism referrals in California has increased by nearly 300% over the past 10 years (California Health and Human Services Agency, 1999; Croen, Grether, Hoogstrate, & Selvin, 2002). The CDC revised its incidence estimates from 1:166 to as high as 1:68 for all disorders on the autism spectrum (CDC, 2014), and the incidence will likely rise as young adults with AS marry and rear children (Baron-Cohen, 2014).

Originally described as "autistic psychopathy" by Hans Asperger in 1944, the syndrome that now bears his name went largely unnoticed until 1981, when Lorna Wing published a paper describing 35 patients whom she classified according to Asperger's earlier description (Wing, 1981). This lack of attention to the syndrome in the English-speaking world may be attributed to the publication, nearly simultaneously with that of Asperger, of a work in English by Leo Kanner (1943) describing children with "early infantile autism." Debate still rages as to whether Kanner's autistic children are the same as or different from those described by Asperger (AS is sometimes alternately identified as high-functioning autism, although this is probably incorrect; Frith, 2004; Gillberg, 1992; Ozonoff, South, & Miller, 2000). Uta Frith's translation (Asperger, 1944/1991) brought Asperger's original monograph to the attention of the wider English-speaking psychiatric community. From there, interest in the United States and abroad increased to the point where in 1994 the disorder was formally codified into standard medical parlance in the United States.

AS has been eliminated in the fifth edition of the *Diagnostic and Statistical Manual of Mental Disorders* (DSM-5; American Psychiatric Association, 2013) and is now included in the autism spectrum. Although somewhat revolutionary at the original discovery, it is now understood that there is a *spectrum of disorders* ranging from severe to mild, with functioning ranging from nonverbal and intellectually disabled with gross relational difficulties at the severe end to near-normal eccentricity at the mildest end (Frith, 2004; Minshew, 2001).

The spectrum disorders all involve impairments in three domains of functioning (the so-called autistic triad; Wing, 1981). First, a deficit in social functioning is arguably the core of the disorder, with significant difficulties in social interaction and reciprocity. Second, language and communication deficits are notable, albeit more subtle in AS than in autism. Lastly, there are clear behavior deficits, including restricted, repetitive, or stereotyped behavior patterns. The varying diagnoses along the spectrum are defined by different combinations of these deficits in different degrees, with or without other identifying developmental or medical histories (American Psychiatric Association, 1994; Frith, 2004; Gillberg, 1992; Minshew, 2001).

As stated previously, AS is at the mildest end of the spectrum of pervasive developmental disorders (PDD), with normal to above normal intelligence and, typically, normal language functioning. Borderline cases range into normal eccentricity and oddness. Individuals with AS often develop into independent adults, including having successful careers and families. AS is believed by most to be neurodevelopmental in origin, most likely with a genetic basis (Bailey et al., 1995), although other etiological theories have been proposed, including obstetrical and perinatal risk factors (Hultman, Sparen, & Cnattingius, 2002), environmental toxins (Evers, Novotny, & Hollander, 2003) and the now-debunked connection between autism and measles–mumps–rubella vaccinations (Fombonne & Chakrabarti, 2001; Taylor et al., 1999; for a more detailed discussion of scientific hypotheses of the etiology of autism, see a review by Herbert, 2004).

Executive Functioning

Neuropsychologists use the term *executive function* (EF) as shorthand for a complex set of behaviors mediated by a widespread network of brain regions including the anterior and subcortical regions of the brain (for reviews, see Wolf & Kaplan, 2007; Wolf & Wasserstein, 2001). These brain regions mature over the lifespan of the individual, supporting the development of behaviors and abilities that adolescents (and college students) use to navigate the complexity of adulthood.

The abilities described as EF include planning, inhibition, shifting, flexibility, and delay of gratification. In other words, the development of EF reflects an emerging capacity for self-control (Barkley, 2004; see also Wolf & Wasserstein, 2001). Tasks such as inhibition, control, and delay are often regarded as "cognitive EFs." However, more recent understanding points to the importance of a parallel system that supports the regulation of affect, motivation, and social–emotional functioning (see Wolf & Kaplan, 2007). We have described students who are impaired in both their cognitive and their social–emotional regulation.

Students with EF deficits may present as disorganized individuals who do not plan ahead, who fail to sustain energy and effort or follow through with tasks, who are rigid or inflexible who have trouble using feedback to modify their approach, and who have difficulties managing and structuring time, materials, and space (Wolf, 2001). Clearly, such students will struggle in college, where success depends on organization, follow-through, and flexibility. Table 4.1 illustrates some of the problem areas for these students.

EF and ASD

Some of the cognitive and behavioral deficits in ASD may be related to difficulties in EF (Russell, 1997). The core cognitive difficulties in ASD may be distilled to deficits in integration and synthesis, resulting in a rigid style that is thought to moderate anxiety (Rosenn, 2002). Persons with AS often fail to integrate details into a whole (Rinehart, Bradshaw, Moss,

---

TABLE 4.1. Executive and Regulatory Functions Relevant to College

• Organizing (space and materials)	• Working memory
• Managing time (planning and prioritizing)	• Monitoring output (especially in relation to future goals)
• Initiating tasks and following through	• Using feedback to adjust performance
• Sustaining energy and effort	• Setting goals and making choices
• Flexible problem solving	• Evaluating social–emotional cues
• Generating alternate solutions	• Regulating emotions
• Switching among tasks	• Maintaining motivation

Note. Based on Wolf (2001).

Brereton, & Tonge, 2000). They may have difficulties planning, shifting, and prioritizing. Finally, difficulties in social functioning, including taking others' perspective, processing social nuances, and understanding motivation (one's own and others') may be related to EF deficits as well (Happé et al., 2006; Hill, 2004; Zelazo & Muller, 2002).

A number of studies have documented deficits in various components of EF in ASD (Happé et al., 2006; Hill, 2004). However, controversy remains as to whether there is a generalized deficit or one that involves selective aspects of EF. One study found deficits in inhibition in youngsters with ASD and hypothesized that problems in sensorimotor gating might explain difficulties in inhibiting repetitive thoughts, speech, and actions (McAlonan et al., 2002). Another study found that individuals with ASD had impairment in task inhibition but not task switching (Manoach, Lindgren, & Barton, 2004). This outcome was interpreted as a selective rather than a generalized EF deficit in ASD.

However, inhibitory deficits are not always reported. Kleinhans, Akshoomoff, and Delis (2005) found that children with ASD were not impaired in their ability to disengage from a behavioral response. Rather, deficits were seen in "complex verbal tasks that require generating and initiating cognitive search strategies and problem solving technique to improve performance" and "cognitive switching between strategies" (Kleinhans et al., 2005). Finally, another recent report (Joseph, Steele, Meyer, & Tager-Flusberg, 2005) found that children with autism do not use language to develop rules to guide behavior. Unlike most children, they do not use internal language or "self-talk" to attempt to regulate their own behavior.

Other authors have hypothesized that deficits in EF in children with ASD underlie their lack of theory of mind, the ability to maintain a representation of another person and to understand that that person possesses motivations and thoughts different from one's own (Joseph & Tager-Flusberg, 2005). This ability is critical to intact social functioning, and it has been hypothesized to be deficient in PDD spectrum disorders (Stuss & Anderson, 2004; Zelazo & Muller, 2002).

Taken together, these studies suggest that ASD may be characterized by selective deficits in EF. In particular, complex verbal tasks that require switching and initiation of efficient retrieval strategies are deficient in adolescent and adult ASD (Kleinhans et al., 2005).

Interventions

Campuses across the country have found different ways to be successful with students on the spectrum. Some campuses have social skills groups.

Others have peer mentors or social mentors. Some campuses have specific programs for students on the spectrum developed to address some of the social and campus concerns for students on the spectrum. These programs may originate from such offices as disability services, counseling services, or an autism treatment center.

We do not encourage families to make their choices based only on the availability of ASD programs. A college might have a very well-designed ASD program in an area the student dislikes or might not provide the special course of study the student is most interested in pursuing.

No ASD program can succeed with an unhappy or unmotivated student, no matter how well conceptualized the program goals. In addition, special programs are subject to the vagaries of funding, as well as the commitment and interest on the part of the campus administration. Table 4.2 outlines some general models found in many of these special ASD programs.

Many college students with ASD require additional services that would be provided by special ASD programs, with or without the involvement of other areas of student support or disability services. Some programs are firmly ensconced on regular campuses, whereas others are residential off-campus support programs that negotiate for students to take courses at local colleges. Special programs—such as specialty housing,

TABLE 4.2. Common Service Models

Types of ASD programs	Services that may be available	Providers
Clinical focus	Counseling, groups, supported living, and transportation	Therapists, psychologists, or students. Some are off-campus residential programs with college as an add-on. Often expensive.
Social skills focus	Peer or other mentors, social skills groups, special programming (activities)	Professors, graduate students, disability services.
Academic skills	Academic coaching, special courses, tutors	Disability services offices, tutoring centers, outside agencies. Often fee based.
Research based	Treatment, testing, support	Researchers and students.
Mixed models	One or more of the above	Often fee based, often external agencies to the college.

Note. From Thierfeld Brown, Wolf, King, and Bork (2012). Copyright by Autism Asperger Publishing Company. Reprinted by permission.

special advising, counseling or therapy, additional academic accommodations, tutoring, or social skills training—may be associated with additional fees, often very costly.

Others are even more specialized. For example, a program may offer supervised or supported living in a shared house or apartment, assistance with daily life skills, and transportation to a local community college (often for an extra fee; see Table 4.3).

The checklist in Figure 4.1 is helpful as families search for and select the best college for their son or daughter with ASD.

For some students, special ASD programs are the best choice. Other students resist labeling and special programming and will not take advantage of the offered supports. It is important to be sure the campus is supportive, regardless of whether the student chooses to partake of the ASD programming or not. It is also important for families to be aware that this

TABLE 4.3. Typical Services Provided by Fee-Based Programs

Area	Assistance provided

Independent living skills	• Supported apartment living:
	  o Meal/prep/grocery shopping
	  o Laundry
	  o Cleaning
	  o Budgeting/managing money

Academic	• Study skills • Time management • Tutoring • Check-ins with instructors • Advising
Social skills	• Relationship development • Communal living • Conflict management • Friendships and dating
Health/wellness	• Exercise and recreation • Healthy lifestyle choices • Mental health, meds management • Stress management • Sensory integration
Careers/employment	• Internships • Mentors • Interviewing skills • Career exploration

Note. From Thierfeld Brown, Wolf, King, and Bork (2012). Copyright by Autism Asperger Publishing Company. Reprinted by permission.

☐ The program is available in support of the course of study that my child is most interested in pursuing.

☐ The program includes the support my child needs (i.e., specialty housing, academic advising, counseling or therapy, additional academic accommodations, tutoring, and/or social skills training).

☐ The program is part of a larger campus supportive of my child's needs.

☐ The program has a track record of success with students with ASD and similar challenges.

☐ The staff members' qualifications and experience are available to me.

☐ The program clearly articulates what it can and cannot provide.

☐ The program can connect us with other families to talk to about their experiences.

☐ The program has options for levels of support if my child's needs change.

FIGURE 4.1. ASD program checklist for parents. From Thierfeld Brown, Wolf, King, and Bork (2012). Copyright by Autism Asperger Publishing Company. Reprinted by permission.

is relatively new territory, with very little critical evaluation to date on the effectiveness of college programming for students with ASD. We advise families to carefully investigate the track records of success, including the professional and nonprofessional training and staffing of postsecondary ASD programs prior to choosing them.

Supported Education

For most students with disabilities, academic accommodations are only part of the formula for success in college. Many students with psychiatric disabilities (and, we argue, all students with ASD) require a more intensive level of service to fully participate in academic life. Such an intervention is "supported education," a psychosocial rehabilitation approach that was initially developed at the Boston University Center for Psychiatric Rehabilitation (Unger, 1998). Supported education was designed to help students with mental illness acquire the necessary skills and supports to succeed in an educational environment. Much research indicates that skills training is most effective when it is carried out within the environment in which the skill will be utilized. Thus supported education works with the student in the normal school setting, fully integrated into campus life (Sullivan-Soydan, 2004).

Supported education was developed originally to meet the needs of older, persistently mentally ill consumers returning to the educational arena after many years of illness and disability (Unger, 1998). However, in response to the needs of an increasing number of undergraduates on the campus, the Office of Disability Services at Boston University recently adapted this model to meet the needs of younger students with less severe mental disorders (Wolf & Legere, 2004). To the best of our knowledge, this program was one of the first applications of this intervention within such an administrative office (Legere, Sullivan-Soydan, & Wolf, 2004; Wolf & Legere, 2004).

The supported education service helps students with mental illness set goals, develop skills, locate and obtain adjunctive supports, and access reasonable and appropriate accommodations so that they can maintain their status as active matriculated students. Some students require assistance with academic skills, such as study skills, pacing and prioritizing tasks, or negotiating with professors or other academic departments. Other students may struggle with issues beyond the classroom and may require work on interpersonal skills to take full advantage of the social and residential aspects of college life. Support is provided on campus and is tailored to the needs of the particular student. Meetings are on a regular (often weekly) basis to provide consistent one-to-one support as the student begins to identify and overcome barriers to success in the academic environment and learns to negotiate the campus as a full member of the academic community. Thus assisting the student to maintain his or her valued student role is a primary goal of the service.

Although it is a proven intervention that has been well validated in older students, supported education does not specifically address campus life or social, executive, and other cognitive deficits in younger students. It also does not address the campuswide understanding of the needs of the student, which is central to our conceptualization of effective service delivery for ASD. For this reason, supported education alone is insufficient to meet the needs of college students with ASD.

Coaching for Students with Attention-Deficit/Hyperactivity Disorder

Attention-deficit/hyperactivity disorder (ADHD) is a common childhood behavior disorder that persists into adulthood and is defined as a variable combination of excessive motor activity, inattention, and impulsivity. Cognitive deficits include diminished attention, poor judgment, poor impulse control, and a lack of organization and planning. Much evidence indicates that ADHD is a disorder of EF (Barkley, 2004; see also Wolf & Wasserstein, 2001). For the reasons just discussed, executive dysfunction in college students requires more than simple academic accommodation. Many campuses have developed expertise in accommodating and supporting the large number of students with ADHD in higher education.

ADHD coaching was developed specifically to address the needs of this population, with the knowledge that college students with ADHD did not benefit from strategy training to the same degree as did their peers with learning disabilities. ADHD coaches work intensively with students, relying on the development of a close personal relationship to solve problems creatively. Typical goals are improved impulse control, time management, paying attention to details, and overall organization. Coaching has been defined as an intervention that involves a "relationship that merges the potential for growth of the individual with the skills of the coach; as a result, the individual achieves more than he or she could have on his or her own" (Quinn, Ratey, & Maitland, 2000, p. 11). The client and the coach develop an intense working relationship in which all areas of the client's life may be fodder for the intervention.

Interventions proven to address executive dysfunction in college students with ADHD should theoretically work with college students with ASD, as we strive to teach both populations "good student skills" through demonstration, scaffolding, and scripting. These skills might include how to avoid becoming overwhelmed, using a syllabus and a planner to develop skills in time management and multitasking, overcoming inertia, dealing with procrastination and deadlines, and taking effective and concise notes. Despite certain similarities in executive dysfunction, however, students with ASD pose somewhat different challenges that may not be amenable to traditional coaching interventions. In order for coaching to be effective, students must feel responsible to their coaches and the coaching relationship. For example, it has been asserted that "the student 'programs' the coach to get her needs met" (Quinn et al., 2000, p. 23) and that coaching is "based on the belief that the person, not the coach, is the expert in the relationship" (Quinn et al., 2000, p. 24). In our experience, this implicit interpersonal demand overwhelms many adolescents and young adults with ASD. Such students frequently do not internalize interpersonal responsibility and are not sophisticated interpersonal communicators. For these reasons, we do not believe that ADHD coaching is the optimal intervention for this population.

Strategic Education for Students with Autism Spectrum Disorders

We have developed a unique intervention designed to address executive, regulatory, and other deficits in college students with ASD. This intervention, termed *strategic education for students with autism spectrum disorders* (SEAD), blends and adapts techniques developed in best practices in disability services, ADHD coaching, strategy tutoring, social skills training, and supported education for students with psychiatric disabilities (Wolf & Thierfeld Brown, 2005b). It is grounded in current research, which finds that adults and adolescents with ASD have deficient use of internal speech and strategy selection. The SEAD intervention guides college students with ASD through direct skills instruction, development of self-awareness, psychoeducation about the nature of their disability, and reasonable and appropriate accommodation. Particular attention is paid to social communication. The SEAD model also emphasizes education, training, and technical assistance to the wider university community in which the student interacts (administration, faculty, and staff).

Beyond Access

The main purpose of Beyond Access (the successor to SEAD) is to provide students with the supports needed to make a seamless transition to university life (see Figure 4.2). Students work with a trained strategy instructor in a one-on-one setting to develop strategies to help students reach established personal and academic goals. Beyond Access aims to provide personalized academic support for students, assists with personal transitions related to college life, and refers students to campus resources as needed. Based on our experience working with students with ASD, we also stress training and/or technical support to the wider campus community, including faculty and staff (such as residential life staff and/or

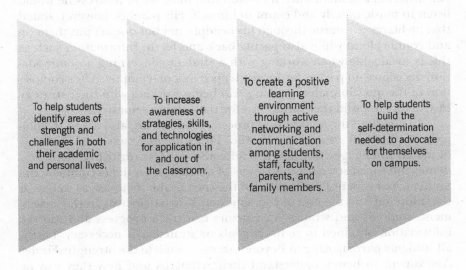

FIGURE 4.2. Goals of Beyond Access.

community standards; see Wolf, Thierfeld Brown, & Bork, 2007). Beyond Access is not a clinical intervention, nor is it coaching or supported education. In contrast, we have developed Beyond Access as a unique model to support students with ASD throughout their higher education experience. One of our main goals is to provide students with the tools and strategies needed to navigate the social and academic facets of university life. It is important to note that many students who are working in Beyond Access are also students who require academic accommodations; therefore our Beyond Access program is housed in the Center for Students with Disabilities.

The Beyond Access model involves a semistructured series of interrelated modules executed over the course of an academic semester (see Table 4.4). Each student's program within Beyond Access is tailored to meet the his or her individual learning and social profile. The concept is to build a program around the student rather than trying to fit a student into a program. Prior to beginning the Beyond Access program, students and their family members are asked to complete an in-depth questionnaire that serves to gather information about how the student responds when he or she is stressed, anxious, angry, and so forth. It also asks students to comment on their learning styles and how they would explain their disabilities to others. Parents and/or family members are asked to complete the questionnaires about the students with the goal of gathering more complete information, as well as to open the doors to discussing with the students different perceptions people have of behaviors. For instance, a student once indicated that in order to destress he would listen to music quietly and count to himself. His parents, however, stated that he blares the music through his headphones but doesn't put them on and counts aloud while also pacing back and forth. Information such as this is invaluable when working with a student concerning accommodation decisions—in particular for students living on campus. After completion of the questionnaire, students will begin working with their strategy instructors to build their programs for the coming semester.

To facilitate the goal-setting process, students are also asked to complete the Student Assessment Profile. The Student Assessment Profile is designed to engage students in a reflective process regarding their academic and social strengths and areas of challenge. Students complete the Student Assessment Profile prior to the start of the semester, as well as at the midpoint and the end of the semester. By participating in this assessment, students and strategy instructors can track progress and use the information obtained to redirect goals or strategies if necessary. Lastly, all students participating in Beyond Access complete the StrengthsFinder Assessment to better understand their strengths and how they can be applied to all aspects of college life and beyond.

TABLE 4.4. Beyond Access Modules

Module One: Relationship Building and Transition
Introduce model to student and family
Campus orientation
Academic preparation
Residential orientation

Module Two: Setting Goals
Academic
Nonacademic

Module Three: Functional Assessment of Strengths and Weaknesses
Academic
Nonacademic

Module Four: Resource Assessment
On campus
Off campus

Module Five: Develop Accommodation Plan
Academic
Nonacademic

Module Six: Build Skills and Strategies
Time management
Organization
ASSET social skills
Self-advocacy

Module Seven: Psychoeducation about ASD
Prepared readings
Peer group learning activities

Module Eight: Evaluation and Planning
Evaluate goals and intervention effectiveness
Plan next semester

As previously noted, students (with some input from professional staff) will be the designers of their programs. Because strategies will be selected based on identified goals, every student's program will be a little different (see Table 4.5). Strategies include, but are not limited to, time management and organization, study strategies, reading and writing strategies, stress management, career exploration and preparation, and breaking down assignments. In addition, students can work with their strategy instructors on social interaction skills, hygiene, health and wellness, finding a social group, and role playing and social scripts. Strategy instructors are also able to assist students in identifying other campus resources that

TABLE 4.5. Beyond Access in Action

- *Goal:* To attend a 4-year residential college.

- *Functional limitations:* Follows semistructured interview, rating scales, and records review. Student has deficits in self-regulation, organization, and social communication.

- *Transition:* Work with student and family regarding residence and room selection, orientation to housing policies and procedures, campus orientation, daily life skills with parent support, differences between high school and college in terms of support versus independence. Work with student advising center on course selection and options, assist with registration as needed. Monitor academic and residential transition with appropriate personnel.

- *Accommodations:* Tailored to student's functional limitations in classroom, course requirements, and fundamental requirements of degree program.

- *Skills:* Geared toward strengthening areas of limitation; might include symptom management, training in organization and time management, social scripting, negotiation and communication (with professors and peers), and psychoeducation about ASD.

- *Support:* Explore and facilitate contacts with on-campus resources, such as student mental health counseling, freshman advising, freshman tutoring center, and residence life. Provide technical support to these resources regarding this student and ASD in general. Provide ongoing support to student regarding procedures and policies (such as conduct code).

- *Planning:* Review past semester, future goals (short and long term), plans for next semester.

---

may be of assistance, such as counseling and mental health services and the writing center, as well as specific tutoring centers. Another main tenet of the Beyond Access program is to work with students to teach them to be good self-advocates and to understand what their disability means to them. Strategy instructors meet with their students for up to 3 hours per week (two different tracks are offered: Track I, 3 hours per week, and Track II, 1 hour per week) in a one-on-one setting.

At the close of each semester, students are given a flash drive containing all strategies and resources used during the course of the semester. Students also receive an end-of-the-semester summary outlining their progress toward the attainment of goals, areas of growth, semester highlights, and areas that still require some work. Students who chose to participate in Beyond Access for subsequent semesters review this summary at the start of each semester and use this information to help create new semester goals.

Offered in conjunction with Beyond Access are two 1-credit courses focused on social interaction, health and wellness, and relationships and dating. Enrollment in these courses is restricted to students who need additional support acquiring these skills. Lastly, a workshop series focusing exclusively on relationships, dating, boundaries, and sex are offered throughout the semester for any interested student.

Case Example of Beyond Access

This hypothetical student is a 17-year-old male who was recently accepted to attend your college or university. His parents contacted disability services regarding support and accommodations for him. This student has been diagnosed with AS and an anxiety disorder and received considerable accommodations and supports in high school. The Beyond Access plan, assuming that the student participated in Track I offering 3 hours of support per week, might look like Figure 4.3.

Technology/Learning Technologies

It seems almost impossible to walk around a college campus without seeing the majority of students using smartphones, listening to music, or carrying around a laptop, iPad, or other tablet. In fact, a study done by Junco and Mastrodicasa (2007) reported that 97% of college students own a cell phone, and a similar study illustrated that 98% of students

Monday	Wednesday	Friday
→Look over all syllabi and plan out assignments for week using Google Calendar.	→Check in on assignment progress and revise if necessary.	→Create work plan for weekend and identify resources needed.
→Break assignments into smaller parts and identify resources needed to complete each assignment.	→Stress management strategies.	→Update grade tracker with any grades.
→Plan out two social activities for the week.	→Problem-solve any issues that may have arisen (e.g., talking with professor, group work).	→Practice social skills and plan social activity for weekend.

FIGURE 4.3. Beyond Access plan for a student in Track I.

own a computer (Cotten, 2008). Given these statistics, it seems rational to explore how technology can be used as another mechanism to provide support for individuals on the spectrum.

New applications and learning tools are generated daily, so it is almost impossible to keep up with every new trend on the market; however, there are several apps for the iPad and smartphones and even programs for laptops and PCs that can prove to be good supplementary supports for students. Students can use myHomework, an app available for the iPhone, Droid, or iPad, to track assignments and due dates, set priorities, and store class information—such as class locations, professors, and professors' office locations. Students can even access their myHomework calendars via the Web when they do not have access to their smartphones or iPads. Organizer Lite, similar to myHomework, provides a platform for students to organize activities and assignments by date and priority. This app has certain features that make it more desirable for some learners—including the ability to record notes within assignments, to attach pictures to entries, and to add maps to pinpoint locations of appointments. There are hundreds of other organization applications available, ranging from simple to-do-list apps such as Primo Do to livelier, animated applications such as Epic Win, which creates a strategy game for users based on tasks to be completed.

Quiz Net and Flashboard, two apps available for a variety of devices, are both used to create flash-cards for students to assist in their studying process. Both apps allow easy access to the material and allow users to import pictures and graphs into the flash cards—very helpful features for visual learners. Stress management applications can range from drawing or word games to guided meditation—obviously dependent on user preference. For some students, it can even be helpful to download an app that will allow them to record their stress busters aloud for easy playback or to create visual reminders of their stress management strategies using uploaded pictures and images. Apps to assist students with managing everyday life tasks, such as financial planning (Envelopes) or healthy eating (Cal Counter), are also readily available.

Specifically for students on the spectrum, or for students for whom social interaction is challenging, a host of social skills applications can be very helpful. Quick Cues is an application designed to provide individuals with suggested step-by-step guidance through communication scenarios ranging from answering the phone to conversation starters to voice control. Social Skills is a similar application and provides instructional steps to navigating certain situations, including dealing with group pressure, expressing affection, and responding to a failure, to name a few. This application is limited, however, in the sense that it does not provide examples or specific scenarios. The Sosh application, created specifically for individuals on the spectrum, provides a range of comprehensive strategies and tools for students. Sosh allows students to create goals and to-do lists and provides various activities under each of the five subcategories (Relax, Relate, Reason, Regulate, Recognize), including guided imaging, a shredder to eliminate negative thoughts, a voice meter, a problem solver to assist students in brainstorming solutions, and strategies for talking and relating to others.

For students who do not own or utilize smartphones or tablets, there are also many options to consider that are accessible using PCs or laptops. Google Calendar, which is widely used by students, can be an excellent tool to help students to organize and plan out assignments—offering students the option of color-coding tasks and setting reminders, as well as the ability to create multiple calendars within one program to keep schoolwork and extracurricular activities organized separately. Many colleges and universities utilize online blackboard systems to disseminate information and offer resources specific for each course. If possible, creating a course for students on the spectrum within this blackboard system is an effective way to make quick tips and information about how to access certain campus resources available 24 hours a day. Based on the complexity of the system, students may also be able to post questions anonymously and connect with other members of the group, which can help students connect with one another and build social networks.

Technology will continue to become more and more entwined in the lives of our college students, and it is therefore advantageous for college personnel to become well versed in student use of these various devices and to examine creative ways to provide students with the information they need using the media they are comfortable using. Specifically with regard to students on the autism spectrum who are so proficient in using technology, these learning tools offer more engaging ways to work with students on strategy development.

Conclusions
• • • • • • •

We have developed a novel intervention for college students with high-functioning ASD that is currently being used. We based this model on our understanding of the core features that characterize students with ASD, coupled with our understanding and experience with other models of intervention for college students with disabilities. We concluded that existing models of support were unlikely to be ideal for students with ASD due to the cognitive and social challenges these students present.

Our review of the literature and our direct experience led to the development of SEAD (now, Beyond Access) as a blend of existing interventions tailored to the unique needs of college students with ASD. Central to our intervention is campus education and liaison so that the community is both welcoming and knowledgeable about ASD. Student intervention is geared toward the student's individual functional limitations in regard to cognitive, academic, and social deficits, course or program of study, and developmental level. Liaison with the family is crucial, as some skill development will not be within the purview of most offices of disability support (activities of daily living, commuting, etc.). Intervention plans are conceptualized as involving a related sequence of modules that pass through the developmental stages of each semester, from transition through accommodation and skill development and planning for subsequent semesters. Study-specific materials and technology are being developed and refined, which will enable us to evaluate the effectiveness of the intervention in the service of developing Beyond Access as an evidence-based practice model that can be disseminated to other campuses and practitioners.

ACKNOWLEDGMENTS

Portions of this chapter are adapted from Thierfeld Brown, Wolf, King, and Bork (2012) and Wolf, Thierfeld Brown, and Bork (2009). Copyright by Autism Asperger Publishing Company. Adapted by permission.

REFERENCES

American Psychiatric Association. (1994). *Diagnostic and statistical manual of mental disorders* (4th ed.). Washington, DC: Author.

American Psychiatric Association. (2013). *Diagnostic and statistical manual of mental disorders* (5th ed.). Arlington, VA: Author.

Asperger, H. (1991). Autistic psychopathy in childhood. In U. Frith (Ed.), *Autism and Asperger syndrome* (pp. 37–92). Cambridge, UK: Cambridge University Press. (Original work published 1944)

Bailey, A., Le Couteur, A., Gottesman, I., Bolton, P., Simonoff, E., Yuzda, E., et al. (1995). Autism as a strongly genetic disorder: Evidence from a British twin study. *Psychological Medicine, 25*(1), 63–77.

Barkley, R. A. (2004). Adolescents with attention-deficit/hyperactivity disorder: An overview of empirically based treatments. *Journal of Psychiatry Practice, 10*(1), 39–56.

Baron-Cohen, S. (2014, February 20). When two minds think alike. *Seed.* Available at *www.seedmagazine.com/news/2006/11/when_two_minds_think_alike. php.* (Original work published 2006)

California Health and Human Services Agency. (1999). *Changes in the population of persons with autism and pervasive developmental disorders in California's developmental services system: 1987 through 1998: A report to the legislature, March 1, 1999.* Sacramento: California Health and Human Services Agency, Department of Developmental Services.

Centers for Disease Control and Prevention. (2014). Prevalence of autism spectrum disorders—Autism and developmental disabilities monitoring network, 14 sites, United States 2002. Available at *www.cdc.gov/ncbddd/autism/data.html.*

Cotten, S. R. (2008). Students' technology use and the impacts on well-being. *New Directions for Student Services, 124,* 55–70.

Croen, L., Grether, J., Hoogstrate, J., & Selvin, S. (2002). The changing prevalence of autism in California. *Journal of Autism and Developmental Disabilities, 32,* 207–215.

Evers, M., Novotny, S., & Hollander, E. (2003). Autism and environmental toxins. *Medical Psychiatry, 24,* 175–198.

Fombonne, E., & Chakrabarti, S. (2001). No evidence for a new variant of measles–mumps–rubella–induced autism. *Pediatrics, 108,* 1–8.

Frith, U. (Ed.). (2004). *Autism and Asperger syndrome.* Cambridge, UK: Cambridge University Press.

Gillberg, C. (1992). Autism and autistic-like conditions: Subclasses among disorders of empathy. *Journal of Child Psychology and Psychiatry and Allied Disciplines, 33,* 813–842.

Gillberg, C., & Wing, L. (1999). Autism: Not an extremely rare disorder. *Acta Psychiatrica Scandinavica, 99,* 399–406.

Happé, F., Booth, R., Charlton, R., & Hughes, C. (2006). Executive function deficits in autism spectrum disorders and attention-deficit/hyperactivity disorder: Examining profiles across domains and ages. *Brain and Cognition, 61,* 25–39.

Herbert, M. R., Ziegler, D. A., Makris, N., Filipek, P. A., Kemper, T. L., Normandin, J. J., et al. (2004). Localization of white matter volume increase in autism and developmental language disorder. *Annals of Neurology, 55*(4), 530–540.

Hill, E. L. (2004). Executive function in autism. *Trends in Cognitive Science, 8,* 26–32.

Hultman, C. M., Sparen, P., & Cnattingius, S. (2002). Perinatal risk factors for infantile autism. *Epidemiology, 13*(4), 417–423.

Joseph, R. M., McGrath, L. M., & Tager-Flusberg, H. (2005). Executive dysfunction and its relation to language ability in verbal school-age children with autism. *Developmental Neuropsychology, 27,* 361–378.

Joseph, R. M., Steele, S. D., Meyer, E., & Tager-Flusberg, H. (2005). Self-ordered pointing in children with autism: Failure to use verbal mediation in the service of working memory? *Neuropsychologia, 43,* 1400–1411.

Junco, R., & Mastrodicasa, J. (2007). *Connecting to the Net generation.* Washington, DC: National Association of Student Personnel Administrators.

Kanner, L. (1943). Autistic disturbances of affective contact. *Nervous Child, 2,* 217–250.

Kleinhans, N., Akshoomoff, N., & Delis, D. C. (2005). Executive functions in autism and Asperger's disorder: Flexibility, fluency, and inhibition. *Developmental Neuropsychology, 27,* 379–401.

Legere, L., Sullivan-Soydan, A., & Wolf, L. (Eds.). (2004). *Boston University Office of Disability Services Supported Education Service Intern Manual.* Boston: Boston University.

Lotter, V. (1966). Epidemiology of autistic conditions in young children: I. Prevalence. *Social Psychiatry, 1,* 124–137.

Manoach, D. S., Lindgren, K. A., & Barton, J. J. S. (2004). Deficient saccadic inhibition in Asperger's disorder and the social-emotional processing disorder. *Journal of Neurology, Neurosurgery, and Psychiatry, 75,* 1719–1726.

McAlonan, G. N., Daly, E., Kumari, V., Critchley, H. D., van Amelsvoort, T., Suckling, J., et al. (2002). Brain anatomy and sensorimotor gating in Asperger's syndrome. *Brain, 125,* 1594–1606.

Minshew, N. J. (2001). The core deficit in autism and autism spectrum disorders. *Journal of Developmental and Learning Disorders. 5,* 107–118.

Ozonoff, S., South, M., & Miller, J. N. (2000). DSM-IV-defined Asperger syndrome: Cognitive, behavioral and early history differentiation from high-functioning autism. *Autism, 4,* 29–46

Quinn, P. O., Ratey, N., & Maitland, T. L. (2000). *Coaching college students with ADHD.* Silver Springs, MD: Advantage Books.

Rinehart, N. J., Bradshaw, J. L., Moss, S. A., Brereton, A. V., & Tonge, B. J. (2000). Atypical interference of local detail on global processing in high-functioning autism and Asperger's disorder. *Journal of Child Psychology and Psychiatry and Allied Disciplines, 41,* 769–778.

Rosenn, D. W. (2002). *Is it Asperger's or ADHD?* Watertown, MA: Aspergers Association of New England. Available at *www.aane.org/asperger_resources/articles/miscellaneous/aspergers_or_adhd.html.*

Russell, J. (1997). *Autism as an executive disorder.* New York: Oxford University Press.

Stratton, K., Gable, A., & McCormick, M. (Eds.). (2001). *Immunization safety review: Measles–mumps–rubella vaccine and autism.* Washington, DC: National Academies Press.

Stuss, D. T., & Anderson, V. (2004). The frontal lobes and theory of mind: Developmental concepts from adult focal lesion research. *Brain and Cognition, 55,* 69–83.

Sullivan-Soydan, A. (2004). Supported education: A portrait of a psychiatric rehabilitation intervention. *American Journal of Psychiatric Rehabilitation, 7,* 227–248.

Taylor, B., Miller, E., Farrington, C. P., Petropoulos, M.-C., Favot Mayaud, I., Li, J., et al. (1999). Autism and measles, mumps and rubella vaccine: No epidemiological evidence for a causal association. *Lancet, 353,* 2026–2029.

Thierfeld Brown, J., Wolf, L. E., King, L., & Bork, G. R. K. (2012). *The parent's guide to college for students on the autism spectrum.* Shawnee Mission, KS: AAPC.

Unger, K. V. (1998). *Supported education: Providing services for students with psychiatric disabilities.* Baltimore: Brookes.

Wing, L. (1981). Asperger's syndrome: A clinical account. *Psychological Medicine, 11,* 115–130.

Wolf, L. E. (2001). College students with ADHD and other hidden disabilities. *Annals of the New York Academy of Sciences, 931*, 385–395.

Wolf, L. E., & Kaplan, E. (2007). Executive functioning and self-regulation in young adults: Implications for neurodevelopmental learning disorders. In L. E. Wolf, H. E. Schreiber, & J. Wasserstein (Eds.), *Current issues in adult learning disorders*. New York: Psychology Press.

Wolf, L. E., & Legere, L. (2004, October). New dimensions on supported education. Paper presented at the Supported Education Conference, Ann Arbor, MI.

Wolf, L. E., & Thierfeld Brown, J. (2005a, April 20). *College transition for students with Asperger disorder.* Paper presented at the Asperger Syndrome Education Network, Short Hills, NJ.

Wolf, L. E., & Thierfeld Brown, J. (2005b, August 4). Managing executive dysfunction in attention disorders and Asperger syndrome. Paper presented at the annual conference of the Association of Higher Education and Disabilities, Milwaukee, WI.

Wolf, L. E., Thierfeld Brown, J., & Bork, G. R. K. (2001, July). *Asperger's syndrome in college students.* Paper presented at the meeting of the Association for Higher Education and Disability, Portland, OR.

Wolf, L. E., Thierfeld Brown, J., & Bork, G. R. K. (2007, July). *Asperger's syndrome in college students.* Paper presented at the annual meeting of the Association for Higher Education and Disability, Charlotte, NC.

Wolf, L. E., Thierfeld Brown, J., & Bork, G. R. K. (2009). *Students with Asperger syndrome: A guide for college professionals.* Shawnee Mission, KS: AAPC.

Wolf, L. E., & Wasserstein, J. (2001). Adult ADHD: Concluding thoughts. *Annals of the New York Academy of Sciences, 931*, 396–408.

Yeargin-Allsopp, M., Rice, C., Larapurkar, T., Doernberg, N., Boyle, C., & Murphy, C. (2003). Prevalence of autism in a U.S. metropolitan area. *Journal of the American Medical Association, 289*, 49–55.

Zelazo, P. D., & Muller, U. (2002). Executive function in typical and atypical development. In U Goswami (Ed.), *Handbook of childhood cognitive development* (pp. 445–469), Oxford, UK: Blackwell Scientific.

PART III
• • • • • •
Instructional and Behavioral Interventions to Promote Quality of Life

CHAPTER 5

• • • • • •

Behavioral Interventions for Complex Communication and Social Skills in Adults with Autism Spectrum Disorders

• Angelica Aguirre, John O'Neill, Ruth Anne Rehfeldt, and Valerie Boyer

Most individuals spend most of their lifetimes in adulthood, yet the majority of research on interventions for individuals with autism spectrum disorders (ASD) is focused on children (Barnhill, 2007; Shattuck et al., 2012). Very few adults with ASD achieve full independence, and many rely primarily on family and government assistance (Howlin, Goode, Hutton, & Rutter, 2004). Current research suggests that the opportunities for adults with ASD to form relationships with others are bleak: Orsmold, Krauss, and Seltzer (2004) surveyed 235 adolescents and adults with ASD and found that 46.4% had no relationships with peers of the same age. Approximately 24% had at least one peer relationship but in pre-arranged settings (e.g., church). Parental reports of 25 adolescents and adults with ASD revealed that they were less likely to rely on their peers to learn about social and romantic relationships and more likely to engage in inappropriate dating behaviors (e.g., stalking) compared with parental reports of their typical peers (Stokes, Newton, & Kaur, 2007). Also, adults with ASD work fewer hours a week and earn less than other groups in vocational programs (Cimera & Cowan, 2009). Attention-deficit/

hyperactivity disorder (ADHD), depression, substance abuse, and anxiety are some common psychological disorders experienced by adults with ASD (Hofvander et al., 2009). Matson and Basjoli (2008) argue that even though early intervention programs for children with ASD are common, comorbid psychopathology in these individuals may not develop until later in their adult lives.

Little research has examined the mediators underlying these poor outcomes for adults with ASD. Hendricks (2010) suggested that communication and social difficulties with supervisors and coworkers can hinder job performance for adults with ASD, possibly leading to job termination. Communication issues in the workplace may include difficulties understanding directions, asking too many questions, not "reading between the lines," and communicating in an inappropriate manner. These communication deficits may also hinder the establishment of social and romantic relationships, as well as participation in community leisure activities. Language and communication are closely intertwined with social skills in more verbally sophisticated individuals with ASD. Although much research has focused on language interventions for preschool children with ASD (Howlin & Moss, 2012), the development and evaluation of such intervention programs for adults with ASD are critical if individuals are to live fulfilling and satisfying lives. For this reason, language and communication continue to require attention from service providers in adult populations, even for those adults with advanced language repertoires.

The purpose of this chapter is to delineate research conducted to date on behavioral interventions for enhancing complex language repertoires in adults with ASD, underscoring the fact that language is developed and maintained in a social environment. Thus language and social goals for intervention are often closely intertwined. We discuss research conducted to date with adults with ASD and also extrapolate from research conducted with adults with intellectual disabilities and children with ASD. We explain how such research can inspire interventions for adults with autism and can contribute to the overarching goal of independent community living, working, and relationship building for adults with the disorder.

Behavioral Skills Training

Behavioral skills training (BST) has been successfully implemented for a number of years with people with and without intellectual disabilities. A substantial body of research has shown BST's efficacy in teaching a variety of behaviors, including communication skills, to persons with intellectual disabilities (e.g., Bates, 1980; Bornstein, Bach, McFall, Friman, &

Lyons, 1980; Kleitsch, Whitman, & Santos, 1983). However, little research has explored the efficacy of BST with individuals with ASD. BST typically consists of six steps in which the clinician or practitioner is to engage: labeling and identifying the target behavior, providing the rationale for engaging in the behavior, describing and demonstrating, practicing, providing feedback, and delivering a consequence (e.g., reinforcement) for an individual's performance on the target behavior (see Table 5.1). BST was first evaluated as part of the teaching family model, a behavior analytic program designed for delinquent adolescents to increase their conversational skills with peers and adults (Maloney et al., 1976; Minkin et al., 1976). In one of the first studies, Minkin and colleagues (1976) implemented BST with four female delinquent and predelinquent adolescents living in a residential group home and focused on teaching the participants to ask questions and provide positive conversation feedback to others (e.g., "That's good," "I understand"). The training procedure

TABLE 5.1. BST Steps and Examples

1. *Label and identify the target behavior.* The behavior analyst describes to the client what reciprocating social information with others (i.e., statements and questions) is about.

2. *Provide the rationale for engaging in the behavior.* The behavior analyst lets the client know that engaging in reciprocating information may create longer interactions with others, provide more information, and establish relationships with family members, peers, and/or coworkers.

3. *Describe and demonstrate.* The behavior analyst explains that, after answering a question from another person, one asks the same question to that person (e.g., "And how was your holiday weekend?"). The analyst demonstrates the behavior by engaging in reciprocal information with a model.

4. *Practice.* The behavior analyst or another model practices the behavior with the client. For example, in a work setting, the consultant can act as a coworker for the client to reciprocate dialogue with or have a model pretend to be the client's coworker.

5. *Provide feedback.* After each practice opportunity, the behavior analyst should provide the client with feedback on specifically what the client did right or what he or she could improve on—for example, "I like that you asked your coworker immediately how was her holiday weekend after she asked you" or "When we practice again, make sure to look at your coworker when you are speaking so he knows you are talking to him."

6. *Deliver a consequence.* The behavior analyst should provide the client with either social praise and/or more contrived reinforcement (e.g., the use of tokens in exchange for preferred items or activities) when the client engages in the target behavior during practice. Fade out the contrived reinforcement to more natural contingencies once the client engages in the behavior more consistently on his or her own.

consisted of the clinician providing the rationale for effective conversation skills, modeling the skills, practicing, and delivering feedback. All four girls increased question asking after the intervention relative to their baseline levels. Results also showed an increase in the girls' delivery of positive conversation feedback when the intervention was implemented. Maloney and colleagues (1976) replicated the previous study with four additional female delinquent adolescents in a residential group home. Sessions were led by trained house parents or by the participants' peers. The research findings also showed that the girls increased their conversational skills after BST, and their new conversational skills were considered socially valid according to adults with whom the participants interacted outside of the group home.

A great deal of research has explored the efficacy of BST in teaching conversational skills to children and adults with intellectual disabilities within groups. Bates (1980) used BST to teach interpersonal skills to a group of adults with intellectual disabilities. Sixteen participants were divided evenly into experimental and control groups. The participants in the experimental group received BST, which included verbal instructions, modeling, role playing, feedback, contingent incentives, and homework, whereas the control group did not receive any instruction. Participants were evaluated based on their introductions and small talk, asking for help, differing with others, and handling criticism during situational role-play assessments after each week of group training. The participants in the experimental group improved during the situational role-play assessment after a 12-session training relative to the control group. However, skills did not generalize to more naturalistic unstructured conversations. This limitation may have been due to participants' not being taught with people with whom they would have had contact in their natural environment (e.g., family, classmates, coworkers). Kleitsch and colleagues (1983) used prompts, practice, and contingent praise to increase the verbal responses of four elderly adult males with intellectual disabilities. The number of instances in which they asked self-initiated questions of others, answered questions independently, and were prompted to ask or answer questions were recorded. Results overall revealed an increase in verbal responses from all participants after instruction, and increases in self-initiated vocalizations generalized to two other settings. Importantly, the group leader faded prompts by the end of the training session in order to transfer stimulus control of the target behaviors to the presence of another person only. The findings also indicated that untrained peers increased their frequency of verbal responses to the participants after training, possibly due to the participants' own improvements in social interactions (Kleitsch et al., 1983). It is important to note that when individuals are taught to answer and ask questions of peers, it is likely that those peers will ask more questions of them, thus sustaining the conversation. Thus it is imperative that instruction include conversation partners and take place in settings in which individuals are likely to have contact outside the context of instruction (see also Haring, Roger, Lee, Breen, & Gaylord-Ross, 1986).

Teaching individuals with ASD to have fluid conversations would greatly aid them in building sustainable relationships with coworkers, friends, family, and people throughout the community. Bornstein and colleagues (1980) used BST with six adults with intellectual disabilities to increase various interpersonal skills such as frequency of words spoken, speech latency, posture, enunciation, loudness, interpersonal effectiveness, intonation of speech, eye contact, and rate of speech. Behaviors that were targeted to decrease were inappropriate hand-to-face gestures, speech content, and hand movements. Four of the preceding behaviors were targeted for each participant, depending on his or her deficits. Overall, all participants showed increases in conversation skills following BST, and skills generalized to novel settings outside of training sessions. Using BST to teach speech fluency, latency, and content to adults with ASD may be helpful when they are interacting with others in fast-paced environments, such as the workplace or busy leisure settings.

BST has also been used to teach job interview skills to adults with intellectual disabilities (Hall, Sheldon-Wildgen, & Sherman, 1980; Kelly, Wildman, & Berler, 1980; Schloss, Santoro, Wood, & Bedner, 1988). Teaching adults with ASD interview skills is essential; although an individual may be highly qualified for a job, how he or she presents him- or herself to an interviewer can affect whether or not he or she is actually hired. Six adults with intellectual disabilities from two community group homes were taught office, application, and interview skills using BST (Hall et al., 1980). Office skills consisted of introducing themselves upon arrival, explaining that they were there for an interview, and following directions after introducing themselves. Participants were taught how to fill out standard job applications, which included providing personal information and job experience. Interview skills included having good posture, appropriate tone of voice and rate of speech, and asking and answering questions appropriately. All participants increased their office, application, and interview skills after BST, and generalization of skills to a novel office setting occurred for three participants. Kelly and colleagues (1980) used BST to teach adolescents with intellectual disabilities to provide information about previous work experience and to ask relevant questions to a job interviewer. Participants were instructed on the rationale of the target behaviors, shown videos of interviews, and role-played with other participants. Instances of positive information about job-related past experiences, positive information about oneself, questions asked to the interviewer, and positive verbal expressions of interest about the position were recorded during posttraining tests. Schloss and colleagues (1988) similarly revealed improvement in interview skills with two adult females with intellectual disabilities using BST taught by their teachers and peers. These findings demonstrate that using participants' peers during instruction may be equally effective and cost-efficient.

Taubman, Leaf, and Kuyumjian (2011) recommend the following prerequisite skills for an individual to benefit from BST: well-developed mands (requests) and tacts (labels), the ability to follow a number of instructions, and tolerance for the presence of others. These researchers also recommend ensuring that the rationale for the skills targeted corresponds to the needs and interests of the particular individual. Practice should occur in contrived and then in more naturalistic settings until mastery is attained, and external reinforcers may motivate the individual to engage in the target behaviors (Taubman et al., 2011). Much research specifying the efficacy of BST to date has been conducted with individuals with intellectual disabilities. More research is needed specifying its efficacy with adults with ASD, and under what conditions it may be most beneficial.

Case Example of BST

Sally was a 28-year-old female with ASD working at a local grocery store. The store's manager reported to Sally's vocational counselor that Sally easily completed all of her duties during her shifts, but continued to make inappropriate statements to other staff members and customers. Sally had already been given two written warnings, and she could have been terminated the next time she said something inappropriate. Sally's vocational counselor decided to try BST with her to increase her use of more appropriate statements and questions, as well as to eliminate her inappropriate statements to coworkers and customers.

Sally and her vocational counselor held meetings at the store's break room three times a week so that they could easily have access to her coworkers and customers. First, the vocational counselor compiled a list of appropriate and inappropriate statements and questions to use at work. Inappropriate statements from Sally consisted of verbal statements spoken in a high tone of voice, such as "Why do I have to bag these groceries?" "Why can't she do it?" "Ugh, why would anyone eat this food?" and "I don't want to work at this stupid store." Appropriate statements from Sally consisted of verbal statements spoken in a low tone of voice, such as "Yes, I will bag these groceries," "How is your day going, sir?" and "I am tired, but I am here at work." Second, the counselor provided Sally with a rationale for using more appropriate statements (e.g., increasing interactions with coworkers, coworkers being more likely to help her when needed, customers possibly giving her a tip). Third, the counselor modeled appropriate statements to a coworker (e.g., accepting verbally a request to help another coworker restock a shelf). Fourth, Sally practiced in the break room with the same two coworkers, one of them role-playing a customer. Fifth, the counselor provided oral feedback to Sally on her performance. If Sally used an appropriate statement or question, she was provided with verbal praise and 1 minute extra during her break time that day. If Sally used an inappropriate statement or question, the counselor provided corrective feedback and had her practice again. The counselor also had Sally practice while in the store.

After 2 weeks of instruction, Sally engaged in appropriate questions and statements with the two coworkers who had helped during practice sessions more frequently and while working (e.g., "How do you like working here?"; "I watched a great movie last night."). She started talking to other coworkers while stocking the shelves and bagging groceries a month after instruction began. Now, customers greet Sally by name and request her help in taking groceries to their car. Sally went to a baseball game with three of her coworkers at the conclusion of the BST intervention.

Modeling, Prompting, and Reinforcement Procedures

Common behavior analytic techniques such as modeling, prompting, and reinforcement have been shown to be effective in teaching conversational skills in a variety of studies with children with ASD (see Table 5.2). It is likely that these same techniques are beneficial in teaching conversational skills to adults with ASD. For example, Secan, Egel, and Tilley (1989) taught four children with autism between the ages of 5 and 9 years to answer *what, how,* and *why* questions about pictures from magazines using modeling and reinforcement. To assess whether children could answer questions about new pictures, generalization probes were used that consisted of asking children to answer *wh-* questions with different storybooks and natural-context stimuli. Some of the target questions were "What is in your lunch?" "Why is she crying?" and "How is he getting to work?" All children answered more *what, how,* and *why* questions after training compared with baseline. However, all participants had difficulty answering *wh-* questions from the storybooks and natural-context stimuli used in the generalization settings. Generalization probes revealed that the participants had more difficulty answering questions such as "Why is Johnny drinking?" if visual cues were not present. In other words, it was more difficult to answer a question about a picture if visual stimuli relating to the questions were not directly visible in the picture .

TABLE 5.2. Modeling, Prompting, and Reinforcement

1. *Modeling.* The behavior analyst or a model demonstrates the target behavior to the client. For instance, when working on how to answer questions at an interview, the model can show each aspect of the behavior(s) at an office, or they could be shown through videotape.

2. *Prompting.* Provide a verbal or written cue for the client to engage in the target behavior. The client could use flash cards containing answers to interview questions during practice sessions. It is important to systematically fade the prompts so that the client is engaging in the behavior according to the naturally occurring antecedents. The behavior analyst may also use a time delay before providing a cue to the client to engage in the behavior.

3. *Reinforcement* The behavior analyst should provide the client with either social praise or access to preferred items or activities when he or she engages in the target behavior. The contrived reinforcement should be faded to more natural contingencies once the client engages in the behavior more independently.

Secan and colleagues (1998) noted that asking questions about unknown stimuli or missing information can be an essential skill in the workplace or other community settings (e.g., looking for food items at a grocery store). Taylor and Harris (1995) also used modeling, prompting, and reinforcement procedures to teach two 9-year-old children and one 5-year-old child with autism to ask, "What is it?" and "What's that?" to unknown stimuli. The experimenter immediately modeled the question at a 0-second delay and gradually progressed to a 10-second delay. All three students attained mastery criteria within four to seven sessions. Asking questions about unknown items can be helpful when looking for a specific destination, such as a restaurant, or even to make small talk with a stranger in an elevator or riding a bus. Taylor and Harris emphasized the necessity of conducting such instruction in the actual settings in which the desired performance is expected to occur.

A variation of this instructional package includes showing participants video recordings of models engaging in the target behavior(s). Video modeling has many benefits; for instance, multiple participants can watch the video model at one time, and watching the video may be interesting for an individual with ASD for whom live social interactions are difficult. Charlop, Dennis, Carpenter, and Greenberg (2010) used video modeling to teach three children with autism between the ages of 7 and 11 socially expressive skills, such as verbal comments, intonation, gestures, and facial expressions. Three individualized videos for each participant were shown during the treatment phase. Each video presented a specific scenario (e.g., a child shown a preferred toy, being tickled, or being denied access to a preferred item), in which the adult in the video displayed the appropriate comments, intonation, gesture, and facial expression. Participants were then taken to a play-room, and the experimenter presented the same setup modeled in the video. If a participant emitted the correct response within 5 seconds, the experimenter reinforced him or her with an appropriate reciprocal interaction. All participants increased their social expressive skills after the video modeling procedure, and skills generalized to other settings and people. Video modeling has been used to teach individuals how to request help in work and classroom settings with adults with severe intel-lectual disability (Morgan & Salzberg, 1992) and children with autism (Reeve, Reeve, Townsend, & Poulson, 2007). In all cases, instruction also included prompting and reinforcement, and in some cases it was not effective until the opportunity for practice in natural environments was arranged (Reeve et al., 2007). Examination of the effects of video model-ing with adults with ASD is still needed.

Case Example of Modeling, Prompting, and Reinforcement

Jason, a 22-year-old male with ASD, recently moved into an assisted living apartment complex for adults with mild to moderate intellectual disabili-ties. Although Jason has strong conversational skills, he had difficulties asking for help when he needed it. For instance, as a requirement for living in his apartment complex, he worked with a behavioral consultant on how to evaluate and ask for help when necessary. The behavioral con-sultant asked Jason to write a list of situations in which he might need to ask for help, starting with items around his apartment. The consultant chose a few items around the apartment to pretend were broken during role play. For the first item, the consultant modeled the target behavior by calling maintenance on the phone to ask for help with changing the light bulb in Jason's bathroom. Jason then called maintenance to come help fix his dryer. If Jason failed to call maintenance within 5 minutes of noticing the broken item, the consultant verbally prompted him to call. He was provided with praise when he called maintenance. Once Jason's accuracy increased around the apartment complex, the consultant had Jason practice asking for help finding items at the nearest grocery store. If Jason could not find an item on his list, he was given 2 minutes before being prompted to ask a salesperson where the item was located. How-ever, Jason started to ignore the consultant's prompts and continued to look for the missing items. The consultant added reinforcement in the form of a $1 food voucher for Jason to use at the store each time he asked a salesperson for help. After a few prompts, Jason started asking for help at the store independently. Jason also practiced at a clothing store. After the third training setting, Jason asked for help when he was at the post office and even at his work site. The consultant was able to transfer the $1 food voucher to Jason's monthly allowance, which was provided by his parents, by the end of his services.

Script Fading

Script fading is a well-researched technique for enhancing spontaneous communication in individuals with autism (Charlop-Christy & Kelso, 2003). Script fading consists of providing written scripts or audio recordings that demonstrate targeted communicative utterances, which are ultimately faded from the last word of the script backward to the first word (Brown, Krantz, McClannahan, & Poulson, 2008). For example, if a script read "How was your day?," it would be faded in five steps to (1) "How was your," to (2) "How was," to (3) "How," to (4) a blank script, and then to (5) no script (see Table 5.3). Brown and colleagues (2008) increased conversational speech with children with autism in a convenience store and a sporting goods store and while watching videos. Scripts such as "Potato chips are salty," "I love to play catch," and "She is wearing purple" were faded one word at a time once each participant began to say the full script independently. Krantz and McClannahan (1993) reported an increase of unscripted initiations with peers for four children with autism following the use of script fading and found that when minimal prompts were present, initiations to peers generalized to different settings. Importantly, three of the four participants maintained these skills after a 2-month follow-up.

TABLE 5.3. Script Fading

1. *Type of scripts.* The behavior analyst can ask the client if he or she would prefer written scripts or audiotaped scripts of the questions or statements, depending on the reading level of the client. This can also depend on the obtrusiveness of the script in the setting in which the script would be used. For example, if the scripts are used to help a client to ask questions while on a date, small written scripts may be less obtrusive than audio recorders.

2. *Presentation of scripts.* The behavior analyst should decide when and how to administer the scripts to the client during practice settings. The scripts could be administered on a fixed time schedule, or the client may be prompted by the consultant to say a script after approximately 30 seconds of no responding.

3. *Fading scripts.* Once the client is saying the script independently when stimuli are presented, each last word of the script is faded until the client is saying the script without the presence of the stimuli.

Script fading has been shown to be easily implemented naturalistically. For example, Sarokoff, Taylor, and Poulson (2001) observed increases in conversational exchanges with two 8- and 9-year-old boys with autism when textual scripts were placed within target stimuli. Likewise, Charlop-Christy and Kelso (2003) employed conversational scripts consisting of seven statements plus a question to be used during training sessions. Generalization was conducted in a playroom and with the participants' parents. All participants increased their conversational skills after scripts were presented. Finally, Brown and colleagues (2008) showed that verbal initiations increased in children with autism when the procedure was implemented by their parents. Mands and joint attention have also been shown to increase in children with autism following script fading (Howlett, Sidener, Progar, & Sidener, 2011; Pollard, Betz, & Higbee, 2012).

Unfortunately, no research to date has explored the efficacy of script fading with adults, although the potential for applications is great. One possible reason for the limited investigation of scripts is that it has been reported that adults with ASD tend to have poor reading repertoires (Howlin et al., 2004). However, textual scripts could be easily embedded within work and home environments to enhance conversation with others. Individuals with autism may often feel like they have run out of conversation topics; using scripts may ensure that they do not run out of things to talk about.

Case Example of Script Fading

Brian was a 32-year-old male with ASD who was interested in dating. Brian is anxious about talking with women because he easily forgets what questions to ask or what follow-up comments to make. This unease results in a lot of long, awkward pauses between statements and the emission of basic questions (e.g., "How are you?") only. A consultant working with Brian suggested script fading as a way of improving his conversation skills in the presence of women. Two women from the consultant's office acted as Brian's dates for instructional sessions. The consultant helped Brian develop five questions to ask the women during their mock sessions. He handed Brian the scripts any time there was a pause in between statements for more than 30 seconds. Once Brian asked the question from the script independently, the counselor systematically faded each word of the question until Brian no longer needed to see the script. Brian practiced with two other women to promote generalization of asking questions outside of the office. After instruction, Brian reported that his anxiety had subsided, and he signed up to go to a speed-dating event.

Peer-Mediated Instruction
• • • • • • • • • • • • • • •

Peer-mediated instruction, or peer tutoring, is an established treatment for increasing communication and social skills with children with ASD, according to the National Standards Project (see Table 5.4). Promising results with children suggest the need for further investigation with adults with ASD (Wilcynski et al., 2009). Peer tutoring consists of having peers teach strategies to facilitate communication and other skills to people with or without disabilities (McGee, Almeida, Sulzer-Azaroff, & Feldman, 1992; Petursdottir, McComas, McMaster, & Horner, 2007). For example, Shafer, Egel, and Neef (1984) observed increases in social interaction skills in four 5- and 6-year-old children with autism when four children with mild intellectual disabilities served as peer trainers. Peer training consisted of providing modeling and feedback to peer trainers for appropriate interactions with participants. Motor movements, vocalizations, and initiations toward peers were measured and recorded. Not only were modeling and feedback shown to be effective in increasing the trained peers' performance, but participants' social interactions toward the peer trainers increased as well. However, social initiations did not generalize to untrained or novel peers until instruction was conducted with an additional peer (see also Pierce & Schreibman, 1997). Farmer-Dougan (1994) evaluated the effects of teaching individuals with intellectual disability and autism to conduct incidental teaching with peers with similar diagnoses. The skill targeted was requesting items. The experimenter taught the peers to recognize opportunities for requests to occur, to remove desired items from the surroundings, to ask for the appropriate response from

---

TABLE 5.4. Peer-Mediated Instruction

1. *Choose peers.* The behavior analyst should determine which of the client's peers would be the most beneficial to train. For instance, if a behavior analyst is teaching a client how to communicate with peers at a work environment, one of the client's own coworkers may be the best peer trainer.

2. *Train peers.* The behavior analyst should meet with the peer trainer(s) to discuss the rationale and to demonstrate the target behavior without the client present. The trainer should also be taught how to provide feedback and reinforcement to the client.

3. *Practice.* The client and the peer trainer(s) practice the target behavior together. For example, a coworker could explain and demonstrate how to exchange more than two questions with the client.

4. *Provide feedback and reinforcement.* After each learning opportunity, the peer trainer(s) may provide the client with feedback and reinforcement on his or her performance (e.g., "I like that you asked me two questions that were different but were still in the same context").

the participant, to wait for the correct response, and then to deliver the item. Not only were peers successful at implementing this form of incidental teaching, but also all three participants showed increases in requesting items during incidental teaching sessions with their peers. Importantly, requesting was maintained once sessions were withdrawn, and increases in requests generalized to two different locations in the residential setting. Peer tutoring thus appears to be an economic and efficient teaching approach, as teaching skills to a subset of peers may result in the production of more skills than actually taught.

It may be beneficial for adults without disabilities to serve as peer tutors for adults with autism, particularly if adults with autism are employed in settings with coworkers without disabilities, as the individual with autism may be more likely to converse with other coworkers following work with a peer mediator. Hughes, Harmer, Killian, and Niarhos (1995) used typically developing peers to teach four adolescent females with moderate intellectual disability, ages 17–21, to increase conversational exchanges with untrained peers. The peer trainers provided each participant with a list of questions and statements that they could say to the trainers during training sessions. The participants were instructed to gain attention from their peer trainers, ask a question, evaluate, and provide feedback on their own interactions with their peers (e.g., "I did a good job"). All four participants increased their conversational exchanges in the gym, classroom, lunchroom, and workroom at their school settings relative to baseline. Peers were also shown to increase their engagement with the participants with disabilities once participants' conversation skills emerged.

If adults with ASD are living in a residential setting, a required "social hour," during which the clients are paired with their peers to interact, may increase more positive interactions with other peers at various periods during their day. To this end, Laushey and Heflin (2000) examined the effectiveness of a "buddy system" approach on positive social interactions in a kindergarten classroom with two 5-year-old male children with autism. Both participants had minimal interaction with peers and engaged in only two or fewer conversational exchanges with peers per day. Positive social interactions consisted of asking for an object and responding according to the answer given from a peer, obtaining attention from a peer, sustaining attention with a peer when speaking, and waiting appropriately for a turn during play activities. Peer training consisted of the researchers' explaining to all the students in the kindergarten class, including the participants, the importance of interacting with peers and that they would be starting a "buddy time" to get to know each other. They were told that during buddy time they would need to stay, talk, and play with their buddy. During 10-minute buddy time sessions, the participants and the rest of the students were assigned a buddy, who changed daily to promote generalization. Overall, both participants increased their positive social interactions when the buddy system was implemented, and follow-up data showed their interactions were maintained 6 weeks into their first-grade class. This approach shows the ease with which the complete procedure could be implemented in an entire classroom or residential setting. This approach could also be easily implemented in a college dormitory for college students with ASD residing alongside students without the disorder, as it provides the opportunity to practice and engage with peers.

In a similar study, Haring and Breen (1992) structured social networks or groups to teach appropriate social interactions to two 13-year-old adolescents with mild to severe disabilities. Each participant was placed into a group with four to five peers without disabilities, and groups met once a week. Groups were instructed on what are considered appropriate conversation topics, how to gain another peer's attention, and how to initiate conversation with peers. When the peer facilitators were instructed to prompt the participants, they demonstrated, modeled, and provided feedback to the participants on their interactions with each other. The experimenter also provided feedback about whether a social interaction was appropriate. The peers without disabilities monitored the participants during training and at other times. Both participants' appropriate social interactions increased once the groups were formed and when they were provided with feedback and prompts. Social networks may be useful in teaching adults with autism problem-solving skills in the work and home settings, as well as creating sustainable work relationships.

Behavior analysts may consider peer training as a supplement to BST when teaching adults with ASD more complex communication skills to promote generalization in other settings and with different people. The behavior analyst could intertwine peer training within the six BST steps or implement peer training after BST is complete (Haring & Breen, 1992; Hughes et al., 1995; Laushey & Heflin, 2000; Pierce & Schreibman, 1997). More research is still needed to determine the efficiency of using peer training with adults with ASD, as well as in which settings this procedure would be the most effective.

Case Example of Peer-Meditated Instruction

Robert, a 25-year-old male with ASD, lived with his parents and 22-year-old brother, Michael. Robert worked part time at a pizza parlor and spent his free time playing video games at home. Robert wanted to live independently but required financial assistance from his parents in order to do so. Robert's parents feared that Robert would become reclusive and engage in solitary activities such as playing video games if he lived independently. They hired a behavioral consultant to help Robert engage in more social activities, and the consultant advised Robert's parents that it might be beneficial for him to have a peer trainer. His parents convinced his brother, Michael, to be Robert's peer trainer and for Robert to spend time with Michael's friends at a few social events. The consultant instructed Michael on how to prompt Robert to ask questions and make statements to his peers when in a social situation. If Robert interacted with Michael's friends five times in 20 minutes, he received money from his parents to allocate toward getting his own apartment, which was highly motivating for Robert. Consequently, the number of interactions required for money increased as Robert's social interactions toward others increased in social settings. After a month of training, Michael's friends started requesting that Robert join them in other activities.

Response Variability

Research on the topic of response variability has received considerable attention during recent years and has inspired interest in interventions for repetitive and perseverative speech in individuals with autism. Not only do individuals with autism often display perseverative or repetitive speech, but also discrete trial teaching protocols may exacerbate speech of this sort, producing restricted, rote responding, which may maintain into adulthood. Repetitive and invariable verbalizations may reduce the likelihood that others will want to engage in conversation with the individual, as well as promote stigma. Consider the following scenario: An adult with autism has attended social skills training and responds "My name is John, I am 31 years old, and I like rock climbing!" in response to "What can you tell me about yourself?" This response may be contextually appropriate in some social settings but inappropriate if John responds with this same answer during a job interview. Likewise, if he responds in this manner each time he is asked a question by relatives or coworkers, his response may be unlikely to produce follow-up questions from his conversation partner. However, if a number of varying responses to "What can you tell me about yourself?" were established in John's repertoire, John might have more response options from which to choose when asked that or similar questions. Consequently, his speech would seem more contextually natural, and social acceptance would be more likely in a variety of situations and settings.

Behavior analytic researchers posit that response variability emerges through the processes of reinforcement and extinction (see Gerhardt, Garcia, & Foglia, Chapter 8, this volume, on applied behavior analysis and skill-building strategies). Differential reinforcement of other behavior (DRO), differential reinforcement of lower rates of behavior (DRL), noncontingent reinforcement (NCR), and extinction have all been shown to increase variability in responding (Lee, McComas, & Jawor, 2002). The lag_n schedule of reinforcement, where n specifies the number of previous responses from which the current response must differ in order for reinforcement to occur, has also been recently shown to increase variability in responding. Lee and colleagues (2002) examined the effects of a lag_1 schedule when combined with differential reinforcement of appropriate verbal responding in two 7-year-old boys and a 27-year-old man with autism. All could speak in full sentences and produced spontaneous speech (i.e., unprompted by an adult). The older participant's spontaneous speech typically consisted of greetings and statements regarding some recent activity, whereas one of the younger participants made spontaneous requests for items or activities, greetings, and descriptive comments about objects in his environment. Social questions that participants answered the same way included "What do you like to do?" for the two 7-year-olds and "How are you?" for the 27-year-old. A varied verbal response was defined as any verbal response that differed in content from the last response to the same question. Sessions consisted of 11 trials in which the question was re-presented 10 times after the initial trial. During baseline, a differential reinforcement of alternative behavior (DRA) procedure was used to reinforce appropriate responses, and during lag_1 phases, appropriate responses that differed from the immediately preceding response were reinforced. Results showed that the lag_1/DRA schedule was effective in increasing varied appropriate responses to a social question ("What do you like to do?") for two of the three participants. For instance, after the lag_1/DRA procedure was implemented for one of the participants, he responded to the question "What do you like to do?" by stating "I like to read" and then "I like to color." The procedure was ineffective for the older participant. One explanation provided by the authors suggested that this participant's resistance was due to a longer reinforcement history for invariant responding. It was also possible that social interaction did not function as a reinforcer for this participant. Lee and Sturmey (2006) conducted a similar study with three 17- to 18-year-old boys with autism who spoke in complete sentences. The experiment was designed to address two limitations of the Lee and colleagues study. The first limitation was an inconsistency in the content of social questions across participants and the second was that the content of participant responses reflected the presence of various environmental stimuli during sessions. The first limitation was addressed by presenting the same question to all three participants. In addition, preference assessments using a multiple stimulus presentation format were conducted on a recurring basis to identify stimuli that would most likely function as reinforcers for each participant. The second limitation was addressed by evaluating the effects of the proportion of preferred tangible stimuli present during the sessions. The authors concluded that the presence of preferred tangible stimuli alone was insufficient to increase varied responding and that the lag schedule was necessary in order to increase varied responding by all participants on a single social question. These findings suggest that response variability may be influenced by operant processes even in older individuals with more extensive learning histories.

Susa and Schlinger (2012) extended the research on lag reinforcement schedules in increasing variability in verbal responses by using a changing criterion design to gradually increase response variability. The participant was a 7-year-old boy who had acquired intraverbal (i.e., a verbal response occasioned by another person's question or comment) responses to 33 social questions but whose repertoire lacked variability (e.g., when asked "How are you?," he always responded with "I'm fine"). Echoic (i.e., repeating the word or words of another person) prompting was used to establish new responses at the beginning of each criterion change. Reinforcers were selected by the participant before each session and took the form of preferred tangible items or access to activities paired with social praise. The lag schedule of reinforcement was shown to increase levels of variability across criteria. At the conclusion of the study, the participant had acquired three novel responses to the social question of "how are you?" ("I'm fine," "I'm good," "I'm okay," and "I'm super") and was successful in varying the delivery of those responses in accordance with the lag schedules of reinforcement.

Research conducted to date reveals that lag reinforcement schedules are effective in increasing the variability of verbal responses to social questions in children and adolescents with autism. These studies are promising for clinical application when an adult with autism exhibits rote or repetitive verbal responses to social questions. These procedures might be incorporated into social and work skills training (O'Neill & Rehfeldt, in press) in order to extend adult verbal repertoires to include complex conversational skills such as variable responding to open-ended questions. These procedures carry the potential to promote the development of fluent, natural-sounding conversation skills.

Case Example of Response Variability

The staff at an educational center for individuals with intellectual disabilities would like to teach interview skills to their incoming cohort of adults with autism. The company is currently short-staffed and would like to decrease the amount of human resources required to effectively teach these skills. Because none of the clients has previously acquired competitive employment, the onsite behavior analyst consults with the head of vocational training in order to identify the most important open-ended questions that the clients might be asked during an interview process. Once these questions are identified, the next step is to formulate multiple appropriate answers to each of the questions (see Figure 5.1). Next, the behavior analyst conducts a baseline mock interview during which each of the target questions is presented and the client's responses are recorded. Questions to which the client has a limited or nonexistent repertoire of responses are then programmed into an automated training that utilizes a lag schedule of reinforcement. The training program consists of a presentation-style format that allows the client to answer questions by selecting from multiple correct responses. When a response is selected, the program provides reinforcement and an audio playback of the onscreen text (e.g., "Yes, you can ask a coworker for help"). Through multiple presentations, the lag reinforcement schedule requires the client

1. What is one way you handle pressure and stress?
   a. *Insert existing response from individual's repertoire.*
   b. Slow down and take a deep breath.
   c. Ask a coworker for help.
   d. Talk to my supervisor.

2. What is one way you handle pressure and stress?
   a. *Existing response from individual's repertoire.*
   b. Slow down and take a deep breath.
   c. Ask a coworker for help.
   d. Talk to my supervisor.

3. What is one way you handle pressure and stress?
   a. *Existing response from individual's repertoire.*
   b. Slow down and take a deep breath.
   c. Ask a coworker for help.
   d. Talk to my supervisor.

4. What is one way you handle pressure and stress?
   a. *Existing response from individual's repertoire.*
   b. Slow down and take a deep breath.
   c. Ask a coworker for help.
   d. Talk to my supervisor.

FIGURE 5.1. Teaching using a lag reinforcement schedule.

to select and listen to each of the appropriate responses. In order for the clients to move on to another question, they are required to meet the lag criterion on 90% of presentations across three sessions. Once the client has completed training on each of the interview questions, the behavior analyst then conducts another mock interview to ensure that the responses learned during training have maintained and will generalize when it comes time for the clients to interview for community employment.

Virtual Environments

Virtual environments (VEs) have been defined as computer-generated three-dimensional simulations of real or imaginary environments that typically involve the use of avatars, or graphical representations of the user and interactive characters (Cobb, Kerr, & Glover, 2001). One advantage to VEs is that they allow the use of automated discrete trial training that can be delivered at the participant's discretion and in the comfort of the individual's home. A second advantage is that users can practice social interaction without experiencing aversive social consequences that may arise from awkward social interactions in natural settings (Trepagnier, Olsen, Boteler, & Bell, 2011). VEs can target differing complexities of skills and also include prompting and prompt fading. They may also prevent fatigue or frustration that may occur over the course of repeated instruction with clinicians (Parsons & Mitchell, 2002). In addition, this technology has the potential to reduce the amount of materials and human resources needed to implement social skills training. For these reasons, VEs have garnered increased attention in recent years and have been utilized in attempts to teach individuals with autism social skills ranging from facial expression recognition to complex conversation skills.

Moore, Cheng, McGrath, and Powell (2005) found that 34 participants with autism (ages 8–16 years) were able to accurately complete VE tasks when facial expressions (happy, angry, sad, and frightened) were depicted by an avatar. The tasks involved recognition of an emotion from an expression, selection of an expression to represent an emotion, prediction of an expression from a simple social scenario, and inference of a causal event from an expression. The authors argued that these skills are all prerequisites to functioning effectively in an interactive VE with expressive avatars. This study provided some evidence to support the notion that VEs might be an effective vehicle for social skills training in persons with autism. Likewise, Mitchell, Parsons, and Leonard (2007) designed interactive three-dimensional computer-generated representations of social environments and targeted the accurate identification of seating in cafes and on buses. Seven adolescents diagnosed with ASD (14–16 years of age) were required to navigate their way through a VE designed to give visual and verbal feedback on how to select an appropriate place to sit under different conditions. The program prompted participants to sit at unoccupied tables if they were available and to ask for permission to sit at occupied tables (e.g., "Is this seat available?"). Programmed responses also prompted the participants to consider the social context and the reason for their selections (e.g., "Sitting at the table is someone you don't know. What should you do?"). Results showed significant improvements in participants' judgments regarding where to sit in the targeted locations. Finally, Trepagnier and colleagues (2011) designed a simulation to teach 16 adolescents and adults with autism in a structured conversational interaction with the goal of teaching the cooperative nature of social conversational interactions. The program engaged participants with video recordings of a real-life conversation partner and utilized algorithms that allowed the program to adjust responses (video clips and a set of response options for the learner) based on the participant's verbal behavior during the session. Essentially, participants interacted with a conversation partner facilitated by a speech recognition system (manual selection of responses by mouse click was also available). Responding was reinforced through a points system for responses that supported the ongoing conversation. Although generalization probes to naturally occurring conversations in natural settings were not conducted, participants reported that they "strongly agreed that a larger simulation would be helpful to them and they would be likely to use it" (Trepagnier et al., 2011, p. 25).

A reasonable objection to the use of VEs for enhancing communication skills is that skills may be unlikely to generalize from the game to naturally occurring social situations. One approach to facilitating generalization might be to gradually introduce natural interactions into the VE through the use of video conferencing technology. In addition, avatars could be modeled to resemble family members, friends, and other important figures in the individual's life and programmed to target specific social interactions, such as vocational training (e.g., interview skills) or more general conversational interactions (e.g., small talk). Considerably more research is necessary to determine whether VEs are effective and efficient for promoting improvements in language in a number of settings for this population. VEs, video games in particular, are an untapped resource in the behavior analytic literature, most likely due to the time and resources involved in their development. This underuse is unfortunate because most popular video games come equipped with in-depth storylines and complex character histories, which would lend themselves quite well to the inclusion of complex communication and social skill building. As companies release open-source software for online games, the development of entertaining and engaging social skills programs becomes increasingly feasible.

Conclusion

The purpose of this chapter was to review evidence for behavioral interventions targeting complex language repertoires of adults with ASD. Complex language use is critical for adults with ASD to establish and maintain social interactions necessary to participate in daily adult activities, including work and independent living. Behavioral interventions have been effectively utilized with individuals to facilitate complex language, although research specific to adults with autism is lacking. Behavioral skills training provides a framework for teaching conversational skills such as asking questions. Modeling, prompting, and reinforcement have been implemented successfully with children with ASD to develop conversational skills, and script fading offers a mechanism to facilitate spontaneous use of language. Spontaneous language may be repetitive and perseverative in individuals with ASD, necessitating the use of procedures such as lag reinforcement schedules to increase response variability. Utilizing peer-mediated instruction enables a focus on natural communication partners, and, with technological improvements, VEs may offer a mechanism to integrate behavioral analytic teaching into a virtual, naturalistic setting.

Research focused on utilization of behavior analytic interventions specifically with adults with ASD is needed. Currently, the foundation for application of the strategies discussed in this chapter is largely based on interventions with children with ASD and adults with intellectual disabilities. Effective intervention with adults with ASD that includes emphasis on generalization will promote enhanced participation for this growing segment of society.

REFERENCES

Barnhill, G. P. (2007). Outcomes in adults with Asperger syndrome. *Focus on Autism and Other Developmental Disabilities, 22*(2), 116–126.

Bates, P. (1980). The effectiveness of interpersonal skills training on the social skill acquisition of moderately and mildly retarded adults. *Journal of Applied Behavior Analysis, 13*(2), 237–248.

Bornstein, P. H., Bach, P. J., McFall, M. E., Friman, P. C., & Lyons, P. D. (1980). Application of social skills training program in the modification of interpersonal deficits among retarded adults: A clinical replication. *Journal of Applied Behavior Analysis, 13*(1), 171–176.

Brown, J. L., Krantz, P. J., McClannahan, L. E., & Poulson, C. L. (2008). Using script fading to promote natural environment stimulus control of verbal interactions among youths with autism. *Research in Autism Spectrum Disorders, 2*, 480–497.

Charlop, M. H., Dennis, B., Carpenter, M. H., & Greenberg, A. L. (2010). Teaching socially expressive behaviors to children with autism through video modeling. *Education and Treatment of Children, 33*(3), 371–393.

Charlop-Christy, M. H., & Kelso, S. E. (2003). Teaching children with autism conversational speech using a cue card/written script program. *Education and Treatment of Children, 26*(2), 108–127.

Cimera, R. E., & Cowan, R. J. (2009). The costs of services and employment outcomes achieved by adults with autism in the US. *Autism, 13*, 285–304.

Cobb, S., Kerr, S., & Glover, T. (2001). The AS Interactive Project: Developing virtual environments for social skills training in users with Asperger syndrome. In K. Dautenhahn (Ed.), *Robotic and virtual interactive systems in autism therapy*. Hatfield, UK: University of Hertfordshire.

Farmer-Dougan, V. (1994). Increasing requests by adults with developmental disabilities using incidental teaching by peers. *Journal of Applied Behavior Analysis, 27*(3), 533–544.

Hall, C., Sheldon-Wildgen, J., & Sherman, J. A. (1980). Teaching job interview skills to retarded clients. *Journal of Applied Behavior Analysis, 13*(3), 433–442.

Haring, T. G., & Breen, C. G. (1992). A peer-mediated social network intervention to enhance the social integration of persons with moderate and severe disabilities. *Journal of Applied Behavior Analysis, 25*(2), 319–333.

Haring, T. G., Roger, B., Lee, M., Breen, C., & Gaylord-Ross, R. (1986). Teach social language to moderately handicapped students. *Journal of Applied Behavior Analysis, 19*(2), 159–171.

Hendricks, D. (2010). Employment and adults with autism spectrum disorders: Challenges and strategies for success. *Journal of Vocational Rehabilitation, 32*, 125–134.

Hofvander, B., Delorme, R., Chaste, P., Nyden, A., Wentz, E., Stahlberg, O., et al. (2009). Psychiatric and psychosocial problems in adults with normal-intelligence autism spectrum disorders. *BMC Psychiatry, 9*(35), 1–9.

Howlett, M. A., Sidener, T. M., Progar, P. R., & Sidener, D. W. (2011). Manipulation of motivating operations and use of a script-fading procedure to teach mands for location to children with language delays. *Journal of Applied Behavior Analysis, 44*(4), 943–947.

Howlin, P., Goode, S., Hutton, J., & Rutter, M. (2004). Adult outcome for children with autism. *Journal of Child Psychology and Psychiatry, 445*(2), 212–229.

Howlin, P., & Moss, P. (2012). Adults with autism spectrum disorders. *Canadian Journal of Psychiatry, 57*(5), 275–283.

Hughes, C., Harmer, M. L., Killian, D. J., & Niarhos, F. (1995). The effects of multiple-exemplar self-instructional training on high school students' generalized conversational interactions. *Journal of Applied Behavior Analysis, 28*, 201–218.

Kelly, J. A., Wildman, B. G., & Berler, E. S. (1980). Small-group behavioral training to improve the job interview skills repertoire of mildly retarded adolescents. *Journal of Applied Behavior Analysis, 13*(3), 461–471.

Kleitsch, E. C., Whitman, T. I., & Santos, J. (1983). Increasing verbal interaction among elderly socially isolated mentally retarded adults: A group language training procedure. *Journal of Applied Behavior Analysis, 16*(2), 217–233.

Krantz, P. J., & McClannahan, L. E. (1993). Teaching children with autism to initiate to effects of a script-fading procedure. *Journal of Applied Behavior Analysis, 26*(1), 121–132.

Laushey, K. M., & Heflin, L. J. (2000). Enhancing social skills of kindergarten children with autism through the training of multiple peers as tutors. *Journal of Autism and Developmental Disorders, 30*(3), 183–194.

Lee, R., McComas, J. J., & Jawor, J. (2002). The effects of differential and lag reinforcement schedules on varied verbal responding by individuals with autism. *Journal of Applied Behavior Analysis, 35*, 391–402.

Lee, R., & Sturmey, P. (2006). The effects of lag schedules and preferred materials on variable responding in students with autism. *Journal of Autism and Developmental Disorders, 36*, 421–428.

Maloney, D. M., Harper, T. M., Braukmann, C. J., Fixsen, D. L., Phillips, E. L., & Wolf, M. M. (1976). Teaching conversation-related skills to predelinquent girls. *Journal of Applied Behavior Analysis*, 9(3), 371.

Matson, J. L., & Boisjoli, J. A. (2008). Autism spectrum disorders in adults with intellectual disability and comorbid psychopathology: Scale development and reliability of the ASD- CA. *Research in Autism Spectrum Disorders, 2*, 276–287.

McGee, G. G., Almeida, C., Sulzer-Azaroff, B., & Feldman, R. S. (1992). Promoting reciprocal interactions via peer incidental teaching. *Journal of Applied Behavior Analysis, 25*(1), 117–126.

Minkin, N., Braukmann, C. J., Minkin, B. L., Timbers, G. D., Timbers, B. J., Fixsen, D. L., et al. (1976). The social validation and training of conversational skills. *Journal of Applied Behavior Analysis, 9*(2), 127–139.

Mitchell, P., Parsons, S., & Leonard, A. (2007). Using virtual environments for teaching social understanding to 6 adolescents with autistic spectrum disorders. *Journal of Autism and Developmental Disorders, 37*, 589–600.

Moore, D., Cheng, Y., McGrath, P., & Powell, N. J. (2005). Collaborative virtual environment technology for people with autism. *Focus on Autism and Other Developmental Disabilities, 20*, 231–243.

Morgan, R. L., & Salzberg, C. L. (1992). Effects of video-assisted training on employment-related social skills of adults with severe mental retardation. *Journal of Applied Behavior Analysis, 25*(2), 365–383.

O'Neill, J., & Rehfeldt, R. A. (in press). Selection-based responding and the emergence of topography-based responses to interview questions. *Analysis of Verbal Behavior.*

Orsmold, G. I., Krauss, M. W., & Seltzer, M. M. (2004). Peer relationships and social and recreational activities among adolescents and adults with autism. *Journal of Autism and Developmental Disorders, 34*(3), 245–257.

Parsons, S., & Mitchell, P. (2002). The potential of virtual reality in social skills training for people with autistic spectrum disorders. *Journal of Intellectual Disability Research, 46*(5), 430–443.

Petursdottir, A., McComas, J., McMaster, K., & Horner, K. (2007). The effects of scripted peer tutoring and programming common stimuli on social interactions of a student with autism spectrum disorder. *Journal of Applied Behavior Analysis, 40*(2), 353–357.

Pierce, K., & Schreibman, L. (1997). Multiple peer use of pivotal response training to increase social behaviors of classmates with autism: Results from trained and untrained peers. *Journal of Applied Behavior Analysis, 30*(1), 157–160.

Pollard, J. S., Betz, A. M., & Higbee, T. S. (2012). Script fading to promote unscripted bids for joint attention in children with autism. *Journal of Applied Behavior Analysis, 45*(2), 387–393.

Reeve, S. A., Reeve, K. F., Townsend, D. B., & Poulson, C. L. (2007). Establishing a generalized repertoire of helping behavior in children with autism. *Journal of Applied Behavior Analysis, 40*(1), 123–136.

Sarokoff, R. A., Taylor, B. A., & Poulson, C. L. (2001). Teaching children with autism to engage in conversational exchanges: Script fading with embedded textual stimuli. *Journal of Applied Behavior Analysis, 34*(1), 81–84.

Schloss, P. J., Santoro, C., Wood, C. E., & Bedner, M. J. (1988). A comparison of peer- directed and teacher-directed employment interview training for mentally retarded adults. *Journal of Applied Behavior Analysis, 21*(1), 97–102.

Secan, K. E., Egel, A. L., & Tilley, C. S. (1989). Acquisition, generalization, and maintenance of question-answering skills in autistic children. *Journal of Applied Behavior Analysis, 22*(2), 181–196.

Shafer, M. S., Egel, A. L., & Neef, N. A. (1984). Training mildly handicapped peers to facilitate changes in the social interaction skills of autistic children. *Journal of Applied Behavior Analysis, 17,* 461–476.

Shattuck, P. T., Roux, A. M., Hudson, L. E., Taylor, J. L., Maenner, M. J., & Trani, J. (2012) Services for adults with an autism spectrum disorder. *Canadian Journal of Psychiatry, 57*(5), 284–291.

Stokes, M., Newton, N., & Kaur, A. (2007). Stalking, and social and romantic functioning among adolescents and adults with autism spectrum disorder. *Journal of Autism and Developmental Disorders, 37*(10), 1969–1986.

Susa, C., & Schlinger, H. D. (2012). Using a lag schedule to increase variability of verbal responding in an individual with autism. *Analysis of Verbal Behavior, 28,* 125–130.

Taubman, M., Leaf, J., & Kuyumjian, A. (2011). Teaching interactions. In M. Taubman, R. Leaf, & J. McEachin (Eds.), *Crafting connections: Contemporary applied behavior analysis for enriching the social lives of persons with autism spectrum disorder.* New York: DRL Books.

Taylor, B. A., & Harris, S. L. (1995). Teaching children with autism to seek information: Acquisition of novel information and generalization of responding. *Journal of Applied Behavior Analysis, 28,* 3–14.

Trepagnier, C. Y., Olsen, D. E., Boteler, L., & Bell, C. A. (2011). Virtual conversation partner for adults with autism. *Cyberpsychology, Behavior, and Social Networking, 14,* 21–27.

Wilczynski, S., Green, G., Ricciardi, J., Boyd, B., Hume, A., Ladd, M., et al. (2009). *National Standards Report: The National Standards Project–addressing the need for evidence-based practice guidelines for autism spectrum disorders.* Randolph, MA: National Autism Center.

CHAPTER 6
• • • • • •
Teaching Functional Communication to Adults with Autism Spectrum Disorders

• **Russell Lang, Jeff Sigafoos, Larah van der Meer, Amarie Carnett, Vanessa A. Green, Giulio E. Lancioni, and Mark F. O'Reilly**

Communication intervention is a major therapeutic priority for individuals with autism spectrum disorders (ASD). Indeed, communication intervention was among the top 10 treatment priorities in a survey of 90 parents of individuals with ASD (Pituch et al., 2011). Specific communication skills prioritized by these 90 parents included (1) asking for information when needed, (2) describing feelings and events, (3) responding appropriately to questions, (4) initiating conversations, (5) naming objects, and (6) expressing wants and needs. The high priority assigned to these skills is not surprising given that communication impairment is a defining feature of ASD (American Psychiatric Association, 2013). However, the extent to which these priority ratings apply to adults with ASD could be questioned because only 14 (16%) of the 90 respondents were parents of older individuals (over 17 years of age) with ASD. Still, Iacono and Caithness (2009) noted that although there have been relatively fewer studies into the communication difficulties of adults with ASD, the few studies that do exist suggest that significant communication impairment—and hence the need for communication intervention—remains prevalent among adults with ASD.

Sturmey and Fitzer (2009) reviewed a number of empirical studies that assessed the nature and severity of communication impairment in individuals with ASD. The collective results of these studies point to three main findings. First, individuals with ASD have delayed language development compared with typically developing peers. Second, individuals with ASD tend to produce less frequent and fewer self-initiated communicative acts than both typically developing peers and individuals with some other types of developmental disabilities (e.g., Down syndrome). Third, ASD is associated with a range of differing types and degrees of communication impairment. At one end of this range are the 30% or so of individuals who fail to develop any appreciable speech (National Research Council, 2001). In addition to ASD, such individuals also have severe communication impairment or complex communication needs (Beukelman & Mirenda, 2013). The remaining 70% of individuals with ASD develop some spoken language, but their speech is often characterized by a number of unusual features. For example, the individual with ASD may simply repeat the speech of others (a condition known as *echolalia*) or speak only when prompted to do so (i.e., lack of spontaneity). In addition, persons with ASD may engage in obsessive, repetitive speech. Their speech might also consist of (1) unusual voice tone and inflection, (2) dysfluency (e.g., stuttering), (3) pronoun reversal, (4) inflexible sentence structuring, and/or (5) immature grammar (Brundage, Whelan, & Burgess, 2013; Scheuermann & Webber, 2002). Although each of these types of deficits—from lack of speech to lack of spontaneous speech to unusual voice tone—represents a potential priority for communication intervention, this chapter focuses on reviewing interventions aimed at developing the functional communication skills of individuals with ASD and severe communication impairment. This population could be viewed as priority candidates for communication intervention (Pituch et al., 2011). Our focus on functional communication includes procedures for establishing speech, as well as the use of one or more and augmentative and alternative communication modes.

In the next sections of this chapter, we define functional communication and describe the major augmentative and alternative communication (AAC) systems that have been incorporated into communication intervention programs for adults with ASD. After this, we provide an overview of research studies that have evaluated general approaches and specific procedures for teaching functional communication to adults with ASD. This overview of research evidence is followed by a summary of the generic instructional steps that appear to be consistently effective for teaching functional communication skills to persons with ASD. A case study is then presented to illustrate the application of these instructional steps for teaching an initial requesting skill to an adult with ASD. We conclude by summarizing the overall evidence base related to teaching functional communication skills to adults with ASD.

Functional Communication

Communication is functional when it enables the individual to express wants and needs and participate in meaningful social interactions (Plavnick & Normand, 2013; Reichle, York, & Sigafoos, 1991). Because opportunities to express wants and needs and to participate socially are pervasive, the communication skills taught to adults with ASD should occur in and be effective across multiple environments (e.g., home, school, work, and community) and with a range of communicative partners (e.g., peers, teachers, family, and general members of the community). Communication skills will be more functional not only when they generalize outside of the training environment but also when they are fluent and readily interpreted by others (Reichle et al., 1991). Some communication modes (e.g., using a speech-generating device to request a meal vs. leading a listener's hand to the desired object) are likely to be more socially acceptable, and hence more functional, across a wider range of settings and listeners (Carr & Kemp, 1989).

Contemporary intervention programs for individuals with ASD and severe communication impairment have tended to concentrate on teaching four basic communicative functions (Fitzer & Sturmey, 2009; Frost & Bondy, 2002; Sundberg & Partington, 1998). These are the mand, the tact, the intraverbal, and the echoic relations first described by Skinner (1957) and later refined by a number of subsequent researchers (Bondy, Tincani, & Frost, 2004; Michael, Palmer, & Sundberg, 2011). Table 6.1 describes the distinguishing features of each of these communicative functions.

Sigafoos and Reichle (1993) outlined a number of more specific communication skills exemplifying each of the four basic functions described in Table 6.1. Skinner (1957) described a *mand* as "the unique relationship between the form of the response and the reinforcement characteristically received in a verbal community" (p. 36). Specific communication skills that exemplify the mand function include (1) requesting preferred objects, (2) requesting help with difficult tasks, and (3) rejecting nonpreferred objects or activities. These communicative behaviors are classified as mands because the contingent consequence is likely to be what was requested. For example, an adult with disabilities might mand for a friend or relative to play cards (i.e., "Will you play cards with me?"), and the resulting reinforcement is likely to be engaging in the card game with that communication partner (i.e., the form of the response predicts

TABLE 6.1. Basic Communication Functions

Function	Definition and example
Mand	The mand is controlled by deprivation or aversive stimulation and reinforced by a characteristic consequence that matches the form of the response. The mand *food*, for example, would be controlled by hunger and reinforced by giving the person a preferred food item. Requesting and rejecting are examples of mands.
Tact	The tact is controlled by a prior nonverbal stimulus, such as some object or event in the environment. The function of the tact is to direct the listener's attention to the object or event. The tact *rain*, for example, would be controlled by water droplets falling from the sky. Reinforcement occurs when the listener thanks the speaker. Naming, labeling, and commenting are examples of tacts.
Intraverbal	An intraverbal is also controlled by the partner's prior communicative behavior, but in this case the form of the response does not match the form produced by the speaker. Instead, the response is contextually related to the prior verbal stimulus. If the parent asks a child what she wants for a birthday present, appropriate intraverbal responses might include *doll*, *bicycle*, and *pony*, for example.
Echoic	An echoic response is controlled by the partner's prior communication behavior, with the form of the echoic response matching the form produced by the speaker. The teacher says *truck*, for example, and the child responds by producing the exact same word. Imitation of speech and manual signs are examples of echoic responding.

Note. Based on Skinner (1957) and reprinted with permission from Sigafoos, O'Reilly, Schlosser, and Lancioni (2007). Copyright 2007 by Pro-Ed, Inc.

the contingent consequence). Although Skinner avoided references to unobservable properties of communication related to internal states (e.g., desires), from a practical perspective, manding is important because these types of communication skills enable the individual to gain access to reinforcing consequences (e.g., mands for preferred stimuli), including escaping from or avoiding aversive stimuli (e.g., requesting food to escape the aversive hunger pains). In lay terms, the types of mands are often referred to as ways of expressing wants and needs.

Second, specific communication skills that exemplify the *tact* function include (1) naming or labeling objects, (2) describing aspects of the environment, and (3) counting objects in the environment. Tacting is important because a number of such skills enable the individual to impart useful information to listeners. A listener benefits when told by a speaker that it is raining or cold outside or that the telephone is ringing.

The speaker benefits in that listeners provide social reinforcement (e.g., "Thank you for telling me that. I really appreciate it"). Tacting is also one way in which the individual might initiate conversational exchanges with others (e.g., "Looks like rain"). Instruction to teach naming or labeling is one way to build vocabulary related to new objects and actions. Tact instruction might also focus on teaching the person to accurately describe what he or she sees, hears, or feels. These skills can be very useful in academic instructional activities and when listeners would benefit from having this type of information.

Third, specific communication skills that exemplify the *intraverbal* function include (1) answering questions, (2) building on the conversation of others, and (3) thematically classifying objects (e.g., "Yogurt, milk, and cheese are all dairy products"). Intraverbals are critical for effective participation in the community, including daily communicative exchanges. For example, persons with ASD must respond accurately to questions such as "Where do you live?" and "Are you okay?". Maintaining a conversation will also typically require intraverbal behavior. For example, if the conversation drifts toward classic movies, intraverbal responses such as *Citizen Kane, Star Wars,* and *The Graduate* are likely to be appropriate ways of contributing to that conversation. As with the tact relation, the reinforcement for intraverbal responses is the resulting social reinforcement from listeners.

Finally, the *echoic* relation can also be thought of as a form of imitation. Specific communication skills that exemplify the echoic relation include repeating the speech of others (e.g., responding with "Hello to you, too" after being greeted with "Hello") or imitating the manual sign greeting of a newly arrived friend. Much conversation is echoic, as the speech of one communicative partner often overlaps with and builds on the prior utterances of the first speaker. For example, the first speaker might say "*Citizen Kane* is a classic movie," and the second person might follow this statement with "Yes, I agree that *Citizen Kane* is a classic movie, and so is *Star Wars*." The echoic relation is often specifically taught in communication interventions for persons with ASD as a way of teaching new response forms (e.g., teaching the person to imitate manual signs), which can then be generalized to serve other communicative functions, such as manding and tacting. The issue for some individuals is too much echoic behavior (i.e., echolalia). Intervention for these individuals has focused on replacing echolalia with tacts and intraverbals (McMorrow & Foxx, 1986).

Although the mand, tact, intraverbal, and echoic relations are often conceptualized as separate and distinct communication functions, Bondy and colleagues (2004) explained that communication responses often represent a blend of different functions. For example, an individual might be taught to name objects when the teacher holds up the object and asks, "What is this?" The naming response in this scenario might in fact be controlled not only by the object but also by the verbal instruction, making the response part tact and part intraverbal. Manding is also often taught in the presence of the preferred objects, which could make the response part mand and part tact. The implication here is that interventionists need to consider the precise antecedent conditions and reinforcing consequences that should evoke and maintain the targeted communication responses so as to ensure that these responses will be functional for the individual.

Augmentative and Alternative Communication

AAC can be used as an alternative to speech when the person develops little or no speech or to augment an existing but limited or unintelligible speech repertoire. AAC includes several alternative modes, such as manual signs, picture-based communication, and electronic speech-generating devices (SGDs). Skinner (1957) recognized that the four classes of basic communicative functions outlined in Table 6.1 could be expressed in a variety of modes. That is, functional communication does not necessarily require speech but can also be expressed through various AAC modes. AAC modes are indicated for adults with ASD who have limited or no speech. This, however, does not mean that efforts to teach speech should necessarily be abandoned when AAC is implemented, as AAC intervention can be used in combination with speech therapy. In fact, this combination might sometimes enhance speech development in persons with ASD and severe communication impairment (Millar, 2009). Millar also noted that AAC intervention does not appear to have any negative effects on speech development. Currently, there is a paucity of research in this area focused on adults with ASD, but, based on the research involving children, it seems likely that AAC use would not hinder and, in some cases, might enhance speech in adults with ASD.

The most common AAC modes taught to individuals with ASD are (1) manual signs or gesture-mode communication, (2) picture-exchange systems and picture-based communication boards, and (3) SGDs (Mirenda, 2003). Thus there are four general intervention approaches that might be implemented in the attempt to teach functional communication skills to an adult with ASD and severe communication impairment (i.e., speech, manual signs or gestures, picture exchange, and SGDs). The evidence base for each of these general approaches is considered next.

Evidence-Based and Promising Practices

This section provides an overview of the four main intervention approaches and associated procedures that have been used to establish functional communication skills in individuals with ASD. An important issue is whether there is in fact sufficient research evidence to support the use of any of these intervention approaches. In line with the guidelines offered by Horner and colleagues (2005), an approach or procedure can be considered evidence based or empirically validated when it has been shown to be effective in at least five high-quality studies involving proper experimental designs, including single-case experimental designs, and with at least 20 individuals with ASD. Of course, as there are fewer studies dealing with adults with ASD than with children with ASD, there might not be five high-quality studies involving 20 adults with ASD for some of these approaches or procedures. Therefore, approaches or procedures with demonstrated effectiveness in fewer than five studies or fewer than 20 individuals or that have been well validated only in studies involving children and adolescents can only be considered as promising, not empirically validated.

Teaching Functional Use of Speech

As mentioned in the introduction, approximately 30% of individuals with ASD present with very limited or no functional speech (National Research Council, 2001). However, previous research has demonstrated that many of these individuals can acquire at least some functional speech via behavioral intervention. In a pioneering study by Lovaas, Berberich, Perloff, and Schaeffer (1966), a shaping procedure was used to teach first words to participants with autism. Shaping involves gradual changes in reinforcement contingencies based on a series of subtle changes in the individual's vocalizations. Specifically, in the first stage of Lovaas and colleagues' intervention, all the participants' vocalizations were reinforced with a small preferred edible. This reinforcement contingency increased the frequency of vocalizations directed at the therapist. In the second stage, the therapist modeled a specific vocalization (e.g., "cookie") and reinforcement was provided only when the participants vocalized within 6 seconds after the therapist spoke; it did not matter what the participants' vocalizations sounded like. In the third stage, after the participants consistently vocalized within this 6-second window, reinforcement was provided only when the vocalizations began to sound similar to the therapist's original vocalization. The similarities between the therapists' vocalizations and those of the participants were then increased by gradually requiring more and more similarity in order to meet the increasingly more precise criteria for reinforcement. For example, the therapist might say "cookie." Initially, reinforcement would be provided for making the hard *c* sound, then *co* or *co-ey*, and, eventually, only for the full word *cookie*. Over time, the participants' speech was brought under the stimulus control of the therapist's spoken (imitative) model, and new words were taught by repeating the final step in the procedure. Although effective in some cases, this procedure is difficult because the subtle distinctions between one vocalization and the next can be hard to determine, and not all individuals with ASD will experience improvement. The validity of this approach also does not seem to have been tested with adults with ASD. The approach is therefore promising, but not empirically validated for adults with ASD.

Another promising approach for teaching speech is known as stimulus–stimulus pairing. Sundberg, Michael, Partington, and Sundberg (1996) demonstrated the potential benefits of this approach for increasing the frequency of vocalizations. In general, pairing is a procedure used to create reinforcing stimuli from neutral stimuli by presenting a neutral stimulus at the same time as (or in close temporal proximity to) a stimulus that already functions as a reinforcer. When used to increase speech, the intent is to condition the sounds produced by speech to be automatically reinforcing. To use this procedure, the therapist first recruits the individual's attention and then produces a target sound (e.g., *wa* or *mmm*). At the very moment the therapist makes the sound, the individual is positively reinforced. When effective, the sound will become a conditioned reinforcer, and the individual with ASD may begin to imitate the sound in an effort to produce this reinforcement independently. It may take as many as 400 such pairings of the sound and reinforcer before the individual with ASD begins to produce the target sound (Miguel, Carr, & Michael, 2002; Yoon & Bennett, 2000). Additional research investigating this procedure is warranted, but this stimulus–stimulus pairing procedure can be considered a promising approach for inducing imitative speech in adults with ASD.

As mentioned earlier, echolalia (i.e., repeating verbatim the verbal behavior of another person) is common among individuals with ASD and has been shown to impede social interactions, cause communication breakdown, and complicate the instruction of new communication skills (Prizant & Duchan, 1981). One approach to intervention aims to replace echolalia with functional speech, such as answering a question. Specifically, the person with echolalia is asked a question, but before he or she has time to echo the question, the therapist provides a model of the correct answer for the person to imitate. For example, the therapist might ask, "What type of animal barks?" and then immediately provide the verbal prompt *dog*. Ideally, the individual receiving treatment would then imitate the word *dog*. This enables the therapist to reinforce the response to the question and, eventually, to fade the verbal prompt for the answer. Although several studies demonstrated that this approach led to a reduction of echolalia and an increase in appropriate responding (e.g., Carr, Schreibman, & Lovaas, 1975), the benefits of this approach may not generalize to untrained verbal stimuli (Carr et al., 1975; McMorrow & Foxx, 1986; Schreibman & Carr, 1978).

A variation of this procedure, called cues–pause–point, involves first prompting the individual to remain silent; for example, the therapist might hold up a finger near his or her lips. If the individual with ASD produces a sound during this pause prompt, the therapist responds by saying "no," "shh," or some other indication to remain quiet. After the participant is able to remain silent in the presence of the pause prompt, the therapist points to a target object and asks, "What is this?" or some equivalent question. The pause prompt is then removed (e.g., finger put down), which signals to the person with ASD to respond. The person is taught to say the name of the object pointed to with the aim of replacing echolalia with tact responses (Foxx, McMorrow, Faw, Kyle, & Bittle, 1987; McMorrow & Foxx, 1986; McMorrow, Foxx, Faw, & Bittle, 1987). This procedure has been shown to generalize to untrained stimuli in studies involving children with ASD, but additional research investigating this approach with adults remains needed (Foxx, Schreck, Garito, Smith, & Wisenberger, 2004)

Teaching Functional Use of Manual Signs and Gestures

Manual signs and gestures have been widely used as a response mode for individuals with ASD and severe communication impairment. In the first such study, Carr, Binkoff, Kologinsky, and Eddy (1978) taught four children with autism to use manual signs to name objects. The children ranged from 10 to 15 years of age. Teaching involved presenting an object and reinforcing the child when the corresponding manual sign was produced. Response prompts were initially used to ensure that the correct sign occurred and could thus be reinforced. After a number of manual signs had been taught in this way, the authors reported that the children also came to use their newly acquired manual signs to mand for (i.e., request) objects. Subsequent research further demonstrated the efficacy of similar instructional tactics (i.e., response prompting, prompt fading, differential reinforcement) for teaching a range of functional communication skills (i.e., mand, tacts, intraverbals) to individuals with a range of developmental disorders (Duker, 1988; Duker, Didden, & Sigafoos, 2004; Sundberg, 1980).

In a systematic review of this research, Wendt (2009) identified 21 intervention studies aimed at teaching manual signs or gestures to a total of 130 individuals with ASD. Of the 21 included studies, 18 used single-case experimental designs and 3 used group designs. The communication skills targeted for intervention were mainly mands for preferred objects, imitative (echoic) responses, and tacts. The intervention procedures used in these studies generally involved the types of behavioral/systematic instructional techniques described by Duker and colleagues (2004). Specific procedures used included: (1) response prompting (i.e., verbal instruction, graduated guidance, modeling), (2) prompt fading, and (3) differential reinforcement. For most studies, the claim for a positive intervention effect was rated as either conclusive or suggestive, based on Simeonsson and Bailey's (1991) guidelines. In only four studies were claims for a positive intervention inconclusive. Overall, these data support the use of behavioral/systematic instructional techniques for teaching functional use of manual signs and gestures to individuals with ASD, but Wendt could not appraise the effectiveness of this approach for adults because the oldest participant in his review was only 16 years of age.

There is one study suggesting that adults with ASD can learn to use manual signs to mand (i.e., request) preferred objects. Specifically, Kee, Casey, Cea, Bicard, and Bicard (2012) provided intervention to a 28-year-old man who was blind and autistic. The aim of the intervention was to teach two manual signs (i.e., EAT and DRINK). These two signs were taught during lunchtime, when it was likely that the man would be hungry and thus motivated to produce the targeted signs to request the available food and drink items. At the beginning of the lunch period, the therapist provided a general verbal cue (i.e., "There is food and drink on the table") and reinforced signing by providing either food or drink. These procedures were in place during an initial baseline phase. After baseline, the intervention procedures were implemented. This involved physically prompting the use of manual signs by lightly touching the man's hand and pushing it in an upward direction. After intervention, signing continued to be monitored during a maintenance and 1-month follow-up phase. The results showed an increase in the number of mands for food from approximately 10 or fewer per session in baseline to between approximately 25 and 40 requests per session in intervention. Mands for food continued at a high and stable level (approximately 40–50 per session) during maintenance and follow-up. The results for the second mand (i.e., DRINK) are more difficult to interpret because the man was already using the sign DRINK at a high rate during baseline (i.e., from 30 to 70 responses per session). In addition, the baseline, intervention, maintenance/follow-up sequence is preexperimental and therefore does not provide conclusive evidence of an intervention effect. Still, this study is unique in its aim to teach manual signs to an adult who was blind and had autism. The results suggested the intervention was effective in increasing the man's use of one of the targeted signs.

Teaching Functional Use of Picture-Exchange Communication Systems

As with manual signs and gestures, picture-based communication boards and the related Picture Exchange Communication System (PECS; Frost & Bondy, 2002) have been widely used as a mode of functional communication for individuals with ASD. With the latter systems, the individual is generally taught to point to or give the listener a line drawing or photograph representing some object, activity, or event. For example, the individual might be taught to exchange a line drawing of a cup of coffee for a real cup of coffee. In one study, Reichle and Brown (1986) provided intervention to a 23-year-old man with autism who reportedly used no "vocal or verbal language to communicate" (p. 68). Intervention focused on teaching the man to use a communication wallet to make a general request and to label objects. For general requesting, a tray of preferred edibles (e.g., cookies, chips) was presented, and the teacher asked "What do you want?" A correct request required the man to touch a line drawing representing WANT. For labeling, the teacher showed the man an object (e.g., a cookie) and asked "What's this?" A correct response required the man to touch the matching line drawing from a choice of two line drawings. Later the man was taught to make explicit requests by touching the WANT symbol and then one of the object symbols (e.g., WANT + COOKIE). These skills were initially assessed in a nonteaching baseline. Intervention was then introduced first to teach general requesting. When progress was obtained with general requesting, intervention began to teach object labeling and, after that, explicit requesting in a delayed multiple baseline design (Kennedy, 2005). The teaching procedures involved physically prompting correct responses using graduated guidance (Duker et al., 2004) and reinforcing correct responses with access to the requested item(s) or by giving an unrelated reinforcer (for correct labeling). The results showed that correct requesting and labeling increased with intervention and that performance was maintained after intervention. The unique aspect of this study was that the man received concurrent instruction on two types of mands (general and explicit requests) and a tacting skill (i.e., object labeling). The delayed multiple baseline design strengthens the authors' claim for a positive intervention effect (Reichle & Brown, 1986). Subsequent work by Reichle and his colleagues (Johnston, Reichle, Feely, & Jones, 2012; Reichle et al., 1991) has provided confirming evidence for picture-based communication approaches for individuals with ASD and other developmental disabilities.

The PECS is a manualized program for teaching functional communication via graphic symbols (Frost & Bondy, 2002). Compared with other picture-based communication approaches, the PECS is unique in that the person is taught to select a graphic symbol (e.g., line drawing, colored picture cards, photographs) and hand it over to a listener, rather than simply touching or pointing to the symbol. For individuals who are ambulatory, this response requirement has the potential advantage of promoting social interaction and gaining the listener's attention. The PECS protocol targets communication skills that are closely aligned with Skinner's (1957) analysis of communicative functions and relies on well-established intervention procedures, such as various response prompting and prompt fading tactics, as well as shaping, chaining, and differential reinforcement. With the PECS, intervention begins by teaching the person to exchange a single picture card to mand (request) a highly preferred object. The person is then taught to seek out the communicative partner before making the exchange. Later, additional mands—requiring symbol discrimination and multisymbol (i.e., sentences) responses—are taught. Additional steps in the PECS protocol target tacts and intraverbals.

Ganz, Davis, Lund, Goodwyn, and Simpson (2012) provided a systematic review and meta-analysis of studies evaluating the effectiveness of the PECS. This team identified 13 studies in which the PECS was implemented with participants with ASD and evaluated them using proper single-case experimental designs (e.g., multiple baseline across participants; Kennedy, 2005). Selected studies also had to have included objective outcome data to enable the calculation of an effect size. These 13 studies included a total of 32 participants, ranging from 3 to 17 years of age. The results of this meta-analysis revealed an overall moderately positive effect, suggesting that there is empirical support for the PECS, at least for teaching functional communication skills to children and adolescents with ASD. Its effectiveness with adults has not yet been sufficiently well researched. However, Ganz and colleagues noted that the results were more positive with younger children versus adolescents. Although speculative, the age trend noted by Ganz and colleagues could suggest that the PECS might be less effective with adults. Conversely, a similar review conducted by Tincani and Devis (2011) found no relationship between PECS acquisition and several learner characteristics, including adult versus child. More research involving the use of the PECS with adults with ASD will likely be needed to elucidate this question.

In another appraisal of the evidence in this area, Lancioni and colleagues (2007) reviewed studies that evaluated the PECS, as well as closely related picture-based communication systems, such as the system used by Reichle and Brown (1986). They identified 17 studies that aimed to teach individuals with ASD and other developmental disabilities to point to, touch, exchange, or otherwise select graphic symbols (e.g., line drawings, picture cards, photographs). These 17 studies included a total of 173 participants ranging from 3 to 40 years of age. Most of these 173 participants were diagnosed with autism (n = 169), but the total participant pool included individuals with other types of developmental disabilities (e.g., Rett syndrome, intellectual disability, and cerebral palsy). Positive results were noted for 170 of the 173 participants, and one of these treatment failures was due to participant illness. The positive results primarily indicate that participants learned to use the PECS or a related picture-based system to request (i.e., mand) preferred objects. This skill equates to Phase I of the PECS protocol. However, some studies taught more complicated requests that required discriminating between picture cards and seeking out the listener before making a request (e.g., Phases II and III of the PECS protocol). Important for this chapter was the fact that two studies evaluated the use of the PECS with adults with ASD (i.e., Bondy & Frost, 1993; Chambers & Rehfeldt, 2003). Both of these studies reported positive outcomes.

Overall, this overview of studies suggests there is sufficient high-quality evidence to support the use of the PECS and related picture-based communication approaches. The data are especially strong for using this approach to teach children with ASD to request (i.e., mand for) preferred objects. The evidence base for adults is less substantial, but the few existing positive reports do suggest that the approach is promising for adults with ASD.

Teaching Functional Use of SGDs

SGDs represent another potential communication option for individuals with ASD (Lancioni, Sigafoos, O'Reilly, & Singh, 2013; Mirenda, 2003; Schlosser, Sigafoos, & Koul, 2009). SGDs typically consist of a visual display that can be configured with various graphic symbols, such as printed words, line drawings, or photographs. These graphic symbols represent the person's available vocabulary. With the vocabulary in place, the SGD is then programmed so that touching or otherwise selecting one of the graphic symbols leads to corresponding digitized or synthesized speech output. For example, selecting a line drawing of an umbrella might lead to some relevant corresponding phrase (e.g., "Looks like rain. Can you get me my umbrella, please?").

Researchers have speculated that SGDs might have several potential advantages as a communication approach for individuals with ASD compared with manual signing or picture-based communication. One potential advantage is that SGDs can be programmed to produce age-appropriate communication with minimal response effort (Mirenda, 2009; Schlosser et al., 2009). The synthesized or digitized speech output might also help to gain the attention of the listener and provide useful feedback that a communication response has occurred (Boesch, Wendt, Subramanian, & Hsu, 2013). An important question is whether functional SGD use can be taught to adults with ASD.

The results of a study by Banda, Copple, Koul, Sancibrian, and Bog-schutz (2010) suggest that the answer to this question might be yes. These researchers investigated the effectiveness of video-based instruction for teaching individuals to request preferred objects using an SGD. The two male participants were 17 and 21 years of age, had been diagnosed with autism, and were described as having no functional speech. Participants received the following sequence of intervention phases: (1) baseline, (2) video modeling, and (3) generalization. These phases were arranged in a multiple-baseline across-subjects design (Kennedy, 2005), and thus the study can be considered to have a high-quality experimental design. At the beginning of the study, a number of preferred (e.g., chips, pudding) and nonpreferred (clipboard, paper napkins) stimuli were identified. The aim of the intervention was to teach the participants to request the preferred stimuli by touching the corresponding photograph of the item from the SGD display. The SGD was available during baseline, but participants were never prompted to request with the device. For the intervention sessions, participants viewed a 10- to 15-second video clip. The clip showed an adult activating the SGD to make a request. After viewing the video, the participants were given the opportunity to use the SGD for up to 30 minutes. After intervention, generalization was assessed with a new set of preferred items. The results were positive in that both participants learned to make requests with the intervention. However, the overall increase in requesting was modest, and one participant never reached the 80% acquisition criteria. It could be that this innovative prompting procedure (i.e., video prompting) might have been more effective if it had been combined with the more direct response prompting procedures that have been used for teaching manual signs and picture-based communication skills.

Lancioni and colleagues (2007) reviewed 16 studies that focused on teaching individuals with developmental disabilities to use SGDs for functional communication purposes. The aim of most of these studies was to teach participants to touch one or more graphic symbols from the SGD display to request corresponding preferred objects. The studies provided intervention to a total of 39 individuals from 3 to 42 years of age, including some adults with ASD. The outcomes from these 16 intervention studies were similar to what Lancioni and colleagues had found for the

PECS studies. Specifically, the vast majority of participants (36 of the 39) acquired the targeted SGD-based communication skills.

In another review, van der Meer and Rispoli (2010) identified 23 studies that aimed to teach individuals with ASD to use SGDs for functional communication. These 23 studies provided intervention to a total of 51 participants, ranging from 3 to 16 years of age. Fourteen different types of SGDs were used in these studies, including (1) GoTalk, (2) BIGmack switch, (3) Vantage, (4) Lightwriter, (5) Tech/Talk, and (6) IntroTalker. The targeted communication skills were not always able to be matched to Skinner's (1957) categories, but included (1) mands—that is, requesting preferred objects or activities; (2) tacts—that is, social commenting; and (3) intraverbals—that is, answering questions. Additional intervention targets included (1) teaching spelling, (2) reducing perseverative speech, and (3) repairing communicative breakdowns. Most studies (70%) focused on one subclass of the mand—specifically requesting preferred objects. The intervention mainly used familiar and well-established instructional tactics derived from principles of applied behavior analysis (i.e., response prompting, prompt fading, and differential reinforcement; Duker et al., 2004; Fitzer & Sturmey, 2009). Van der Meer and Rispoli classified the outcomes from these 23 studies as (1) positive, if all participants in the study learned the targeted communication skill(s); (2) negative, if none of the participants in the study learned the targeted communication skill(s); or (3) mixed, if some but not all of the participants in the study learned the targeted communication skill(s). Using this classification system, 87% of the studies reported positive outcomes, and 13% reported mixed outcomes. None of the studies reported negative outcomes. This review supports Lancioni and colleagues' (2013) conclusion that SGDs can be taught as a mode of functional communication. However, no adults were included in these 23 studies, and so a more cautious conclusion is warranted with respect to the use of SGDs with adults with ASD.

Common Steps in Teaching Functional Communication

The research covered in this chapter points to the general efficacy (and perhaps the explicit need for) careful implementation of well-established systematic instructional tactics. The effective instructional tactics common to the studies reviewed herein can, in turn, be closely associated with the field of applied behavior analysis. Showing and telling a person how to communicate with the PECS or an SGD, for example, appears insufficient. Instead, intervention success appears to depend on the four generic intervention steps.

1. Creating frequent opportunities and motivation for communication—for example, by withholding highly preferred objects until the person makes a request.
2. Using effective response prompting strategies to ensure that the person makes frequent correct responses, which can then be reinforced.
3. Using procedures to fade out the need for prompting, so as to ensure that the person becomes more independent in communicating.
4. Providing immediate (listener-mediated) reinforcement. This step would seem critical for teaching and maintaining the person's communication skills. Listeners need to be highly responsive to the person's communicative attempts and provide the right type of reinforcement at the right time.

Interestingly, the studies reviewed in this chapter reveal that these steps have been successfully used for teaching functional communication skills regardless of whether the mode of communication involved manual signs, picture exchange, or SGD-based communication. For example, the therapist might use the same prompting procedure (e.g., perhaps using the least amount of physical guidance necessary or graduated guidance) to prompt the targeted manual sign, to prompt the person to exchange the correct line drawing from a PECS board, or to prompt the person to touch the correct graphic symbol from the display of an SGD. In addition, after a number of correct communication responses have been prompted, successful interventions include implementing a procedure to fade out the use of response prompts, such as by gradually waiting longer and longer before delivering a prompt (i.e., a time-delay procedure) and/or by reducing the amount of prompt given. These prompt-fading strategies have also been successfully applied whether in teaching manual signs, picture exchange, or SGD use. However, such procedures might not be directly applicable for teaching speech because speech cannot be so easily prompted, except perhaps by first establishing some imitative speech. As noted before, this latter objective has been accomplished using shaping procedures similar to those described by Lovaas and colleagues (1966).

Overall, the generic steps or procedures that appear to represent the keys to intervention success have also been successfully used for teaching a wide range of other adaptive skills to individuals with ASD (Duker et al., 2004; Fitzer & Sturmey, 2009). So although these general intervention procedures may not yet have been widely applied to the teaching of functional communication skills to adults with ASD, they must still be seen as having considerable generality and as being empirically validated

(Horner et al., 2005). Given the extensive evidence base supporting the use of these procedures, successful intervention outcomes for any given adult with ASD are perhaps likely to depend more on the application skills of the therapist than on the specific age of the participant.

Case Example

This case study illustrates the application of the empirically validated steps outlined herein to teach an initial mand to an adult with ASD. The case is taken from a larger study that included a 16-year-old and a 20-year-old (Sigafoos et al., 2004). The adult in this study (Megan) was a female diagnosed with autism, intellectual disability, and bilateral hearing loss. Megan had no speech, and her vocal output was restricted to occasional whining and humming. She had no formal method of alternative communication prior to her participation in the study. An initial assessment was undertaken to identify whether Megan had any current way of indicating when she wanted something. This assessment revealed that Megan would reach for and/or lead a person's hand to objects that she wanted. We also conducted a systematic preference assessment (Duker et al., 2004) to identify a number of preferred foods that we could then teach Megan to request using a single general request form (WANT). Starting with a single general request that can be used to request a number of highly preferred objects is consistent with Reichle and colleagues' (1991) approach for beginning an AAC intervention.

The study that Megan participated in involved a baseline phase and then the intervention. These two phases were arranged in a multiple-baseline across-participants design (Kennedy, 2005). The AAC mode selected for her was a BIGmack switch (AbleNet, Inc.). We put a single graphic symbol (WANT) on the switch, which was programmed with the message "I want more." During each baseline and intervention session, Megan received six opportunities to make a request for a number of preferred foods that were offered. During baseline, she gained access to the foods through reaching or leading or by pressing the BIGmack switch to activate the recorded message "I want more." We reinforced whichever response occurred first with a preferred food, except in one of the five trials, in which we ignored the use of reaching or leading. This was done to assess what, if anything, Megan would do in an attempt to repair the communicative breakdown. Specifically, we were interested in seeing whether she would switch from reaching and leading to using the SGD. We discovered that even when reaching and leading were ignored, Megan never used the SGD in baseline.

Getting her to use the SGD when reaching and leading were ignored thus became the intervention objective. To teach this, we implemented a set of teaching procedures when a communicative breakdown occurred (i.e., when the listener temporarily ignored Megan's reaching and leading). The teaching procedures consisted of (1) ignoring reaching and leading for 10 seconds; (2) reinforcing SGD use by giving her access to preferred foods, if SGD use occurred independently within the 10-second period; (3) prompting SGD use, using the least amount of physical guidance necessary, if correct SGD use did not occur within 10 seconds; and (4) reinforcing any prompted SGD use by giving her access to preferred foods.

The results suggested that the procedures were effective in getting Megan to use the SGD to repair communicative breakdowns. Specifically, SGD use did not occur during baseline but reached the 80–100% correct level within three teaching sessions. This finding suggests that SGD use might represent a viable communicative repair strategy. This is an important finding because communicative breakdowns are frequently experienced by individuals with ASD, making effective repair strategies highly functional (Brady & Halle, 2002).

Summary and Conclusion

Overall, the studies summarized in this chapter reported generally positive results. Although some participants failed to show much progress, most of the participants in these studies did acquire the targeted communication skills. However, most studies focused mainly on teaching one type of mand (i.e., requesting preferred objects), and few adults with ASD were included in most of the studies. Still, the general intervention approaches and specific teaching procedures that were used in the studies reporting positive results shared a number of common elements, and these common elements have wide generality and considerable empirical support. There are therefore good reasons to suspect that these types of procedures would also be effective for teaching functional communication skills to adults with ASD.

ACKNOWLEDGMENTS

Preparation of this chapter was supported by a grant from the New Zealand Government through the Marsden Fund Council, administered by the Royal Society of New Zealand, and by Victoria University of Wellington.

REFERENCES

American Psychiatric Association. (2013). *Diagnostic and statistical manual of mental disorders* (5th ed.). Arlington, VA: Author.

Banda, D. R., Copple, K. S., Koul, R. K., Sancibrian, S. L., & Bogschutz, R. J. (2010). Video modelling interventions to teach spontaneous requesting using AAC devices to individuals with autism: A preliminary investigation. *Disability and Rehabilitation, 32,* 1364–1372.

Beukelman, D. R., & Mirenda, P. (2013). *Augmentative and alternative communication: Supporting children and adults with complex communication needs* (4th ed.). Baltimore: Brookes.

Boesch, M. C., Wendt, O., Subramanian, A., & Hsu, N. (2013). Comparative efficacy of the Picture Exchange Communication System (PECS) versus a speech-generating device: Effects on requesting skills. *Research in Autism Spectrum Disorders, 7,* 480–493.

Bondy, A., & Frost, L. (1993). Mands across the water: A report on the application of the Picture Exchange Communication System in Peru. *Behavior Analyst, 16,* 123–128.

Bondy, A., Tincani, M., & Frost, L. (2004). Multiply controlled verbal operants: An analysis and extension to the Picture Exchange Communication System. *Behavior Analyst, 27,* 247–261.

Brady, N. C., & Halle, J. W. (2002). Breakdowns and repairs in conversation between beginning AAC users and their partners. In J. Reichle, D. R. Beukelman, & J. C. Light (Eds.), *Exemplary practices for beginning communicators: Implications for AAC* (pp. 323–351). Baltimore: Brookes.

Brundage, S. B., Whelan, C. J., & Burgess, C. M. (2013). Brief report: Treating stuttering in an adult with autism spectrum disorder. *Journal of Autism and Developmental Disorders, 43,* 483–489.

Carr, E. G., Binkoff, J. A., Kologinsky, E., & Eddy, M. (1978). Acquisition of sign language by autistic children: I. Expressive labeling. *Journal of Applied Behavior Analysis, 11,* 489–501.

Carr, E. G., & Kemp, D. C. (1989). Functional equivalence of autistic leading and communicative pointing: Analysis and treatment. *Journal of Autism and Developmental Disorders, 19,* 561–578.

Carr, E. G., Schreibman, L., & Lovaas, O. I. (1975). Control of echolalic speech in psychotic children. *Journal of Abnormal Child Psychology, 3,* 331–351.

Chambers, M., & Rehfeldt, R. A. (2003). Assessing the acquisition and generalization of two mand forms with adults with severe developmental disabilities. *Research in Developmental Disabilities, 24,* 265–280.

Duker, P. C. (1988). *Teaching the developmentally handicapped communicative gesturing.* Berwyn, PA: Swets.

Duker, P. C., Didden, R., & Sigafoos, J. (2004). *One-to-one training: Instructional procedures for individuals with developmental disabilities.* Austin, TX: Pro-Ed.

Fitzer, A., & Sturmey, P. (Eds.). (2009). *Language and autism: Applied behavior analysis, evidence, and practice.* Austin, TX: Pro-Ed.

Foxx, R. M., McMorrow, M. J., Faw, G. D., Kyle, M. S., & Bittle, R. G. (1987). Cues-pause-point language training: Structuring trainer statements to provide students with correct answers to questions. *Behavior Residential Treatment, 2*, 103–115.

Foxx, R. M., Schreck, K. A., Garito, J., Smith, A., & Wisenberger, S. (2004). Replacing echolalia of children with autism with functional use of verbal labeling. *Journal of Developmental and Physical Disabilities, 16*, 307–320.

Frost, L., & Bondy, A. (2002). *The Picture Exchange Communication System training manual.* Newark, DE: Pyramid Educational Products.

Ganz, J. B., Davis, J. L., Lund, E. M., Goodwyn, F. D., & Simpson, R. L. (2012). Meta-analysis of PECS and individuals with ASD: Investigation of targeted versus non-targeted outcomes, participant characteristics, and implementation phase. *Research in Developmental Disabilities, 33*, 406–418.

Horner, R. H., Carr, E. G., Halle, J., McGee, G., Odom, S., & Wolery, M. (2005). The use of single-subject research to identify evidence-based practice in special education. *Exceptional Children, 71*, 165–179.

Iacono, T., & Caithness, T. (2009). Assessment issues. In P. Mirenda & T. Iacono (Eds.), *Autism spectrum disorders and AAC* (pp. 23–48). Baltimore: Brookes.

Johnston, S. S., Reichle, J., Feely, K. M., & Jones, E. A. (2012). *AAC strategies for individuals with moderate to severe disabilities.* Baltimore: Brookes.

Kee, S. B., Casey, L. B., Cea, C. R., Bicard, D. F., & Bicard, S. E. (2012). Increasing communication skills: A case study of a man with autism spectrum disorder and vision loss. *Journal of Visual Impairment and Blindness, 106*, 120–125.

Kennedy, C. H. (2005). *Single-case designs for educational research.* Boston: Allyn & Bacon.

Lancioni, G. E., O'Reilly, M. F., Cuvo, A. J., Singh, N. N., Sigafoos, J., & Didden, R. (2007). PECS and VOCAs to enable students with developmental disabilities to make requests. An overview of the literature. *Research in Developmental Disabilities, 28*, 468–488.

Lancioni, G. E., Sigafoos, J., O'Reilly, M. F., & Singh, N. N. (2013). *Assistive technology interventions for individuals with severe/profound and multiple disabilities.* New York: Springer.

Lovaas, O. I., Berberich, J. P., Perloff, B. F., & Schaeffer, B. (1966). Acquisition of imitative speech by schizophrenic children. *Science, 151*, 705–707.

McMorrow, M. J., & Foxx, R. M. (1986). Some direct and generalized effects of replacing an autistic man's echolalia with correct responses to questions. *Journal of Applied Behavior Analysis, 19*, 289–297.

McMorrow, M. J., Foxx, R. M., Faw, G. D., & Bittle, R. G. (1987). Cues-pause-point language training: Teaching echolalics functional use of their verbal labeling repertoires. *Journal of Applied Behavior Analysis, 20*, 11–22.

Michael, J., Palmer, D. C., & Sundberg, M. L. (2011). The multiple control of verbal behavior. *Analysis of Verbal Behavior, 27*, 3–22.

Miguel, C. F., Carr, J. E., & Michael, J. (2002). The effects of a stimulus–stimulus pairing procedure on the vocal behavior of children diagnosed with autism. *Analysis of Verbal Behavior, 18*, 3–13.

Millar, D. C. (2009). Effects of AAC on natural speech development of individuals with autism spectrum disorders. In P. Mirenda & T. Iacono (Eds.), *Autism spectrum disorders and AAC* (pp. 171–192). Baltimore: Brookes.

Mirenda, P. (2003). Toward functional augmentative and alternative communication for students with autism: Manual signs, graphic symbols, and voice output communication aids. *Language, Speech, and Hearing Services in Schools, 34,* 203–216.

Mirenda, P. (2009). Promising interventions in AAC for individuals with autism spectrum disorders. *Perspectives on Augmentative and Alternative Communication, 18,* 112–113.

National Research Council. (2001). *Educating children with autism.* Washington, DC: National Academy Press.

Pituch, K. A., Green, V. A., Didden, R., Lang, R., O'Reilly, M. F., Lancioni, G. E., et al. (2011). Parent reported treatment priorities for children with autism spectrum disorders. *Research in Autism Spectrum Disorders, 5,* 135–143.

Plavnick, J. B., & Normand, M. P. (2013). Functional analysis of verbal behavior: A brief review. *Journal of Applied Behavior Analysis, 46,* 349–353.

Prizant, B. M., & Duchan, J. F. (1981). The functions of immediate echolalia in autistic children. *Journal of Speech and Hearing Disorders, 46,* 241–249.

Reichle, J., & Brown, L. (1986). Teaching the use of a multipage direct selection communication board to an adult with autism. *Journal of the Association for Persons with Severe Handicaps, 11,* 68–73.

Reichle, J., York, J., & Sigafoos, J. (1991). *Implementing augmentative and alternative communication: Strategies for learners with severe disabilities.* Baltimore: Brookes.

Scheuermann, B., & Webber, J. (2002). *Autism: Teaching does make a difference.* Belmont, CA: Wadsworth/Thomson Learning.

Schlosser, R. W., Sigafoos, J., & Koul, R. K. (2009). Speech output and speech-generating devices in autism spectrum disorders. In P. Mirenda & T. Iacono (Eds.), *Autism spectrum disorders and AAC* (pp. 141–169). Baltimore: Brookes.

Schreibman, L., & Carr, E. G. (1978). Elimination of echolalic responding to questions through the training of a generalized verbal response. *Journal of Applied Behavior Analysis, 11,* 453–463.

Sigafoos, J., Drasgow, E., Halle, J. W., O'Reilly, M., Seely-York, S., Edrisinha, C., et al. (2004). Teaching VOCA use as a communicative repair strategy. *Journal of Autism and Developmental Disorders, 34,* 411–422.

Sigafoos, J., O'Reilly, M. F., Schlosser, R. W., & Lancioni, G. E. (2007). Communication intervention. In P. Sturmey & A. Fitzer (Eds.), *Autism spectrum disorders: Applied behavior analysis, evidence, and practice* (pp. 109–128). New York: Springer.

Sigafoos, J., & Reichle, J. (1993). Establishing spontaneous verbal behavior. In R. A. Gable & S. F. Warren (Eds.), *Strategies for teaching students with mild to severe mental retardation* (pp. 191–230). Baltimore: Brookes.

Simeonsson, R., & Bailey, D. (1991). Evaluating programme impact: Levels of certainty. In D. Mitchell & R. Brown (Eds.), *Early intervention studies for young children with special needs* (pp. 280–296). London: Chapman & Hall.

Skinner, B. F. (1957). *Verbal behavior.* Englewood Cliffs, NJ: Prentice-Hall.

Sundberg, M. L. (1980). *Developing a verbal repertoire using sign language and Skinner's analysis of verbal behavior.* Unpublished doctoral dissertation, Western Michigan University.

Sundberg, M. L., Michael, J., Partington, J. W., & Sundberg, C. A. (1996). The role of automatic reinforcement in early language acquisition. *Analysis of Verbal Behavior, 13,* 21–37.

Sundberg, M. L., & Partington, J. W. (1998). *Teaching language to children with autism or other developmental disabilities.* Danville, CA: Behavior Analysts.

Sturmey, P., & Fitzer, A. (2009). Language problems in autism spectrum disorders. In A. Fitzer & P. Sturmey (Eds.), *Language and autism: Applied behavior analysis, evidence, and practice* (pp. 3–21). Austin, TX: Pro-Ed.

Tincani, M., & Devis, K. (2011). Quantitative synthesis and component analysis of single-participant studies on the Picture Exchange Communication System. *Remedial and Special Education, 32,* 458–470.

van der Meer, L., & Rispoli, M. (2010). Communication intervention involving speech-generating devices for children with autism: A review of the literature. *Developmental Neurorehabilitation, 13,* 294–306.

Wendt, O. (2009). Research on the use of manual signs and graphic symbols in autism spectrum disorders. In P. Mirenda & T. Iacono (Eds.), *Autism spectrum disorders and AAC* (pp. 83–139). Baltimore: Brookes.

Yoon, S., & Bennett, G. M. (2000). Effects of a stimulus–stimulus pairing procedure on conditioning vocal sounds as reinforcers. *Analysis of Verbal Behavior, 17,* 75–88.

CHAPTER 7

• • • • • •

Positive Behavior Support for Adults with Autism Spectrum Disorders

• **Matt Tincani and Shannon Crozier**

Positive behavior support (PBS) is an empirically driven approach to prevent challenging behavior and improve quality of life. This chapter presents an overview of PBS and its extension to adults with autism spectrum disorders (ASD). First, we define PBS, providing a brief overview of its history within the broader fields of ASD and intellectual disabilities, including the relationship of PBS to applied behavior analysis. Next, we describe special considerations for applying PBS with adults with ASD, including differences in adult service delivery systems, autonomy and choice, and medical and health issues. We conclude with specific examples of primary, secondary, and tertiary supports for adults followed by directions for future research.

Overview of PBS

• • • • • • • • • •

PBS is an applied science that uses comprehensive behavior support to enhance an individual's quality of life and reduce problem behavior (Carr & Sidener, 2002; Dunlap, Sailor, Horner, & Sugai, 2009; Horner, 2000). PBS is a systematic, evidence-based approach with two goals. The primary goal of PBS is to help individuals change their lifestyles and enjoy an improved quality of life; the secondary goal of PBS is to make problem behavior irrelevant, inefficient, and ineffective (Carr et al., 2002; Dunlap et al., 2009; Tincani, 2011). Prosocial behaviors are all behaviors that increase an individual's likelihood of success and satisfaction in educational settings, work, community, recreational activities, and social and family life. Problem behaviors are those that impede success in these areas, as they tend to result in isolation of the individual and exclusion from community settings, activities, and other typical environments (Buschbacher & Fox, 2003; Carr & Sidener, 2002) and to have negative impacts on those around the individual, including his or her family (Fox, Vaughn, Wyatte, & Dunlap, 2002). Fundamentally, PBS aims to strengthen prosocial behaviors, thereby removing challenging behaviors as an impediment to important lifestyle goals and improved quality of life.

PBS also relies heavily on prevention and early intervention to create a collaborative model to implement effective behavior support (Colvin Kame'enui, & Sugai, 1993; Powell, Dunlap, & Fox, 2006, Sugai, Sprague, Horner, & Walker, 2000). This comprehensive support focuses on instructional strategies to increase the prosocial behavior repertoires of target individuals and environmental redesign to improve quality of life, as well as behavior interventions aimed at reducing problem behavior (Carr & Sidener, 2002). Schall (2010) describes the positive effects of a team approach to support a 25-year-old man with autism at the coffee shop where he was employed. The team identified and implemented preventative and instructional strategies to enable him to be a more successful staff member by increasing his appropriate and productive behaviors and reducing his challenging behaviors. West and Patton (2010) describe the use of a PBS approach to find appropriate employment opportunities in a variety of settings for adults with a range of severe disabilities. They used functional behavioral assessments and a team planning process to identify potential jobs, to identify skills and challenging behaviors to overcome, and to appropriately match clients with jobs. The teams used instruction on routines and expectations for required tasks and job coaches to facilitate successful employment.

Importantly, behavior change cannot be accomplished unless the systems surrounding the individual, including family, residential, vocational, and community supports, are designed and implemented to sustain prosocial behavior and make problem behaviors irrelevant, inefficient, and ineffective (Carr, Horner, et al., 1999; Gage, Fredericks, Johnson-Dorn, & Lindley-Southard, 2009; McCart, Wolf, Sweeney, Markey, & Markey, 2009; Schall, 2010). PBS is therefore a systems approach that emphasizes identifying and working with the community systems relevant to the focus individual to scale up interventions and supports to create broader, more widespread impact.

As a cornerstone of PBS, a focus on prevention means that environments are designed so that low-level problem behaviors do not become high-intensity problem behaviors that must be treated with intensive, intrusive individualized behavior intervention programs. This emphasis on prevention is no more evident than in schoolwide positive behavior support (SWPBS), which utilizes a three-tiered model to prevent challenging behavior at primary, secondary, and tertiary levels (Sugai & Horner, 2002, 2009). Adult service delivery systems must also be designed to prevent challenging behavior utilizing this multi-tiered logic, though differences in human services organizations that support adults necessitate a distinct approach (Freeman et al., 2005). We explore systems approaches to prevent challenging behavior within adult service delivery systems later in the chapter.

Carr and colleagues (2002) codified these elements by identifying nine critical features that define PBS as a cohesive philosophy and practice of science:

1. Comprehensive lifestyle change and improved quality of life result, based on the values of the individual receiving support.
2. Supports are implemented with a lifespan perspective.
3. The interventions selected possess ecological validity.
4. Support teams include all relevant stakeholders, who participate actively in the development of behavior support plans.
5. Interventions and behavior plans have strong social validity.
6. Intervention support plans include attention to systems change procedures and include multicomponent intervention plans.
7. Plans are developed with a focus on preventing problem behavior from occurring and addressing the functional supports that can be put in place when problem behavior is not occurring.
8. Practitioners of PBS have a flexible, pragmatic approach to scientific practice in order to apply behavior change practices in the real world, with real problems of real clients in need of behavior analytic support.
9. Practitioners understand the multiple theoretical perspectives that contribute to effective intervention plans (e.g., systems analysis and environmental psychology).

History of PBS and Relation to Applied Behavior Analysis

During the 1980s and 1990s the development of PBS as a distinct approach started as a quest for nonaversive behavior support for individuals with severe disabilities and serious challenging behavior (Horner et al., 1990).

The initiative that eventually led to the development of PBS began with the professional assertion that aversive procedures that were considered unacceptable for people without disabilities were also unacceptable for people with disabilities (Brown, Gothelf, Guess, & Lehr, 1998). In the 1980s and 1990s it was widely held that aversive intervention procedures were a necessary component of behavior change programs for individuals with intellectual disabilities (ID) whose severe challenging behaviors proved difficult to treat (e.g., Mudford, 1995; Van Houten et al., 1988). However, by the late 1990s, a substantial, robust body of research emerged documenting the effectiveness of nonaversive interventions for individuals with ID and a variety of serious challenging behaviors (Carr, Horner, et al., 1999). Moreover, there began a movement to distinguish emergency procedures and so-called behavior management techniques from proactive programming that was intended to have broad implementation with preventative and educational effects.

In addition to its roots in the nonaversive intervention movement and person-centered values, the development of PBS was strongly influenced by the science of applied behavior analysis (ABA) and shares a common heritage with it (Carr et al., 2002; Dunlap, Carr, Horner, Zarcone, & Schwartz, 2008; Tincani, 2011). Several of the founders of PBS were also early pioneers of ABA and contributed substantially to the early development of ABA's conceptual and empirical foundation (Dunlap, 2006). Indeed, a close examination of PBS reveals many common features with ABA, including a strong adherence to science and data-based decision making, the use of principles of behavior (e.g., stimulus control, reinforcement) to strengthen and build new behavioral repertoires, and a commitment to socially valid or meaningful outcomes for consumers (Dunlap, 2006; see also Gerhardt, Garcia, & Foglia, Chapter 8, this volume). In many instances, the practices of PBS and of ABA look highly similar, as PBS practitioners and applied behavior analysts share many (if not most) common techniques, in addition to the overarching goal of helping individuals achieve desired behavior change.

However, even as the practice of PBS and ABA maintain substantially common features, it is clear that there are core distinctions that define PBS as a separate discipline. Foremost, PBS is a values-based science. For PBS practitioners, the primary purpose of intervention is not simply to increase or decrease behavior but to accomplish behavior change that leads to improved quality of life and happiness for the focus person and significant stakeholders (Carr, 2007; Carr et al., 2002). Therefore, incorporation of the focus persons' and significant stakeholders' values and preferences into the design, selection, and implementation of specific techniques is a central and necessary tenet of intervention and is essential to sustaining desired outcomes (e.g., Lucyshyn et al., 2007).

Systems change is also a distinguishing feature of PBS. On the one hand, an examination of research articles published in the *Journal of Applied Behavior Analysis* shows many carefully controlled experiments conducted in analog settings with highly trained experts implementing interventions. Although these studies often exemplify eloquent demonstrations of experimental control, the extent to which treatment effects extend to natural situations in the presence of multiple, complex contingencies and typical stakeholders is not always clear (Poling, 2010). By contrast, a defining feature of PBS interventions, as is evident in articles published in *Journal of Positive Behavior Interventions,* the field's flagship journal, is successful behavior change in the natural environment in the context of natural systems of support, including interventions that are implemented and sustained by typical intervention agents (Carr, 2007; Tincani, 2007).

Prevention and multicomponent interventions are also unique and defining characteristics of PBS. Leaders within PBS looked toward the fields of community psychology and preventative medicine to identify strategies for creating environments that encourage skill development and discourage challenging behavior (Carr, 2007; Carr et al., 2002; Sugai & Horner, 2002). Just as primary health care professionals seek to encourage universal "wellness" behaviors (e.g., healthy eating, regular exercise) to prevent lifestyle-related diseases (e.g., diabetes, heart disease), PBS practitioners seek to create universal systems that encourage prosocial behavior and prevent negative side effects that accompany challenging behavior (e.g., academic failure, dropout, unemployment, incarceration) (Sugai & Horner, 2002; Scott et al., 2002; Scott & Eber, 2003). When practitioners collaborate with stakeholders to create effective primary and secondary prevention systems, they reduce the need for intensive, individualized interventions and reactive disciplinary strategies that are often ineffective in ameliorating challenging behavior (Anderson & Kincaid, 2005). Finally, multicomponent interventions are those that incorporate multidisciplinary strategies into comprehensive behavior intervention programs (Carr et al., 2002). Therefore, perspectives from positive psychology (e.g., Steed & Durand, 2013), medicine (Carr, 2007), and the disability rights movement (Doody, 2009) are integral and necessary components of successful multicomponent interventions for adults with ASD.

Importantly, these distinctions do not imply that PBS is better than ABA, or vice versa. As PBS sought to define and establish itself as a distinct approach, there arose a subsequent backlash from the ABA community (Dunlap, 2006; Dunlap et al., 2008; Tincani, 2007). Some critics sought to question the distinctiveness of PBS from ABA (Carr & Sidener, 2002), whereas others attacked PBS and alleged that PBS was a threat to the field of ABA and its consumers (Johnston, Foxx, Jacobson, Green, &

Mulick, 2006). Over several years, there was much debate and dissension in the ABA community regarding the substance and distinctness of PBS. However, a dispassionate analysis reveals that the dichotomy between ABA and PBS is false (Dunlap et al., 2008; Tincani, 2007). For example, Filter, Tincani, and Fung (2011) found that practitioners who affiliated themselves exclusively with PBS or ABA were largely similar in their views on the value of core components of both PBS and ABA in their intervention practices. Although today there is little doubt that PBS and ABA are separate disciplines with unique defining features, behavioral practitioners can and should incorporate components of both, as it is clear that both PBS and ABA contribute greatly to successful outcomes for consumers of our services (Dunlap et al., 2008).

Special Considerations for PBS and Adults with ASD

PBS is widely associated with young children with ASD (Benedict, Horner, & Squires, 2007; Buschbacher & Fox 2003), schoolwide applications (Sugai & Horner, 2002), and people with ID and serious challenging behavior (Carr, Horner, et al., 1999). However, PBS is a valid approach for persons with ASD across the lifespan, although implementation of PBS with adults has distinct differences from implementation with children. These differences raise challenges, including differences in adult service delivery systems, balancing rights to autonomy and choice with access to effective intervention, medical and health issues, entrenchment of behaviors and history of reinforcement, work environments, questions of independent living, and independence of the individual, to name only a few. We explore substantive issues of PBS with adults with ASD in the following section.

Adult Service Delivery Systems

Applying PBS with children and adults requires certain assumptions about service delivery systems. For young children who participate in center-based programs, universal systems of prevention can be arranged across children within the same preschool (Carter & Van Norman, 2010), and for elementary, middle, and high school students, schoolwide systems can be created to prevent challenging behavior across all students and settings (Horner & Sugai, 2002). Staff who develop PBS systems in center-based and school programs typically work for the same school or for the same service provider in the same "host" environment, which facilitates creation of a common set of practices for each level of prevention.

In contrast, adult service delivery systems comprise a complex web of different settings, service providers, agencies, and funding sources, all of which complicate successful provision of PBS. Moreover, unlike school-based services for children with ASD that are universally mandated by federal law, there is no common legal framework for providing services to adults with ASD, and states vary significantly in the type and level of supports they provide and the ease with which consumers can identify and obtain them. And even though it is apparent that adults with ASD have unique needs in comparison with adults with ID and other types of disabilities (Müller, Schuler, Burton, & Yates, 2003), specialized services to support people with ASD may not be available, and individuals with high-functioning ASD (HFASD) may not qualify for services that are available to people with intellectual or other types of disabilities. One indicator of this inconsistent service delivery is the finding that adults with ASD are unlikely to be competitively employed (see Wehman, Targett, Schall, & Carr, Chapter 11, this volume). For instance, Taylor and Seltzer (2011) found that less than 20% of young adults with ASD in their sample participated in competitive or supported employment and that adults who displayed challenging behavior were significantly more likely to receive services in noninclusive settings (e.g., sheltered workshops).

An additional factor affecting service delivery for adults with ASD relates to professional training. Staff who support adults with disabilities frequently lack the education, experience, and credentialing of their counterparts in PreK-through-21 education, and service delivery providers must rely heavily on short-term workshops and inservices to teach intervention skills. Although workshops that accompany field-based, on-the-job training are likely to be more effective than workshops only, training formats vary considerably and may not include follow-ups with on-the-job training (van Oorsouw, Embregts, Bosman, & Jahoda, 2009).

Despite the challenges associated with adult service delivery systems, there is an emerging and promising training literature in PBS that may be applied to adult service delivery systems for people with ASD. For example, Reid and colleagues (2003) evaluated a training program for residential supervisors that involved classroom and on-the-job training in core aspects of PBS for adults with intellectual disabilities, including person-centered planning, effective teaching strategies, and providing feedback to staff. Participants improved their performance of PBS techniques during role plays and demonstrated a high degree of satisfaction with the training. Freeman and colleagues (2005) describe a statewide PBS training and support network for Kansas, one of many such statewide PBS networks in North America and the world (*www.apbs.org/network_preview. aspx*), which seeks to embed and sustain PBS within human services organizations across the state. Elements of this model include online training and field-based learning activities that can be delivered to geographically distant locations, development of a mentor network of professionals who have completed a year-long training, availability of a toolkit of resources to support ongoing program development and evaluation, and support for parents and families. Importantly, a team-based approach is the hallmark of PBS interventions; in this approach diverse stakeholders, including professionals, parents, and the focus person her- or himself collaborate in developing PBS plans (Ballard-Krishnan, et al., 2003; Boettcher, Koegel, McNerney, & Koegel, 2003). A desirable by-product of this process is that participants gain experience, knowledge, and skills they can bring to bear on future cases. Despite these promising practices, clearly more research is needed to imbed PBS within complex adult service delivery systems for people with ASD.

Case Example: Bryn

Consider Bryn, a 24-year-old woman with ASD whose verbal outbursts and physical aggression have limited her friendships and strained her relationship with her parents. Bryn lives in a community residence maintained by one agency but participates in a supported employment program maintained by a different agency. Bryn has two behavior analysts, one from each agency, in addition to a case manager who works for the state. Additionally, Bryn's parents, whom she visits on the weekend, receive assistance from a third agency that helps parents of adult children with disabilities. Collectively, staff of four agencies, along with Bryn and her parents, must collaborate to develop effective behavior support.

Bryn's residential behavior analyst heard about a state-funded program to support teams of individuals, family members, and professionals in implementing PBS. To participate, Bryn's team agreed to attend six day-long workshops on PBS over a 6-month period, which included onsite support from a PBS facilitator with expertise in the process (Anderson, Russo, Dunlap, & Albin, 1996) and access to online training resources (Freeman et al., 2005). The workshop facilitator guided Bryn's team through a process that began with person-centered planning (PCP) to identify goals for Bryn's plan, a functional behavioral assessment (FBA) to identify environmental variables affecting Bryn's behavior, development of function-based interventions that Bryn's parents and professionals had the capacity to implement, and a system of data collection for ongoing monitoring and, if needed, changing the plan to meet Bryn's evolving needs (see the later section on primary, secondary, and tertiary supports). After several weeks of implementing the plan, the team found that Bryn's verbal outbursts and physical aggression decreased dramatically, she made new friends in the community, and her once-strained relationship with her parents improved. As a result, Bryn and her parents went on a weekend trip together, the first such trip they had taken together in 10 years.

Autonomy and Choice

As discussed, PBS began in response to highly restrictive, aversive intervention procedures applied to people with ID (Horner et al., 1990). In light of this history, we must carefully consider the autonomy and human rights of adults with ASD in the PBS process. School personnel routinely implement behavior support procedures with children that could be construed as highly restrictive with adults. For example, a critical component of SWPBS is developing schoolwide reward systems (Sugai & Horner, 2002). However, applying such reward systems with adults necessarily involves limiting choices by withholding desirable things that most adults access freely. Conversely, adults with ASD who engage in challenging behavior are likely to experience negative consequences of their behavior (e.g., few meaningful social relationships, unemployment), which limit their life choices. Consequently, professionals must carefully balance the rights of adults with ASD to habilitative programming against their most basic rights as human beings (Bannerman, Sheldon, Sherman, & Harchik, 1990).

Incorporating the principles and practices of self-determination (Wehmeyer & Schwartz, 1998), including PCP (Flannery et al., 2000), is central to developing PBS programming that is habilitative and maximizes individual autonomy. PCP describes a collection of strategies to enhance the focus person's input and control in the selection of supports and design and implementation of programming (Flannery et al., 2000; Hagner et al., 2012; Kincaid & Fox, 2002). PCP is consistent with the values-based perspective of PBS; however, successful PCP is not simply a philosophy but a set of evidence-based practices that leads to better outcomes for the focus person and stakeholders. Successful PCP, therefore, involves systematic and carefully facilitated processes in which professionals assist individuals and their families in identifying priorities, selecting goals, and implementing supports (e.g., Hagner et al., 2012).

Case Example: Paul

Paul is a 32-year-old-man with ASD who receives vocational supports through a private agency funded by the state. Last year, the agency's job developer identified a supported employment position that she thought would be an excellent fit for Paul: working as a bagger at a local grocery store. Though initially Paul was enthusiastic about the job, after a few weeks he complained about feeling sick before work and missed several days of work per week. On the days he went to work, he was often rude to customers and would complain to the cashier that she was ringing up items too quickly. After consulting with the store manager, Paul's job developer and his behavior specialist decided that the position was not a good fit for Paul and that he would be better off with a different job. Disappointed, Paul spent the next few months at home waiting for a new job to become available.

Then the agency adopted a PCP process to help individuals to successfully participate in supported employment. Paul's job developer and behavior specialist facilitated a series of planning sessions in which Paul, his parents, and his job coach collaborated to identify Paul's strengths, desires, and the kind of job that would be best for him. They listened carefully to Paul as he discussed his past experiences and learned that his job as a bagger had made him anxious because it was noisy and because he was often very close to customers and felt that his personal space was violated. They helped Paul to identify a different job stocking shelves at a local department store. Paul really liked this new job because he enjoyed working at his own pace and could move about freely without needing to be in close proximity to staff or customers. Paul and his job coach identified a "quiet" area of the store where Paul could take a brief break if he was feeling anxious. He was also allowed to wear headphones with his favorite music, blocking out uncomfortable noise. Paul was productive and polite with customers, and Paul's manager considered him to be an exemplary employee. After several months, his job coach faded herself completely from the store, and Paul worked independently, with minimal contact between Paul's manager and the agency. Paul's story exemplifies how PCP can be used to identify and incorporate individual preferences into supports, a process that minimizes challenging behaviors and promotes successful outcomes.

Medical and Health Issues

ASD accompanies a variety of special medical and health-related concerns that we must consider in developing PBS programming. First, individuals with ASD may be diagnosed with one or more comorbid conditions (Filipek, 2005). Often, these conditions accompany unique behavioral challenges in addition to those associated with ASD. For example, Turygin, Matson, MacMillan, and Konst (2013) found a positive relationship between symptoms of depression and challenging behavior in adults with ASD served by two state-run developmental centers. Professionals who implement PBS programming must carefully review records and consider the effects of additional diagnoses on challenging behavior and how supports can be adapted accordingly. Professionals should also consider how medication side effects and interactions may affect an individual's behavior. Obviously, such evaluations assume the presence and full involvement of competent medical professionals on the PBS team.

Second, specific medical and health conditions increase the probability of challenging behavior in individuals with ASD (Kring, Greenberg, & Seltzer, 2010). For instance, an ear infection may increase the likelihood of challenging behaviors in the presence of loud noises and environmental events that cause vibrations within the individual's eardrum (May & Kennedy, 2010). Advancing age accompanies increasing risk of health problems for all of us; therefore, it is logical to conclude that adults with ASD are more prone to health-related challenging behaviors as they age. Effective primary medical care, including regular checkups, dental and specialist care, preventative screenings, and healthy diet and exercise, are central to preventing health-related challenging behaviors. Currently, little research is available on how adults with ASD obtain health care services; however, there is overwhelming evidence to suggest that people with ID have poorer access to health care services than people without disabilities (Krahn, Hammond, & Turner, 2006), and few physicians have specialized training in providing care to adults with ASD (Bruder, Kerins, Mazzarella, Sims, & Stein, 2012). These problems create a special burden for PBS professionals who must carefully consider the role of health and medical problems in development of problem behaviors.

Additionally, because adults with ASD frequently have limited communication skills, they may not be able to tell others about the symptoms of a specific medical condition (e.g., pain), and therefore the underlying condition may remain undiagnosed, and problem behavior caused by the condition may be inappropriately treated. Smith, Graveline, and Smith (2012) present a case report on Shannon, a 24-year-old woman with autism and ID who lived at home with assistance from a caregiver. Shannon experienced increases in screaming, aggression, and oppositional behavior, which were treated with a combination of psychotropic medication and behavioral interventions. Following a period of behavioral deterioration and worsening physical symptoms, Shannon was unsuccessfully treated with different psychotropic medications and electroconvulsive therapy. Finally, 36 months after initial onset of symptoms, Shannon was accurately diagnosed with multiple sclerosis. By this time, she was incontinent, bound to a wheelchair, and required nursing home care. Smith and colleagues identify lack of doctor–patient communication, inability of doctors to develop rapport with the patient, and presence of challenging behavior as barriers to the ability of people with ASD to obtain adequate medical treatment. Shannon's story, though tragic, underscores the importance of thorough medical assessment in understanding the function of challenging behavior (May & Kennedy, 2010).

Case Example: Allie

Allie is a 22-year-old woman with ASD and severe ID who receives residential and vocational supports through a private agency. She does not speak and communicates basic wants and needs through use of a picture-based AAC system (see Lang et al., Chapter 6, this volume). Allie recently transitioned to the agency from a school-based program focusing on life skills. She had a history of severe challenging behavior in the school, including self-injury and aggression. Two years ago, Allie kicked a teaching assistant; the resulting serious injury caused a week-long hospitalization. Following the incident, the school placed no instructional demands on Allie, and she was constantly monitored by two teaching assistants. When she transitioned to the adult agency, they continued to place no demands on her, and she was continuously monitored by two support staff members.

Upon Allie's admission to the adult services agency, Allie's psychologist reviewed her medical records and noted that there was no dental history in her report. The psychologist followed up with Allie's parents, who confirmed that her teeth had not been examined in 8 years due to behavioral difficulties she exhibited at the dentist's office. Reviewing Allie's behavioral data, her psychologist noticed a spike in aggression and self-injury around mealtimes. After consulting with the agency's nurse, they arranged for Allie to receive a dental exam under sedation. The dentist discovered serious infections that resulted in extractions of seven of Allie's teeth. In the weeks following these extractions, her team noted a gradual yet significant decrease in Allie's self-injury and aggression, as the pain from the infections presumably subsided. After 6 months with low levels of challenging behavior, they faded the second staff person from Allie's program, and she began to participate in community-based supported employment.

Primary, Secondary, and Tertiary Supports

Now that we have examined the defining characteristics of PBS and special considerations for adults with ASD, we turn our attention to the three-tiered model of prevention. Table 7.1 includes examples of primary, secondary, and tertiary prevention, described as follows.

TABLE 7.1. Examples of Primary, Secondary, and Tertiary Prevention for Adults with ASD

Primary prevention
    Person-centered planning (PCP)
    Preferred home, community, and work environments
    Choice making
    Preventative health care

Secondary prevention
    Communication programming, augmentative
        and alternative communication (AAC)
    Social skills instruction
    Sexuality education
    Activity schedules and visual supports

Tertiary prevention
    Functional behavioral assessment (FBA)
    Antecedent interventions
    Behavior teaching interventions (e.g., functional
        communication training)
    Consequence interventions

Primary Prevention

The fundamental purpose of primary prevention is to reduce the occurrence of new cases of problem behavior (Sugai & Horner, 2002). For adults with ASD, primary prevention means ecological and lifestyle arrangements that create and maintain a high quality of life for the individual, such as availability of preferred leisure activities and social networks, the opportunity to make choices, and the ability to freely communicate wants and needs (Freeman et al., 2005). Preventative measures for leisure and socializing include knowing the individual's activity preferences and with whom he or she prefers to socialize. With this information, family and staff can assist the person with making choices and gaining access to preferred activities with preferred individuals. As illustrated by Paul's case study, PCP is an essential first step in arranging environments that incorporate individual preferences (Kincaid & Fox, 2002). PCP lessens the likelihood of challenging behavior by identifying residential, vocational, and community arrangements that are important to the focus person, that contain a high density of positive reinforcers, and that limit exposure to aversive stimuli. In Paul's case, PCP translated into identifying a preferred work environment in which Paul could remain in his own personal space while completing the essential tasks of his job, free of loud, distracting noises.

Choice making prevents challenging behavior by enhancing the focus person's control over his or her environment; therefore, it is critical to arrange host environments with opportunities for the individual to make choices that most adults make, such as selecting the order in which daily living activities are completed (Watanabe & Sturmey, 2003) or the order in which job-related tasks are performed (Schall, 2010). Choice making also means helping to arrange the people, activities, and living arrangements that are important to the focus person by taking into account the individual's preferences as to where, how, and with whom he or she would like to live and what details about his or her home are important to him or her, and helping the person to achieve a living arrangement that is a good fit for him or her, where he or she feels comfortable and welcome. This also includes ensuring that he or she has adequate skills and resources to maintain daily life (e.g., doing laundry, cleaning the house, navigating the neighborhood).

Health and medical problems increase the likelihood of challenging behavior (May & Kennedy, 2010); therefore, effective preventative health care is critical to primary prevention. Preventative health care means attention to maintaining an adequate level of health and regular access to health care services, as well as systems to manage existing health care needs. Specific steps to establish adequate health care include medication procedures and schedules to ensure that the focus person takes medication regularly and appropriately, scheduling regular physicals and dental exams, as well as maintaining medical records to support continuity of care, and ensuring that staff, friends, and family know how to help manage existing medical conditions (e.g., information on allergens, what to do if a seizure occurs, understanding and managing diabetes).

This is not an exhaustive list of primary preventative strategies. There can be no exhaustive list, as the needs of individuals vary greatly. It is most important to understand the general principles and strategies behind primary prevention, namely, identifying lifestyle arrangements that are important to the focus person, facilitating access to preferred activities, facilitating important social relationships, and creating and maintaining health and wellness. Primary prevention is about creating a life that the individual values and finds fulfilling, as well as minimizing challenging behavior.

Secondary Prevention

Secondary prevention involves identifying and providing targeted interventions to individuals who are at risk for serious challenging behavior due to an underlying condition. ASD is characterized by impairments in social communication and social interaction and restricted, repetitive patterns of behavior, interests, or activities (American Psychiatric Association, 2013). Each of these impairments places adults with ASD at risk for problem behavior in different ways. Consequently, secondary supports involve targeted strategies to enhance appropriate communication and social interaction and to create environments that capitalize on needs for sameness, structure, and consistency. Importantly, ASD is a heterogeneous condition, and individuals have different levels of impairment, ranging from mild to severe. The nature of targeted secondary intervention strategies will vary greatly across individuals based on needs. The following description of evidence-based and promising secondary prevention strategies is, therefore, only a partial list of potentially effective supports.

Communication breakdowns can lead to challenging behavior. Consequently, creating environments in which to teach and actively support communication is critical. Many adults with ASD and ID lack the ability to vocally communicate; therefore, we must teach communication using augmentative and alternative strategies, including picture-based systems (e.g., Conklin & Mayer, 2011) and speech-generating devices (Rispoli, Franco, van der Meer, Lang, & Camargo, 2010; see Lang et al., Chapter 6, this volume). Simply providing devices is insufficient to maintain ongoing, functional communication. Professionals must actively support communication by using effective teaching strategies based in the principles of ABA (Bondy & Frost, 2001), by ensuring that devices are maintained and continuously available across settings, and by arranging explicit opportunities to communicate throughout the day, such as by requesting preferred leisure items, work materials, and breaks, commenting on the salient aspects of the environment, and engaging in conversations with family members, peers, coworkers, and staff.

Adults with HFASD typically have sophisticated language skills; however, deficits in social interactions limit their ability to succeed in post-secondary education, to obtain and keep competitive employment, and to navigate meaningful personal relationships. Consequently, strategies to enhance social and communicative functioning are a necessary component of targeted interventions for individuals with HFASD (see Myles, Coffin, Owens, & Yantes, Chapter 1, this volume). Barnhill, Cook, Tebbenkamp, and Myles (2002) employed social skills groups to increase the nonverbal communication skills of eight adolescents with HFASD. The groups' activities targeted nuanced social and communicative skills, such as understanding tones and emphases of speech and identifying and responding to facial expressions. Although promising recent studies have confirmed the benefits of using social skills groups to enhance a variety of social skills for adolescents with HFASD (e.g., Laugeson, Frankel,

Gantman, Dillon, & Mogil, 2012), clearly more research is needed to expand these promising practices to adults.

Professionals increasingly recognize the importance of sexuality education to individuals with ASD (Travers & Tincani, 2010). Alarmingly, Sutton and colleagues (2013) found that 60% of adolescents adjudicated for sexually related crimes in a state treatment facility met the diagnostic criteria for ASD. The study was limited by a small sample size of 37 individuals; however, the finding highlights the need to provide early and ongoing sexuality education as part of secondary prevention. Unfortunately, although a variety of sexuality education curricula are available, there is very little research to support effectiveness of any specific curriculum, particularly for individuals with ASD (Travers, Tincani, Whitby, & Boutot, in press). More research is urgently needed to establish evidence-based practices for teaching sexuality and relationship skills to people with ASD (see Travers & Whitby, Chapter 9, this volume).

Finally, the tendency of adults with ASD to exhibit restricted, repetitive patterns of behavior and interests translates into a need for structure and predictability in the environment. Many individuals benefit from individualized pictorial or written activity schedules to promote structure and predictability in home, work, and community settings (McClannahan & Krantz, 2010; Schall, 2010). Increasingly, software is available to enable tablet computers and smartphones to function as activity schedules (Carlile, Reeve, Reeve, & DeBar, 2013). Electronic devices as activity schedules lessen stigma associated with traditional systems, as they incorporate technology that most people use. Additionally, activity schedules can be an excellent way to incorporate choice into daily routines (Watanabe & Sturmey, 2003).

Tertiary Prevention

Given the genesis of PBS in helping persons with severe disabilities, there has been a substantial focus on interventions for individuals with chronic, intensely challenging behavior (LaVigna & Willis, 2012). Consequently, tertiary interventions are perhaps the most well understood of the three intervention tiers. This is unfortunate, in a sense, as more emphasis on high-fidelity primary and secondary interventions would obviate the need for individualized, function-based supports in many cases. On the other hand, much is known about how to help individuals who exhibit severe challenging behavior through individualized behavior interventions (Carr, Levin, et al., 1999; LaVigna & Willis, 2012; Tiger, Hanley, & Bruzek, 2008).

FBA is a necessary and essential component of tertiary PBS plans. FBA describes a variety of strategies to identify motivating operations, triggering antecedents, skill deficits, and consequences that maintain challenging behavior (Crone & Horner, 2003). This assists PBS teams in creating multicomponent interventions that address behavior function(s). For example, if it is understood that an individual's aggression is maintained by attention from caregivers, the team can use functional communication training (FCT) to teach the individual to gain attention in more socially acceptable, nondestructive ways (Tiger et al., 2008). Function-based interventions are more likely to have good contextual fit and durability if they are designed with input from critical stakeholders, including parents and staff (Carr et al., 1999; Lucyshyn et al., 2007). Therefore, FBA should be viewed as a team-based process in which information from multiple sources is incorporated into assessment. Data collection in FBA is composed of two general strategies: indirect assessment, including interviews and rating scales, and direct assessments, including A–B–C assessments, scatterplots, and other strategies for taking data directly on the individual's behavior as it happens in the environment in relation to antecedent and consequent events (see Crone & Horner, 2003, and Tincani, 2011, for a more detailed description of FBA techniques).

Once the team understands the problem behavior's function(s), they can design function-based interventions to alter the specific environmental variables producing the behavior. As with primary and secondary interventions, the goal of tertiary supports is not simply to alter the environment but to change the behavior of individuals around the focus person in ways that enhance the focus person's lifestyle and quality of life. Broadly, function-based interventions can be divided into three categories: antecedent interventions, alternative behavior teaching interventions, and consequence interventions.

Antecedent interventions involve altering motivating operations and discriminative stimuli preceding challenging behavior to lessen or prevent the behavior's occurrence (Wacker, Berg, & Harding, 2006). For example, if the FBA reveals that aggression is more likely when demands are presented to the focus person following an unplanned change in the daily schedule, staff could "neutralize" the effects of losing the preferred activity by providing choice of an alternative preferred activity or by temporarily lessening demands following disruptions in the daily schedule (Horner, Day, & Day, 1997). If the FBA suggests that a particular activity increases the likelihood of escape-maintained problem behavior, staff could alter the activity by providing assistance during the activity, offering a choice of materials or locations for the activity, interspersing easier tasks into the activity, or increasing the predictability of the activity by adding written or visual cues (Miltenberger, 2006). Alternatively, if challenging behavior is maintained by attention from others, staff could "enrich" the environment by providing attention to the focus person noncontingently on a predetermined schedule (Carr & LeBlanc, 2006).

Alternative behavior teaching interventions lessen challenging behavior by strengthening the focus person's adaptive skills. Perhaps the best known of these interventions is FCT (Carr & Durand, 1985; Tiger et al., 2008). FCT involves teaching the focus person a more acceptable, appropriate communicative response that produces the same consequences as the challenging behavior. For instance, if an FBA suggests that the focus person's screaming is maintained by attention from staff who provide assistance following the behavior (e.g., "Are you okay?"), then FCT could involve teaching the focus person a more acceptable way to obtain attention from staff, such as by exchanging a picture symbol for "help." For FCT to be successful, the alternative response must be more efficient and effective than the problem behavior in producing reinforcing consequences. Therefore, staff must select an alternative response that is easy for the focus person to perform, they must lessen or eliminate reinforcement when the problem behavior occurs, and they must provide a rich schedule of reinforcement for each alternative communicative response.

Finally, consequence interventions involve altering the arrangement of reinforcers for challenging and prosocial behaviors. All tertiary interventions involve some degree of consequence interventions, as staff must effectively use reinforcement to increase the focus person's performance of alternative skills (e.g., West & Patton, 2010). For example, if an FBA reveals that staff demands increase the focus person's engagement in escape-maintained problem behaviors, the PBS team may create an individual activity schedule for the focus person, offer a choice of activities, and implement FCT. In implementing these strategies, staff must diligently provide reinforcement in the form of praise or tangible or other reinforcers when the focus person follows the activity schedule, appropriately chooses activities, and engages in adaptive communicative responses. At the same time, they must minimize reinforcement for problem behaviors and implement crisis management strategies, as necessary.

Conclusions and Recommendations for Future Research

PBS is a science-based approach to preventing challenging behavior and improving quality of life. From its genesis in the nonaversive intervention movement and strong roots in ABA, PBS has evolved into a distinct science with a continually expanding empirical base. Although the core concepts of PBS, such as primary, secondary, and tertiary prevention, are now well understood, the field has only recently begun to explore how PBS maps onto adults with ASD, a unique population whose needs are intrinsically different from those of children and people with other types of disabilities.

A scan of the field reveals two broad, yet critical, areas for future research. First, although the concepts of primary, secondary, and tertiary prevention are well understood through the application of SWPBS with children, the large majority of adult research focuses on tertiary supports for individuals with severe challenging behavior. More research is needed to understand how the continuum of prevention applies to adults with ASD and how primary, secondary, and tertiary interventions can be arranged across complex adult service delivery systems. Second, there is virtually no research on how PBS applies to adults with HFASD, including those traditionally labeled with Asperger syndrome. Given that individuals with HFASD often reside outside of traditional adult service delivery systems, research that focuses on identifying and providing effective supports to individuals with HFASD is especially critical.

REFERENCES

American Psychiatric Association (2013). *Diagnostic and statistical manual of mental disorders* (5th ed.). Washington, DC: Author.

Anderson, C. M., & Kincaid, D. (2005). Applying behavior analysis to school violence and discipline problems: Schoolwide positive behavior support. *Behavior Analyst, 28*(1), 49–63.

Anderson, J. L., Russo, R., Dunlap, G., & Albin, R. W. (1996). A team training model for building the capacity to provide positive behavioral supports in inclusive settings. In L. K. Koegel, R. L. Koegel, & G. Dunlap (Eds.), *Positive behavioral support: Including people with difficult behavior in the community* (pp. 467–490). Baltimore: Brookes.

Ballard-Krishnan, S., McClure, L., Schmatz, B., Travnikar, B., Friedrich, G., & Nolan, M. (2003). The Michigan PBS Initiative: Advancing the spirit of collaboration by including parents in the delivery of personnel development opportunities. *Journal of Positive Behavior Interventions, 5*(2), 122–126.

Bannerman, D. J., Sheldon, J. B., Sherman, J. A., & Harchik, A. E. (1990). Balancing the right to habilitation with the right to personal liberties: The rights of people with developmental disabilities to eat too many doughnuts and take a nap. *Journal of Applied Behavior Analysis, 23*, 79–89.

Barnhill, G. P., Cook, K., Tebbenkamp, K., & Myles, B. (2002). The effectiveness of social skills intervention targeting nonverbal communication for adolescents with Asperger syndrome and related pervasive developmental delays. *Focus on Autism and Other Developmental Disabilities, 17*(2), 112–118.

Benedict, E. A., Horner, R. H., & Squires, J. K. (2007). Assessment and implementation of positive behavior support in preschools. *Topics in Early Childhood Special Education, 27*(3), 174–192.

Boettcher, M., Koegel, R. L., McNerney, E. K., & Koegel, L. (2003). A family-centered prevention approach to PBS in a time of crisis. *Journal of Positive Behavior Interventions, 5*(1), 55–59.

Bondy, A., & Frost, L. (2001). The Picture Exchange Communication System. *Behavior Modification, 25*(5), 725–744.

Brown, F., Gothelf, C. R., Guess, D., & Lehr, D. H. (1998). Self-determination for individuals with the most severe disabilities: Moving beyond Chimera. *Journal of the Association for Persons with Severe Handicaps, 23*(1), 17–26.

Bruder, M., Kerins, G., Mazzarella, C., Sims, J., & Stein, N. (2012). Brief report: The medical care of adults with autism spectrum disorders: Identifying the needs. *Journal of Autism and Developmental Disorders, 42*(11), 2498–2504.

Buschbacher, P. W., & Fox, L. (2003). Understanding and intervening with the challenging behavior of young children with autism spectrum disorder. *Language, Speech, and Hearing Services in Schools, 34*(3), 217–227.

Carlile, K. A., Reeve, S. A., Reeve, K. F., & DeBar, R. M. (2013). Using activity schedules on the iPod touch to teach leisure skills to children with autism. *Education and Treatment of Children, 36*, 33–57.

Carr, E. G. (2007). The expanding vision of positive behavior support: Research perspectives on happiness, helpfulness, hopefulness. *Journal of Positive Behavior Interventions, 9*(1), 3–14.

Carr, E. G., & Durand, V. M. (1985). Reducing behavior problems through functional communication training. *Journal of Applied Behavior Analysis, 18*, 111–126.

Carr, E. G., Horner, R. H., Turnbull, A. P., Marquis, J. G., McLaughlin, D., McAtee, M. L., et al. (1999). *Positive behavior support for people with developmental disabilities: A research synthesis.* Washington, DC: American Association on Mental Retardation.

Carr, E. G., Levin, L., McConnachie, G., Carlson, J. I., Kemp, D. C., Smith, C. E., et al. (1999). Comprehensive multisituational intervention for problem behavior in the community: Long-term maintenance and social validation. *Journal of Positive Behavior Interventions, 1*(1), 5–25.

Carr, J. E., & LeBlanc, L. A. (2006). Noncontingent reinforcement as antecedent behavior support. In J. K. Luiselli (Ed.), *Antecedent assessment and intervention: Supporting children and adults with developmental disabilities in community settings* (pp. 147–164). Baltimore: Brookes.

Carr, J. E., & Sidener, T. M. (2002). On the relation between applied behavior analysis and positive behavioral support. *Behavior Analyst, 25*(2), 245–253.

Carter, D., & Van Norman, R. K. (2010). Class-wide positive behavior support in preschool: Improving teacher implementation through consultation. *Early Childhood Education Journal, 38*(4), 279–288.

Colvin, G., Kame'enui, E. J., & Sugai, G. (1993). Reconceptualizing behavior management and schoolwide discipline in general education. *Education and Treatment of Children, 16*, 361–381.

Conklin, C. G., & Mayer, G. (2011). Effects of implementing the Picture Exchange Communication System (PECS) with adults with developmental disabilities and severe communication deficits. *Remedial and Special Education, 32*(2), 155–166.

Crone, D. A., & Horner, R. H. (2003). *Building positive behavior support systems in schools: Functional behavioral assessment.* New York: Guilford Press.

Doody, C. (2009). Multi-element behaviour support as a model for the delivery of a human rights based approach for working with people with intellectual disabilities and behaviours that challenge. *British Journal of Learning Disabilities, 37*(4), 293–299.

Dunlap, G. (2006). The applied behavior analytic heritage of PBS: A dynamic model of action-oriented research. *Journal of Positive Behavior Interventions, 8*(1), 58–60.

Dunlap, G., Carr, E. G., Horner, R. H., Zarcone, J. R., & Schwartz, I. (2008). Positive behavior support and applied behavior analysis: A familial alliance. *Behavior Modification, 32*(5), 682–698.

Dunlap, G., Sailor, W., Horner, R. H., & Sugai, G. (2009). Overview and history of positive behavior support. In W. Sailor, G. Dunlap, G. Sugai, & R. H. Horner (Eds.), *Handbook of positive behavior support* (pp. 3–16). New York: Springer.

Filipek, P. A. (2005). Medical aspects of autism. In F. R. Volkmar, R. Paul, A. Klin, & D. Cohen (Eds.), *Handbook of autism and pervasive developmental disorders: Vol. 1. Diagnosis, development, neurobiology, and behavior* (3rd ed., pp. 534–578). Hoboken, NJ: Wiley.

Flannery, B. K., Newton, S., Horner, R., Slovic, R., Blumberg, R., & Ard, W. (2000). The impact of person centered planning on the content and organization of individual supports. *Career Development of Exceptional Individuals, 23*, 124–137.

Fox, L., Vaughn, B. J., Wyatte, M., & Dunlap, G. (2002). "We can't expect other people to understand": Family perspectives on problem behavior. *Exceptional Children, 68*(4), 437–450.

Freeman, R., Smith, C., Zarcone, J., Kimbrough, P., Tieghi-Benet, M., Wickham, D., et al. (2005). Building a statewide plan for embedding positive behavior support in human service organizations. *Journal of Positive Behavior Interventions, 7*(2), 109–119.

Gage, M., Fredericks, H., Johnson-Dorn, N., & Lindley-Southard, B. (2009). In-service training for staffs of group homes and work activity centers serving developmentally disabled adults. *Research and Practice for Persons with Severe Disabilities, 34*(2), 49–58.

Hagner, D., Kurtz, A., Cloutier, H., Arakelian, C., Brucker, D. L., & May, J. (2012). Outcomes of a family-centered transition process for students with autism spectrum disorders. *Focus on Autism and Other Developmental Disabilities, 27*(1), 42–50.

Horner, R. H. (2000). Positive behavior supports. *Focus on Autism and Other Developmental Disabilities, 15*, 97–105.

Horner, R. H., Day, H. M., & Day, J. R. (1997). Using neutralizing routines to reduce problem behaviors. *Journal of Applied Behavior Analysis, 30*, 601–614.

Horner, R. H., Dunlap, G., Koegel, R. L., Carr, E. G., Sailor, W., Anderson, J., et al. (1990). Toward a technology of "nonaversive" behavioral support. *Journal of the Association for Persons with Severe Handicaps, 15*, 125–132.

Johnston, J. M., Foxx, R. M., Jacobson, J. W., Green, G., & Mulick, J. A. (2006). Positive behavior support and applied behavior analysis. *Behavior Analyst, 29*(1), 51–74.

Kincaid, D., & Fox, L. (2002). Person-centered planning and positive behavior support. In S. Holburn & P. M. Vietze (Eds.), *Person-centered planning: Research, practice, and future directions* (pp. 29–49). Baltimore: Brookes.

Krahn, G. L., Hammond, L., & Turner, A. (2006). A cascade of disparities: Health and health care access for people with intellectual disabilities. *Mental Retardation and Developmental Disabilities Research Reviews, 12*(1), 70–82.

Kring, S. R., Greenberg, J. S., & Seltzer, M. (2010). The impact of health problems on behavior problems in adolescents and adults with autism spectrum disorders: Implications for maternal burden. *Social Work in Mental Health, 8*(1), 54–71.

Laugeson, E. A., Frankel, F., Gantman, A., Dillon, A. R., & Mogil, C. (2012). Evidence-based social skills training for adolescents with autism spectrum disorders: The UCLA PEERS program. *Journal of Autism and Developmental Disorders, 42*(6), 1025–1036.

LaVigna, G. W., & Willis, T. J. (2012). The efficacy of positive behavioural support with the most challenging behaviour: The evidence and its implications. *Journal of Intellectual and Developmental Disability, 37*(3), 185–195.

Lawrence, L. R., Hughes, T. L., Huang, A., Lehman, C., Paserba, D., Talkington, V., et al. (2013). Identifying individuals with autism in a state facility for adolescents adjudicated as sexual offenders: A pilot study. *Focus on Autism and Other Developmental Disabilities, 28*, 175–183.

Lucyshyn, J. M., Albin, R. W., Horner, R. H., Mann, J. C., Mann, J. A., & Wadsworth, G. (2007). Family implementation of positive behavior support for a child with autism: Longitudinal, single-case, experimental, and descriptive replication and extension. *Journal of Positive Behavior Interventions, 9*(3), 131–150.

May, M. E., & Kennedy, C. H. (2010). Health and problem behavior among people with intellectual disabilities. *Behavior Analysis in Practice, 3*(2), 4–12.

McCart, A., Wolf, N., Sweeney, H. M., Markey, U., & Markey, D. J. (2009). Families facing extraordinary challenges in urban communities: Systems-level application of positive behavior support. In W. Sailor, G. Dunlap, G. Sugai, & R. H. Horner (Eds.), *Handbook of positive behavior support* (pp. 257–277). New York: Springer.

McClannahan, L. E., & Krantz, P. J. (2010). *Activity schedules for children with autism: Teaching independent behavior* (2nd ed.). Bethesda, MD: Woodbine House.

Miltenberger, R. (2006). Antecedent interventions for challenging behaviors maintained by escape from instructional activities. In J. Luiselli (Ed.), *Antecedent assessment and intervention* (2nd ed., pp. 101–124). Baltimore: Brookes.

Mudford, O. C. (1995). An intrusive and restrictive alternative to contingent shock. *Behavioral Interventions, 10*(2), 87–99.

Müller, E., Schuler, A., Burton, B. A., & Yates, G. B. (2003). Meeting the vocational support needs of individuals with Asperger syndrome and other autism spectrum disabilities. *Journal of Vocational Rehabilitation, 18*(3), 163–175.

Poling, A. (2010). Looking to the future: Will behavior analysis survive and prosper? *Behavior Analyst, 33*, 7–17.

Powell, D., Dunlap, G., & Fox, L. (2006). Prevention and intervention for the challenging behaviors of toddlers and preschoolers. *Infants and Young Children, 19*, 25–35.

Reid, D. H., Rotholz, D. A., Parsons, M. B., Morris, L., Braswell, B. A., Green, C. W., et al. (2003). Training human service supervisors in aspects of PBS: Evaluation of a statewide, performance-based program. *Journal of Positive Behavior Interventions, 5*(1), 35–46.

Rispoli, M., Franco, J. H., van der Meer, L., Lang, R., & Camargo, S. (2010). The use of speech generating devices in communication interventions for individuals with developmental disabilities: A review of the literature. *Developmental Neurorehabilitation, 13*(4), 276–293.

Schall, C. M. (2010). Positive behavior support: Supporting adults with autism spectrum disorders in the workplace. *Journal of Vocational Rehabilitation, 32*(2), 109–115.

Scott, T. M., & Eber, L. (2003). Functional assessment and wraparound as systemic school processes: Primary, secondary, and tertiary systems examples. *Journal of Positive Behavior Interventions, 5*(3), 131–143.

Scott, T. M., Nelson, C., Liaupsin, C. J., Jolivette, K., Christle, C. A., & Riney, M. (2002). Addressing the needs of at-risk and adjudicated youth through positive behavior support: Effective prevention practices. *Education and Treatment of Children, 25*(4), 532–551.

Smith, M., Graveline, P. J., & Smith, J. (2012). Autism and obstacles to medical diagnosis and treatment: Two case studies. *Focus on Autism and Other Developmental Disabilities, 27*(3), 189–195.

Steed, E. A., & Durand, V. (2013). Optimistic teaching: Improving the capacity for teachers to reduce young children's challenging behavior. *School Mental Health, 5*(1), 15–24.

Sugai, G., & Horner, R. (2002). The evolution of discipline practices: Schoolwide positive behavior supports. *Child and Family Behavior Therapy, 24*(1–2), 23–50.

Sugai, G., & Horner, R. H. (2009). Responsiveness-to-intervention and school-wide positive behavior supports: Integration of multi-tiered system approaches. *Exceptionality, 17*(4), 223–237.

Sugai, G., Sprague, J., Horner, R., & Walker, H. (2000). Preventing school violence: The use of office discipline referrals to assess and monitor schoolwide discipline interventions. *Journal of Emotional and Behavioral Disorders, 8*, 94–101.

Sutton, L. R., Hughes, T. L., Huang, A., Lehman, C., Paserba, D., Talkington, V., et al. (2013). Identifying individuals with autism in a state facility for adolescents adjudicated as sexual offenders: A pilot study. *Focus on Autism and Other Developmental Disabilities, 28*, 175–183.

Taylor, J., & Seltzer, M. (2011). Employment and post-secondary educational activities for young adults with autism spectrum disorders during the transition to adulthood. *Journal of Autism and Developmental Disorders, 41*(5), 566–574.

Tiger, J. H., Hanley, G. P., & Bruzek, J. (2008). Functional communication training: A review and practical guide. *Behavior Analysis in Practice, 1*(1), 16–23.

Tincani, M. (2011). *Preventing challenging behavior in your classroom: Positive behavior support and effective classroom management.* Waco, TX: Pruforck Press.

Travers, J., & Tincani, M. (2010). Sexuality education for individuals with autism spectrum disorders: Critical issues and decision making guidelines. *Education and Training in Autism and Developmental Disabilities, 45,* 284–293.

Travers, J., Tincani, M., Whitby, P., & Boutot, A. (in press). Alignment of sexuality education and self-determination for people with significant disabilities: A review of research and future directions. *Education and Training in Autism and Developmental Disabilities.*

Turygin, N. C., Matson, J. L., MacMillan, K., & Konst, M. (2013). The relationship between challenging behavior and symptoms of depression in intellectually disabled adults with and without autism spectrum disorders. *Journal of Developmental and Physical Disabilities, 25*(4), 475–484.

Van Houten, R., Axelrod, S., Bailey, J. S., Favell, J. E., Foxx, R. M., Iwata, B. A., et al. (1988). The right to effective behavioral treatment. *Journal of Applied Behavior Analysis, 21*(4), 381–384.

van Oorsouw, W. J., Embregts, P. M., Bosman, A. T., & Jahoda, A. (2009). Training staff serving clients with intellectual disabilities: A meta-analysis of aspects determining effectiveness. *Research in Developmental Disabilities, 30*(3), 503–511.

Wacker, D. P., Berg, W. K., & Harding, J. W. (2006). Evolution of antecedent-based interventions. In J. K. Luiselli (Ed.), *Antecedent assessment and intervention: Supporting children and adults with developmental disabilities in community settings* (pp. 3–28). Baltimore: Brookes.

Watanabe, M., & Sturmey, P. (2003). The effect of choice-making opportunities during activity schedules on task engagement of adults with autism. *Journal of Autism and Developmental Disorders, 33*(5), 535.

Wehmeyer, M. L., & Schwartz, M. (1998). The relationship between self-determination, quality of life, and life satisfaction for adults with mental retardation. *Education and Training in Mental Retardation and Developmental Disabilities, 33,* 3–12.

West, E. A., & Patton, H. (2010). Positive behaviour support and supported employment for adults with severe disability. *Journal of Intellectual and Developmental Disability, 35*(2), 104–111.

CHAPTER 8

• • • • • •

Skill-Building Interventions for Adolescents and Adults with Autism Spectrum Disorders

• Peter F. Gerhardt, Maria Fernanda Garcia, and Anthony Foglia

Over the past three decades interventions based on the principles of applied behavior analysis (ABA) have become increasingly sophisticated, naturalistic, socially valid, and applicable across diverse cohorts of individuals. As noted by Gerhardt and Weiss (2011), ABA-based interventions are the most robustly verified treatment for individuals with autism spectrum disorders (ASD) (e.g., Matson, Benavidez, Compton, Paclawskyj, & Baglio, 1996; Wolery, Barton, & Hine, 2005).

For adults with autism, unfortunately, beyond intervention for challenging behavior (e.g., Sturmey, Seiverling, & Ward-Horner, 2008) and interventions targeting specific social (e.g., Weiss, 2013), vocational (e.g., Lattimore, Parsons, & Reid, 2009), academic (e.g., Burton, Anderson, Prater, & Dyches, 2013), and functional living skills (Smith, Ayres, Mechling, & Smith, 2013), there is a limited body of research. In some skill domains this deficit of research may not represent a significant challenge. For example, discrimination training provided to a young child with ASD to teach the distinctions between boys and girls is potentially different for older individuals only in the stimuli presented (e.g., men's room vs. women's room). However, in areas such as community living, personal safety, sexuality, self-advocacy, travel/community navigation, health care, aging, residential supports, and quality of life the research base is limited or, in some cases, nonexistent (Agency for Healthcare Quality Research, 2013), and studies that have focused on young children have little, if any, applicability in these domains. Although there is a growing body of descriptive studies including studies using archival data focusing on outcomes of adults with ASD (e.g., Mazurek, Shattuck, Wagner, & Cooper, 2012; Narendorf, Shattuck, & Sterzing, 2011; Parish, Thomas, Rose, Kilany, & Shattuck, 2012; Roux et al., 2013; Shattuck, Orsmond, Wagner, & Cooper, 2011), intervention studies are sorely lacking.

Although the absence of an extensive body of intervention research is troubling, it is not wholly unexpected. Despite an accumulated record of over 40 years of behavior analytic research, there continues, at least in some quarters, to be a belief that interventions based on the principles of ABA are ineffective with, and inapplicable to, adolescents and adults with ASD. For example, Autism Speaks (2014) reported that 36 states and the District of Columbia mandate insurance coverage for behavior analytic intervention in ASD. However, a small percentage of these mandates include interventions directly relevant to adults on the spectrum. This bias may, in part, be related to the potential for "recovery" via intensive behavior analytic early intervention (e.g., Lovass, 1987), which has been heavily promoted in the field of behavior analysis and autism. Similarly, it also may be due to the prevalent misconception that ABA is synonymous with early intervention and discrete trial instruction (DTI) and, therefore, of little use with older individuals. Perhaps the absence of substantial research may be related to the fact that school-age children with ASD can readily be found in schools and so are easily accessible to researchers, whereas after graduation many, though certainly not all, adults with ASD are without services and therefore are beyond the reach of researchers (Gerhardt & Lainer, 2011; Gerhardt & Weiss, 2011). Whatever the reason, this lack of research is worrying in that it significantly limits our ability to provide adults with ASD with the opportunity to acquire new skills that are useful across the complex domains and environments associated with adulthood.

Adaptive Behavior Interventions

A basic challenge facing individuals with ASD transitioning from school to the adult world is that they tend to graduate with skills that were highly useful in the classroom but have little or no utility in the adult world. This misalignment is most likely the result of our focus on traditional academics (e.g., reading, math) as appropriate individualized education program (IEP) goals rather than on life skills in the form of adaptive behavior as

IEP goals. Unfortunately, although adaptive behavior deficits are recognized as a core diagnostic symptom of intellectual disability, they are not recognized as diagnostic for an ASD (although communication and social skills are components of adaptive behavior). Despite the fact that adaptive behavior deficits are recognized as important intervention targets, they are not addressed effectively in many programs for individuals with ASD (Matson, Dempsey, & Fodstad, 2009).

Although research on adaptive behavior is limited, there has long been recognition of the critical importance of certain isolated skills (e.g., toilet training). As noted by Gerhardt and Weiss (2011), research suggests that individuals with ASD have significant deficits in adaptive behavior, including basic communication (Anderson, Oti, Lord, & Welch, 2009; Liss et al., 2001), social skills (Bölte & Poustka, 2002; Kenworthy, Case, Harms, Martin, & Wallace, 2010; Liss et al., 2001; Rodrigue, Morgan, & Geffken, 1991), and general adaptive functioning (Kenworthy et al., 2010).

Adaptive behavior has been described as skills and abilities that allow an individual to meet standards of independence as exemplified by typical peers (Heward, 2005). Furthermore, these skills change according to an individual's interests and environmental demands. Adaptive behavior deficits are so problematic that they have been discussed as the central challenge to the development of more positive outcomes in adults with ASD (e.g., Mazefsky, Williams, & Minshew, 2008). One component of adaptive behavior, the development of self-care skills, may have long-term implications for individual inclusion, independence, and quality of life. Anderson (2013) provides a comprehensive overview of behavior analytic interventions and the development of self-care skills in younger learners on the autism spectrum. Among those evidence-based practices are stimulus control procedures, chaining, shaping, prompting, stimulus transfer, and generalization programming (discussed later in this chapter).

The adaptive behavior challenges recognized in youth with ASD remain very much evident in adolescence and adulthood and have a more direct impact on such desirable outcomes as employment, community living, safety, and self-care. The larger physical size of adults may make the continued display of challenging behavior more problematic (e.g., aggression by a 21-year-old is more dangerous than that by a 7-year-old), and some skill deficits are no longer easily accommodated (e.g., a lack of socially acceptable "table manners" limits social inclusion of adults). As such, the need for effective, easily implemented, and generalizable adaptive behavioral interventions for older individuals cannot be overstated. As noted by Gerhardt and Lainer (2011), "There exists a significant need to further identify and research potential evidence-based and socially valid interventions for adults with autism in the community" (p. 46).

Adaptive behavior, as a skill domain, is extremely broad and often complex. Take, for example, street crossing (see Table 8.1). Safely crossing the street in a rural environment may be a relatively easy skill for an individual to acquire given (1) the limited risk associated with minimal traffic flow and (2) that the entire universe of potential streets to cross is both small and finite. Instruction in the same skill in an urban environment involves a much larger universe of exemplars, greater risk due to increased traffic, and instruction in the ability to assess multiple variables that are not wholly under the stimulus control of the traffic light (bicyclists, other pedestrians, late traffic, etc.). A comparison of the two skill sets necessary to safely cross the street in each environment is given in Table 8.1.

Although no one would argue that the skill competencies associated with either environment are simple, the demands of the urban environment require a longer, more complex task analysis to be in place, and at least some of the component skills involve fairly complex discriminations. Although important adaptive behavior skills may be easily identifiable (e.g., street crossing), the component skills required therein may be less obvious, more complex, and directly determined by a specific set of environmental conditions. This lack of specificity is problematic given that the limited skill acquisition research with adolescents or adults with ASD (e.g., McClannahan, McGee, MacDuff, & Krantz, 1990; Smith & Belcher,

TABLE 8.1. Skill Competencies for Street Crossing as a Function of Location

Rural county (low risk)	Manhattan (high risk)
Leave house and proceed to street.	Leave building and proceed to street.
	Watch for pedestrians and active driveways—stop as necessary.
Stop at curb.	Stop at curb.
	Identify and wait for "Walk" sign to light.
Look for cars.	Look for cars and bicycles.
	Respond only to combined stimulus of lit "Walk" sign, no turning cars or bicycles, and other individuals crossing the street.
If clear, proceed with caution.	If above conditions are met, proceed with caution.
Repeat only as necessary.	Repeat the entire process for the next block.

1985) has tended to focus on relatively isolated skills with little attention to context in which the skill is to be used, to social validity (i.e., the relationship of the acquired skills to community living), and to generalization into the natural environment.

As noted earlier, there are a number of behavioral interventions, such as prompting, shaping, chaining, and the systematic use of positive reinforcement, that have been extensively documented as being effective with youth with ASD. Although these interventions are viewed as effective across the lifespan, much of the research with adults has targeted adults with intellectual disabilities without ASD (National Research Council, 2001). It must be understood that effectively teaching skills to adults with ASD requires significant consideration of their individual needs, including the unique contexts in which skills are taught. For example, independently purchasing 10 items at the supermarket requires more complex skills than just matching sample items to words on a grocery list and identifying money. Grocery shopping in context also requires (1) physically navigating the store without running into people, (2) offering and responding to verbal prompts (e.g., "excuse me") to/from other shoppers, (3) asking for help if necessary, (4) patiently waiting in line, and (5) putting items on the conveyer belt and paying for and bagging purchases in a relatively fluent manner so as not to inconvenience other customers. In providing instruction on adaptive responding, this is where intervention is both lacking and sorely needed.

Social Skill Interventions

Deficits in social engagement are considered hallmarks of ASD. In practice, however, there appears to be little consensus on the definition of social skills (e.g., Matson & Wilkins, 2007; Mayville, 2013), and what research there is indicates that improvements in social functioning, even when demonstrated, are moderate (Rao, Beidel, & Murray, 2008). In their review of the social skill interventions for older individuals, Walton and Ingersoll (2013) found only 17 studies that covered a fairly broad set of interventions (e.g., social skill groups, social stories, video modeling, computer-based interventions) and target skills. Though many were reported to have emerging research support, the vast majority of interventions were targeted for individuals with Asperger syndrome/high-functioning autism (Bellini & Peters, 2008). Furthermore, the defining variables of typical social skill interventions (e.g., social skill groups, social stories, role plays) appear to suffer from challenges in treatment fidelity (e.g., What practices actually constitute an effective social skill group?) and reliability across trainers (e.g., Koenig, 2013), significantly limiting their evidence-based application.

Hoch, Taylor, and Rodriquez (2009) adopted an understanding of social skills tied directly to the context in which the skills occur. Working in the community, the authors taught three nonverbal adolescents with ASD to (1) recognize when they were lost, (2) answer their cell phones, (3) comply with verbal directions to locate a nearby adult, and (4) hand their cell phones to another individual, along with a card stating, "I am lost. I cannot speak. My teacher/parent is on this phone. Please listen to the phone. My name is _____. I have autism" (p. 17).

Interestingly, although all three individuals acquired the skills taught by the intervention, the naive community members who were approached generally did not respond to the cards and speak on the phone, as requested. However, compliance of naive community members increased when students were taught to present only the card and not the phone, though the reason for this outcome is unclear. Results support the contention that young adults with ASD who present with significant language and social challenges can acquire fairly complex safety skills when taught in context.

The reaction of naive community members is worth discussion, as it highlights the importance of providing instruction in the natural context (thereby eliminating the need for generalization training) as a function of community response. For social skills to be effective, they require a sender, in this case the student, and a receiver, in this case the naive community member. The skill initially taught in the Hoch and colleagues (2009) study was ineffective in that it did not result in the desired response on the part of the receiver. With subsequent modifications, however, an increase in receiver responding was reported, indicating that the new skill was effective in that it resulted in the desired social response.

Recently, Walton and Ingersoll (2013) investigated the effectiveness of reciprocal imitation training (RIT) with adolescents with autism. RIT is a "naturalistic behavioral intervention that teaches imitation skills within a social context" (p. 248), the basic components of which include context-based modeling, delayed prompting, positive reinforcement, and attention to individual language competencies and interests. Four adolescents with autism and an intellectual disability living in a residential treatment facility participated in the study. Utilizing a multiple-baseline across-subjects design, the authors reported improvements in spontaneous social imitation in all four and improvements in joint engagement in two of the four. In addition, two of the four participants experienced reductions in stereotypy during treatment. Although these results are promising, their applicability is limited, as the authors used a very restricted definition of social skills as including only social reactions and not social initiations.

In addition, generalization was not assessed in any significant manner, potentially limiting the functionality of the noted behavior change in more typical environments.

With the current emphasis on integrated community living, there appears to be a growing interest in the development of functional repertoires of social skills in adults with ASD. Unfortunately, the research on the teaching skills within community arrangements lags considerably behind. As noted by Walton and Ingersoll (2013), although "a variety of social skills may be amenable to treatment in youth and adults with ASD this body of literature suffers from many weaknesses in measurement and research design that need to be addressed to confirm the utility of these interventions for this population" (p. 608).

Vocational Skills Training

Perhaps the ultimate barometer of successful community integration is employment (see also Wehman, Targett, Schall, & Carr, Chapter 11, this volume). Being employed is generally recognized as an important universal characteristic of adulthood, and it is often considered a critical measure of positive adult outcomes. Employment is associated with social and financial status and provides access to a broad social community. Despite the potential value of employment, Roux and colleagues (2013) reported that only 50% of young adults with ASD have ever worked for pay in the 7 years after they left high school. Furthermore, when they do work, they earn significantly lower wages than do age-referenced peers with other educational disabilities. Those who obtained employment at any given time since graduation tended to be individuals who were higher functioning, had graduated from high school, had greater adaptive behavior and social repertoires, and whose families had greater financial resources (Chiang, Cheung, Li, & Tsai, 2013; Roux et al., 2013).

There is general agreement that employment should be a goal for all individuals who wish to work, and there should be an effort to match the preferences of the individual with the programmatic choices offered (Hendricks & Wehman, 2009; Lattimore, Parsons, & Reid, 2003). Given that adults with ASD are increasingly being considered as future employees, vocational skills training is becoming a more essential component of preparation for adult life (Sheridan & Raffield, 2008). Yet research into this particular area of adult life is limited (e.g., Bennett & Dukes, 2013).

Little behavior analytic research looks at increasing vocational or employment-related skills (taking a coffee break, for example), so much of what we do know comes from studies targeting individuals with intellectual disabilities (e.g., Reid, Green, & Parsons, 2003; Reid, Parsons, & Green,

1998; Wallace & Knights, 2003; Worsdell, Iwata, & Wallace, 2002). Some recent research, however, has targeted the specific needs of adults with ASD in this arena. For example, Graff, Gibson, and Galliatsatos (2006) compared the effectiveness of pictorial and tangible paired-stimulus preference assessments on the vocational and academic performance of four adolescents with severe disabilities, two of whom were diagnosed with autism. The results indicated that both assessments resulted in similar preference hierarchies and that when noted preferences were taken into account, high rates of responding on mastered tasks (including vocational tasks) were noted. The process by which individual tasks and environmental preferences are "matched" with employment variables is referred to as the development of a "job match" in the supported employment literature (e.g., Menchetti & Garcia, 2003).

Lattimore, Parsons, and Reid (2009) investigated the utility of training job tasks in the natural environment alone versus training in the natural environment plus task simulation training away from the job in an adult day program for four adults with autism. Job tasks included clerical and cleaning tasks. The results indicated that training in the natural environment plus task simulation resulted in greater skill acquisition than did training in the natural environment alone for three of the four individuals. Instructional time was not controlled across conditions, however, which somewhat influences the significance of these results.

Some behavior analytic research can be discovered in journals outside of those that typically publish behavior analytic research (e.g., *Journal of Applied Behavior Analysis, Behavior Modification*). As one example, Hagner and Cooney (2005) interviewed supervisors of 14 successfully employed individuals on the spectrum to determine effective supervisory practices. A qualitative analysis found that a specific set of supervisory strategies was associated with employment success. The authors discuss these strategies in non–behavior analytic terms, but all of the strategies are either established behavior analytic interventions or are consistent with the principles and applications of ABA. The authors report that supervisors who met with success provided a consistent and predictable schedule, along with clearly outlined job responsibilities; in behavior analytic terms, this can be interpreted as supporting the use of activity schedules to increase the predictability of tasks and the clarity of expectations (e.g., McClannahan & Krantz, 1999; Watanabe & Sturmey, 2003). In the workplace, activity schedules may also be useful in facilitating independent work with reduced supervision and coaching (Stromer, Kimball, Kinney, & Taylor, 2006). Providing precise and clear job responsibilities overlaps considerably with the concept of task analysis, in which the steps of a complex task are broken down into its many components to facilitate instruction (e.g., Stokes, Cameron, Dorsey, & Fleming, 2004).

Successful supervisors, it was reported, also used organizers to structure the job and improve job performance. This strategy is consistent with the widespread use of visual supports to improve performance in individuals with ASD (see Tincani & Crozier, Chapter 7, this volume, on secondary prevention in positive behavior support). Such supports might include steps of a task, reminders to check work, or a visual timer to inform the individual of how much longer he or she needs to work before a break. Minimizing unstructured time was noted as being an effective supervisory practice. Behavior analysts might modify the environment to ensure that productive (or preferred) tasks are always available and, as indicated, provide instruction in a chained set of behaviors that constitute "break skills."

Successful employees, it was noted, had supervisors who communicated directly and clearly with them. This technique is commonly used by behavior analysts to facilitate the emergence of stimulus control. Assuming, as indicated below, that supervisors reinforced responses to the clearly stated cues, behavior analysts would say that these supervisors provided discriminative stimuli (SD) for the display of a variety of work-related behaviors. By providing "frequent reminders and reassurance," the supervisors seem to be using the principles of prompting, shaping, and the delivery of positive reinforcement.

With a comprehensive understanding of behavior analytic principles, non–behavior analytic research can, at times, be translated into established behavior analytic interventions designed to promote skill acquisition. Certainly not all non-ABA research would fall easily or readily into this category. However, a willingness of behavior analysts to look beyond the few established behavior analytic journals will, most likely, be frequently reinforced.

Leisure and Recreation Skills Training

In the area of leisure skills, Miller and Neuringer (2000) reinforced the variable responding of five adolescents with autism when playing a video game, and the increases they showed were maintained during postintervention probes. Variable responding is considered important in that it may facilitate the acquisition of new, more complex behaviors or behavior chains later on. For example, producing variable responses may serve as a prerequisite for the acquisition of more complex behavior chains that require choosing from a series of preferred options as a function of changing stimuli (e.g., street crossing). Other researchers (Lee, McComas, & Jawar, 2002; Page & Neuringer, 1985) have investigated the potential of lag schedules of reinforcement to increase response variability (see also Aguirre, O'Neill, Rehfeldt, & Boyer, Chapter 5, this volume). Lag schedules deliver reinforcement for responses that differ from previous responses emitted on a specified number of previous trials. For example, Lee and Sturmey (2006) investigated an intervention to teach adolescents with ASD to emit novel responses to questions. The procedure was successful in increasing novel responses for two of three participants.

Generalization of Acquired Skills in Older Individuals

A challenge associated with much of the available literature is that generalization and maintenance probes, when conducted, are relatively short lived or done across only one other environment. When young adults with ASD transition from school to the adult services system, they encounter a number of significant changes that may directly affect the extent to which skills acquired in school generalize to the new environment and, subsequently, that may be maintained under vastly different instructional conditions. Although it is not uncommon for a school-age individual to have been provided with a 1:1 instructional aide, that level of staffing is virtually nonexistent in the adult system (where the norm can be anywhere from 4–8:1). In school, services are provided via a team of certified professionals (i.e., board-certified behavior analysts,, speech and language pathologists, special education teachers, school psychologists, and occupational therapists). After graduation, however, professional credentialing is no longer a mandate, and the only certified professional who may be available if the individual engages in significantly challenging behavior is a board-certified behavior analyst (BCBA). Staff attrition in programs serving adults with developmental disabilities is approximately 50% on an annual basis (U.S. Department of Health and Human Services, 2004). And although there is a nationwide shortage of special education teachers (Billingsley, 2003), the rate of attrition combined with continued staff vacancies is still far less than that in the adult system. Given the significant differences in context, staff-to-learner ratios, credentialing of personnel, and attrition rates, the critical importance of providing intervention in a way that promotes generalization and maintenance of acquired skills postgraduation would seem to be a critical variable.

Beginning with Kanner's (1943) seminal article, individuals with autism have been understood as having deficits in the area of generalization of acquired skills. Although generalization deficits have been a significant focus of research (Dunlap, 1993), the mechanism resulting in lack of generalization remains poorly understood (Brown & Bebko, 2012). One possible explanation, and one over which we may exercise some control, can be found in behavior analysis and matching theory.

Matching theory states that behavior is distributed across response alternatives in the same proportion in which reinforcement is distributed across those alternatives (Herrnstein, 1970; McDowell, 1988, 2013) In other words, behavior that produces high rates of positive reinforcement (SR+) will be displayed more frequently than behavior that produces lower rates of SR+, given availability of concurrent schedules of reinforcement for a specific response. In terms of generalization, a behavior that is acquired in one environment via high rates of SR+ may not generalize to other environments in which the availability of SR+ is significantly less. Therefore, many of the adaptive behavior skills acquired under dense schedules of SR+ in the classroom may not generalize to home or community, where such dense levels of reinforcement are not available.

The matching law also allows us to predict which skills might generalize on the basis of the natural reinforcement that occurs when a particular skill is performed. For example, a skill that in and of itself provides an individual with high rates of SR+ (e.g., opening a package of cookies) may generalize more readily than a skill that does not (e.g., brushing teeth). With regard to our earlier example of street crossing, generalization might occur more readily in an urban, rather than a rural, environment given the assortment of potentially reinforcing items (a doughnut shop) or activities (seeing a movie) that are available contingent on crossing the street in an urban environment. This concept, with attention to response effort, is depicted in Figure 8.1.

The role matching law plays in the generalization of new skills acquired by individuals with ASD is still theoretical and, therefore, remains an empirical question. The argument is presented here solely as an attempt to shift the discussion away from generalization deficits being intrinsic to autism to the same deficits being at least partially due to our choice of reinforcement schedule, coupled with a tendency to target skills that, once mastered, produce little in the form of naturally occurring SR+.

In other words, does toothbrushing fail to generalize from school to home because of a neurological characteristic of autism or because the SR+ available for the skill, which is fairly complex, is insufficient at home? Further complicating the question is that SR+ that maintains toothbrushing in typical learners (e.g., white teeth, fresh breath, social approach, a kiss) may be of little or no value to the learner on the spectrum. If it is the former factor, there may be little we can do other than providing additional intervention in the untrained environment. If, on the other hand, it is the latter factor, there may be alternative ways of providing the initial intervention that may result in greater generalization. For example, if intervention were provided utilizing a self-reinforcement protocol (thereby maintaining high rates of SR+ independent of the rate of external, or teacher-delivered, SR+), we might see greater generalization

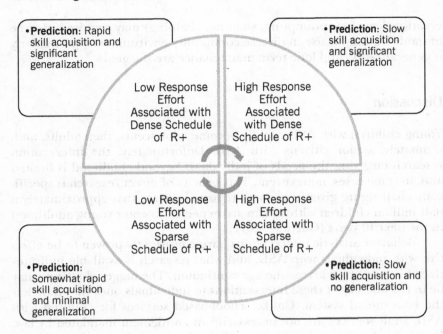

FIGURE 8.1. The matching law and acquisition and generalization of high versus low response effort skills.

evidenced. There are other potential examples, but space limits their discussion here.

As individuals grow up and age out of the educational system, how we approach effective behavioral intervention needs to be reconsidered. Intervention targets should include a variety of skills that have significant functional relevance (i.e., the degree to which a skill, once acquired, can be used to access individual preferences, interests, or desires, and meet specific community-referenced standards of behavioral competence). Contextual variables begin to play a major role, particularly given the reality that once a student leaves the classroom at age 21, he or she will never again inhabit that space. Adult discriminations become more complex (e.g., "Which urinal do I use?"), and the skills required for community living are both relatively complex and context-specific. When an instructor is providing intervention in a classroom, many of the instructional variables are under his or her direct control, but when he or she is working in the community, far fewer variables are amenable to such control. As such, the systems that have proven to be so effective in the classroom (e.g., discrete trial training, token economies, activity schedules, errorless learning, prompting, shaping, chaining) may require a degree of modification for use in diverse community environments, particularly if generalization and long-term maintenance are the goals.

Discussion

Young children with ASD rapidly become adolescents, then adults, and, ultimately, senior citizens with ASD. Unfortunately, the intervention research targeting the needs of individuals beyond childhood is limited and, in some cases, nonexistent. This paucity of direct research is specifically challenging given that some reports indicate that approximately a half million children with autism are expected to enter young adulthood in the next 10 years (Goehner, 2011).

Behavior analytic interventions have consistently proven to be effective with individuals with ASD, and what research is available indicates that this holds true across the age continuum. The bigger challenge may lie in the delivery of these interventions to individuals once they have left the educational system. Unlike school-based services for children with ASD, adult services are not necessarily an entitlement mandated by law. Nancy Thaler, executive director of the National Association of State Directors of Developmental Disabilities Services, has stated, "We are facing a crisis of money and workforce. The cohort of people who will need services—including aging baby boomers—is growing much faster than the cohort of working-age adults that provide care" (cited in Goehner, 2011). Unfortunately, if this critical need is not met, the documented promise of interventions based on the principles of applied behavior analysis will not be fully, or even partially, realized, and many of the educational gains evidenced in younger individuals with ASD will, potentially, be lost in the process of transitioning to adulthood.

REFERENCES

Agency for Healthcare Quality Research. (2013). *Comparative Effectiveness Review Number 65: Interventions for adolescents and young adults with autism spectrum disorders.* Washington, DC: Author. Retrieved from *http://effectivehealthcare. ahrq.gov/index.cfm/search-for-guides-reviews-and- reports/?productid=1197&page action=displayproduct.*

Anderson, D. K., Oti, R. S., Lord, C., & Welch, K. (2009). Patterns of growth in adaptive social abilities among children with autism spectrum disorders. *Journal of Abnormal Child Psychology, 37*(7), 1019–1034.

Anderson, S., (2013). The development of self-help skills in children with autism.

In P. F. Gerhardt & D. Crimmins (Eds.), *Social skills and adaptive behavior in learners with autism spectrum disorders* (pp. 133–158). Baltimore: Brookes.

Autism Speaks. (2014). State initiatives. Retrieved from *www.autismspeaks.org/advocacy/states*.

Bellini, S., & Peters, J. K. (2008). Social skills training for youth with autism spectrum disorders. *Child and Adolescent Psychiatric Clinics of North America, 17*(4), 857–873.

Bennett, K. D., & Dukes, C. (2013). Employment instruction for secondary students with autism spectrum disorder: A systematic review of the literature. *Education and Training in Autism and Developmental Disabilities, 48*(1), 67–75.

Billingsley, B. S. (2003). *Special education teacher retention and attrition: A critical analysis of the literature* (COPSSE Document No. RS-2). Gainesville: University of Florida, Center on Personnel Studies in Special Education.

Bölte, S., & Poustka, F. (2002). The relation between general cognitive level and adaptive behavior domains in individuals with autism with and without comorbid mental retardation. *Child Psychiatry and Human Development, 33*(2), 165–172.

Brown, S. M., & Bebko, J. M. (2012). Generalization, overselectivity, and discrimination in the autism phenotype: A review. *Research in Autism Spectrum Disorders, 6*(2), 733–740.

Burton, C. E., Anderson, D. H., Prater, M. A., & Dyches, T. T. (2013). Video self-modeling on an iPad to teach functional math skills to adolescents with autism and intellectual disability. *Focus on Autism and Other Developmental Disabilities, 28*(2), 67–77.

Chiang, H.-M., Cheung, Y. K., Li, H., & Tsai, L. Y. (2013). Factors associated with participation in employment for high school leavers with autism. *Journal of Autism and Developmental Disorders, 43*(8), 1832–1842.

Dunlap, G. (1993). Promoting generalization: Current status and functional considerations. In R. Van Houten & S. Axelrod (Eds.), *Behavior analysis and treatment* (pp. 269–296). New York: Plenum Press.

Gerhardt, P. F., & Lainer, I. (2011). Addressing the needs of adolescents and adults with autism: A crisis on the horizon. *Journal of Contemporary Psychotherapy, 41*(1), 37–45.

Gerhardt, P. F., & Weiss, M. J. (2011). Behavior analytic interventions for adults with autism spectrum disorders. In E. A. Mayville & J. A. Mulick (Eds.), *Behavioral foundations for effective autism treatment* (pp. 217–232). Baltimore: Brookes.

Goehner, L. (2011, April 13). A generation of autism, coming of age. *New York Times.* Retrieved from *www.nytimes.com/ref/health/healthguide/esn-autism-reporters.html*.

Graff, R. B., Gibson, L., & Galiatsatos, G. T. (2006). The impact of high- and low-preference stimuli on vocational and academic performances of youths with severe disabilities. *Journal of Applied Behavior Analysis, 39*, 131–135.

Hagner, D., & Cooney, B. F. (2005). "I do that for everybody": Supervising employees with autism. *Focus on Autism and Other Developmental Disabilities, 20*, 91–97.

Hendricks, D. R., & Wehman, P. (2009). Transition for school to adulthood for youth with autism spectrum disorders: Review and recommendations. *Focus on Autism and Other Developmental Disabilities, 24,* 77–88.

Herrnstein, R. J. (1970). On the law of effect. *Journal of the Experimental Analysis of Behavior, 13*(2), 243–266.

Heward, W. L. (2005). *Exceptional children: An introduction to special education.* Uppers Saddle River, NJ: Prentice Hall.

Hoch, H., Taylor, B. A., & Rodriquez, A. (2009). Teaching teenagers with autism to answer cell phones and seek assistance when lost. *Behavior Analysis in Practice, 2,* 14–20.

Ingersoll, B., Walton, K., Carlsen, D., & Hamlin, T. (2013). Social intervention for adolescents with autism and significant intellectual disability: Initial efficacy of reciprocal imitation training. *American Journal on Intellectual and Developmental Disabilities, 118*(4), 247–261.

Kanner, L. (1943). Autistic disturbances of affective contact. *Nervous Child, 2,* 217–250.

Kenworthy, L., Case, L., Harms, M. B., Martin, A., & Wallace, G. L. (2010). Adaptive behavior ratings correlate with symptomatology and IQ among individuals with high-functioning autism spectrum disorders. *Journal of Autism and Developmental Disorders, 40*(4), 416–423.

Koenig, K. (2013). Interpreting the efficacy research on group-delivered social skills intervention for children with autism spectrum disorders. In P. F. Gerhardt & D. Crimmins (Eds.), *Social skills and adaptive behavior in learners with autism spectrum disorders.* Baltimore: Brookes.

Lattimore, L. P., Parsons, M. B., & Reid, D. H. (2003). Assessing preferred work among adults with autism beginning supported jobs: Identification of constant and alternating task preferences. *Behavioral Interventions, 18,* 161–177.

Lattimore, L. P., Parsons, M. B., & Reid, D. H. (2009). Rapid training of a community job skill to nonvocal adults with autism: An extension of intensive teaching. *Behavior Analysis in Practice, 2*(1), 34–42.

Lee, R., McComas, J., & Jawar, J. (2002). The effects of differential reinforcement on varied verbal responding by individuals with autism. *Journal of Applied Behavior Analysis, 35,* 391–402.

Lee, R., & Sturmey, P. (2006). The effects of lag schedules and preferred materials on variable responding in students with autism. *Journal of Autism and Developmental Disorders, 36,* 421–428.

Liss, M., Harel, B., Fein, D., Allen, D., Dunn, M., Feinstein, C., et al. (2001). Predictors and correlates of adaptive functioning in children with developmental disorders. *Journal of Autism and Developmental Disorders, 31*(2), 219–230.

Lovaas, O. I. (1987). Behavioral treatment and normal educational and intellectual functioning in young autistic children. *Journal of Consulting and Clinical Psychology, 55,* 3–9.

Matson, J., Benavidez, D., Compton, L., Paclawskyj, J., & Baglio, C. (1996). Behavioral treatment of autistic persons: A review of research from 1980 to the present. *Research in Developmental Disabilities, 17,* 433–465.

Matson, J., & Wilkins, J. (2007). A critical review of assessment targets and methods for social skills excesses and deficits for children with autism spectrum disorders. *Research in Autism Spectrum Disorders, 1,* 28–37.

Matson, J. L., Dempsey, T., & Fodstad, J. C. (2009). The effect of autism spectrum disorders on adaptive independent living skills in adults with severe intellectual disability. *Research in Developmental Disabilities, 30,* 1203–1211.

Mayville, E. (2013). The assessment of social skills. In P. F. Gerhardt & D. Crimmins (Eds.), *Social skills and adaptive behavior in learners with autism spectrum disorders* (pp. 17–32). Baltimore: Brookes.

Mazefsky, C. A., Williams, D. L., & Minshew, N. J. (2008). Variability in adaptive behavior in autism: Evidence for the importance of family history. *Journal of Abnormal Child Psychology, 36,* 591–599.

Mazurek, M. O., Shattuck, P. T., Wagner, M., & Cooper, B. P. (2012). Prevalence and correlates of screen-based media use among youths with autism spectrum disorders. *Journal of Autism and Developmental Disorders, 42*(8), 1757–1767

McClannahan, L. E., & Krantz, P. J. (1999). *Activity schedules for children with autism: Teaching independent behavior.* Bethesda, MD: Woodbine House.

McClannahan, L. E., McGee, G. G., MacDuff, G. S., & Krantz, P. J. (1990). Assessing and improving child care: A personal appearance index for children with autism. *Journal of Applied Behavior Analysis, 23,* 469–482.

McDowell, J. J. (1988). Matching theory in natural human environments. *Behavior Analyst, 11*(2), 95–109.

McDowell, J. J. (2013). On the theoretical and empirical status of the matching law and matching theory. *Psychological Bulletin, 139*(5), 1000–1028.

Menchetti, B. M., & Garcia, L. A. (2003). Personal and employment outcomes of person-centered career planning. *Education and Training in Developmental Disabilities, 38*(2), 145–156.

Miller, N., & Neuringer, A. (2000). Reinforcing variability in adolescents with autism. *Journal of Applied Behavior Analysis, 33,* 151–165.

Narendorf, S. C., Shattuck, P. T., & Sterzing, P. R. (2011). Mental health service use among adolescents with an autism spectrum disorder. *Psychiatric Services, 62*(8), 975–978

National Research Council. (2001). *Educating children with autism.* Washington, DC: National Academies Press.

Page, S., & Neuringer, A. (1985). Variability is an operant. *Journal of Experimental Psychology: Animal Behavior Processes, 11,* 429–452.

Parish, S. L., Thomas, K. C., Rose, R., Kilany, M., & Shattuck, P. T. (2012). State Medicaid spending and financial burden of families raising children with autism. *Intellectual and Developmental Disabilities, 50*(6), 441–451.

Rao, P., Beidel, D., & Murray, M., (2008). Social skills interventions for children with Asperger's syndrome or high-functioning autism: A review and recommendations. *Journal of Autism and Developmental Disorders, 38,* 355–361.

Reid, D. H., Green, C. W., & Parsons, M. B. (2003). An outcome management program for extending advances in choice research into choice opportunities for supported workers with severe multiple disabilities. *Journal of Applied Behavior Analysis, 36,* 575–578.

Reid, D. H., Parsons, M. B., & Green, C. W. (1998). Identifying work preferences among individuals with severe multiple disabilities prior to beginning supported work. *Journal of Applied Behavior Analysis, 31*, 281–285.

Rodrigue, J. R., Morgan, S. B., & Geffken, G. R. (1991). A comparative evaluation of adaptive behavior in children and adolescents with autism, Down syndrome, and normal development. *Journal of Autism and Developmental Disorders, 21*(2), 187–196.

Roux, A. M., Shattuck, P. T., Cooper, B. P., Anderson, K. A., Wagner, M., & Narendorf, S. C. (2013). Postsecondary employment experiences among young adults with an autism spectrum disorder. *Journal of the American Academy of Child and Adolescent Psychiatry, 52*(9), 931–939.

Shattuck, P. T., Orsmond, G. I., Wagner, M., & Cooper, B. P. (2011). Participation in social activities among adolescents with an autism spectrum disorder. *PLoS ONE, 6*(11), e27176.

Sheridan, K., & Raffield, T. (2008). Teaching adaptive skills to people with autism. In J. Matson (Ed.), *Clinical assessment and intervention for autism spectrum disorders* (pp 327–350). London: Academic Press.

Smith, M., Ayres, K., Mechling, L., & Smith, K. (2013). Comparison of the effects of video modeling with narration vs. video modeling on the functional skill acquisition of adolescents with autism. *Education and Training in Autism and Developmental Disabilities, 48*(2), 164–178.

Smith, M. D., & Belcher, R. (1985). Teaching life skills to adults disabled by autism. *Journal of Autism and Developmental Disorders, 15*, 163–175.

Stokes, J. V., Cameron, M. J., Dorsey, M. F., & Fleming, E. (2004). Task analysis, correspondence training, and general case instruction for teaching personal hygiene skills. *Behavioral Interventions, 19*(2), 121–135.

Stromer, R., Kimball, J. W., Kinney, E. M., & Taylor, B. A. (2006). Activity schedules, computer technology, and teaching children with autism spectrum disorders. *Focus on Autism and Other Developmental Disabilities, 21*, 14–24.

Sturmey, P., Seiverling, L., & Ward-Horner, J. (2008). Assessment of challenging behavior in people with autism spectrum disorders. In J. Matson (Ed.), *Clinical assessment and intervention in autism spectrum disorders* (pp. 131–164). Burlington, MA: Academic Press.

United States Department of Health and Human Services. (2004). *The supply of direct service professionals serving individuals with intellectual disabilities and other developmental disabilities.* Washington, DC: Author. Available at *www. ancor.org/issues/shortage/aspe_dsp_11-09-04.doc.*

Wallace, M. D., & Knights, D. J. (2003). An evaluation of a brief functional analysis format within a vocational setting. *Journal of Applied Behavior Analysis, 36*, 125–128.

Walton, K. M., & Ingersoll, B. R. (2013). Improving social skills in adolescents and adults with autism and severe to profound intellectual disability: A review of the literature. *Journal of Autism and Developmental Disorders, 43*(3), 594–615.

Watanabe, M., & Sturmey, P. (2003). The effect of choice-making opportunities during activity schedules on task engagement of adults with autism. *Journal of Autism and Developmental Disorders, 33*, 535–538.

Wolery, M., Barton, E. E., & Hine, J. F. (2005). Evolution of applied behavior analysis in the treatment of individuals with autism. *Exceptionality, 13,* 11–23.

Worsdell, A. S., Iwata, B. A., & Wallace, M. D. (2002). Duration-based measures of preference for vocational tasks. *Journal of Applied Behavior Analysis, 35,* 287–290.

Weiss, M. J. (2013). Behavior analytic interventions for developing social skills in individuals with autism. In P. F. Gerhardt & D. Crimmins (Eds.), *Social skills and adaptive behavior in autism spectrum disorders* (pp. 33–51). Baltimore: Brookes.

CHAPTER 9
• • • • • •
Sexuality and Relationships for Individuals with Autism Spectrum Disorders

• **Jason C. Travers and Peggy Schaefer Whitby**

Autism spectrum disorders (ASD) negatively affect social development. This simple statement does not adequately convey the complexity of human social development. Social development encompasses every nuance of behavior we learn to use when interacting with other people. The intricacies of our environment compound the complexity of human social development. For example, layers of cultural influence (e.g., ethnic, familial, gender, locality) and the idiosyncratic history of the individual are manifested in our social behavior. Whereas many social skills are expected to be formally and informally learned, the taboo nature of sexuality education in the United States makes teaching sexuality daunting for parents and professionals. Educators and other support professionals must identify and deliver supports to ensure that individuals with ASD successfully navigate social situations, acquire and maintain relationships, and become sexually healthy adults. Attaining desired sexuality-related outcomes requires all stakeholders to understand the rationale for sexuality education for people with ASD and the components of comprehensive sexuality education and to prepare to provide evidence-based interventions to support sexuality-related skills for people with ASD. This chapter addresses each of these topics.

Sexuality is often misperceived as referring only to sexual behavior (e.g., masturbation, intercourse) and reproductive health, but sexuality is more accurately characterized by broad physical, emotional, and social development (National Commission on Adolescent Sexual Health [NCASH], 1995). Precise definitions of sexuality are elusive, perhaps because culture and social development are so deeply entwined. The NCASH explained that sexuality encompasses knowledge, attitudes, beliefs, values, and behaviors of individuals. The NCASH further describes sexuality as having to do with anatomy, physiology, biochemistry, identity, personality, and roles that are manifested in our thoughts, feelings, behaviors, and relationships with others. Understanding one's own sexuality is a lifelong learning process that forms attitudes, beliefs, and values about our identity, relationships, and intimacy (Sexuality Information and Education Council of the United States [SIECUS], 2004). Given these characteristics of human sexuality, it is clear that people with ASD will need supports that extend beyond those specific to supporting appropriate sexual behaviors such as masturbation.

Rationale for Sexuality Education for People with ASD

People with ASD have a right to sexuality education (Haracopos & Pederson, 1992). The rationale for sexuality education, however, can be articulated in more specific ways. For example, people with ASD are entitled to have relationships, get married, and be parents. Furthermore, individuals with ASD are at risk for sexual abuse because of their poor communication skills and frequent dependence on others for various types of support (Mandell, Walrath, Manteuffel, Sgro, & Pinto-Martin, 2005; Mansell, Sobsey, Wilgosh, & Zawallich, 1996). People with ASD likely require highly specialized instruction in order to learn sexuality-related skills (Travers &Tincani, 2010). Sexuality education leads to better overall health and hygiene throughout the lifespan and increases longevity, as well as socially appropriate sexual behavior (Stokes & Kaur, 2005). Lastly, sexuality education for people with ASD aligns well with the concept of self-determination of people with disabilities (Travers, Tincani, Whitby, & Boutot, 2014).

The Right to Relationships, Marriage, and Parenthood

Relationships are central to the lives of human beings. Through relationships, we learn about families, friendships, love, romance, and commitment (SIECUS, 2004). It is through our relationships that we learn about what we value, how to communicate abstract concepts (e.g., feelings), and to advocate for ourselves and what we believe in (SIECUS, 2004). It is a fundamental human right to have various types of relationships, participate in consensual romantic and sexual behavior, marry a life partner, and conceive and care for a child. Individuals with autism often have been excluded from these activities because they are perceived as being sexually immature or asexual (Konstantareas & Lunsky, 1997; Ludlow, 1991; Stokes & Kaur, 2005). To the contrary, there have been reports in the professional and popular media that people with ASD want to have social and sexual relationships, but they lack the skills necessary to initiate and sustain them (Ashkenazy & Yergeau, 2013; Attwood, 1998; Harmon, 2011; Ousley & Mesibov, 1991). Not every individual with ASD is capable of giving consent to sexual behavior and may not, even with extensive supports, have the skill set to safely care for a child. The existence of a disability, including ASD, does not exempt the person from these rights. People with ASD are therefore entitled to specialized sexuality education in order to maximize quality of life.

The Right to Prevent and Report Sexual Abuse

People with disabilities are at an increased risk of sexual abuse (Putnam, 2003; Sobsey, Randall, & Parrila, 1997; Westcott & Jones, 1999). Some evidence suggests that people with ASD are especially prone to sexual abuse because they (1) often cannot report the abuse due to communication deficits and (2) do not know that what is being done to them is wrong (Howlin & Clements, 1995; Mansell et al., 1996). The traumatic effects of isolated and/or repeated sexual abuse can lead to a variety of short- and long-term problems ranging in severity, including depression, anxiety, generalized fear, problem behavior, sexual dysfunction, sleep disturbances, eating problems, self-injury, and relationship problems (American Psychological Association, n.d.). Furthermore, because people with ASD are less likely to report sexual abuse, the probability of repeated offenses against the same or other individuals with autism is even more concerning. If sexual predators are not caught, charged, and convicted, then the prevalence of sexual abuse of people with ASD will be maintained or will increase. Given the increased risk of sexual abuse among people with ASD and the serious impact it has on every aspect of development, people with ASD have the right to sexuality education to learn to prevent and/or report sexual crimes.

Preventing Inappropriate and Supporting Appropriate Behavior

People with ASD often use contextually inappropriate behavior for a variety of reasons. In response, professionals may design interventions that suppress behavior (e.g., using rewards for competing behaviors) rather than addressing the underlying cause(s) of inappropriate behavior. For example, a young man with ASD may begin to touch his genitals while in the grocery store. A common response would be to suppress the behavior with redirection or a punishment procedure across all environments. Although this may be an effective short-term solution, it fails to address the underlying need to learn where and when it is okay to touch one's own genitals. Also, consider that many men quickly and covertly "adjust" their genitals in public spaces without serious social or criminal repercussions. Failing to address social needs can lead to obsessions and other inappropriate behavior (e.g., public disrobing, touching other people, sexual aggression) that compromises quality of life (Ray, Marks, & Bray-Garretson, 2004; Stokes & Kaur, 2005; Walsh, 2000). Sexuality education is therefore warranted as a means of preventing inappropriate and supporting appropriate sexual behavior.

The Right to Sexual Health and Hygiene

People with disabilities are less likely to regularly access quality medical care (Krauss, Gulley, Sciegaj, & Wells, 2003). People with ASD who have poor sexual health and hygiene can experience physical pain, contract preventable illnesses and diseases, experience unwanted/unplanned pregnancy, or die. One historical response to addressing the sexual health needs of people with ASD and other developmental disabilities was forced sterilization (removal of ovaries, cervix, testes; American Academy of Pediatrics, 1999). Despite the progression away from these practices in the United States, there remain indications that the sexual health needs of people with ASD are not being met. For example, women with intellectual disabilities (ID) are significantly less likely to access basic gynecological services (Rivera Drew, & Short, 2010). Poor sexual health and hygiene act as a barrier to developing and maintaining social relationships and thereby negatively affect quality of life. Conversely, comprehensive sexuality education that includes specialized instruction in health and hygiene can instill a positive sense of physical and mental well-being as well as lead to a long and healthy life.

The Right to Be Self-Determined

Self-determination is a construct that can be interpreted as an individual's right to have control over aspects of his or her life and fate (Wehmeyer, 1998). Attainment of self-determination exists on a continuum and is influenced by the capacity of the individual, opportunities and experiences provided by the environment, and perceptions the person has about him- or herself (Wehmeyer, 2001; Wehmeyer & Garner, 2003; Wehmeyer, Kelchner, & Richards, 1996; Wehmeyer & Schwartz, 1997). The degree to which a person is self-determined is related to his or her mastery of such skills as choice making, decision making, problem solving, goal setting, self-monitoring, self-instruction, self-advocacy, leadership, and resiliency, to name a few (Taylor, Richards, & Brady, 2005). A person with ASD may have more or better capacity, opportunities, and self-perceptions in some areas of self-determination while experiencing deficits in others. Travers and colleagues (2014) suggested that specialized sexuality education for people with ASD complements self-determination because it confers greater autonomy and control over one's own life. Thus sexuality education for people with ASD can be justified in terms of promoting self-determination.

The Right to Specialized Sexuality Instruction

People without disabilities typically learn about sexuality through a variety of informal social experiences in community, family, and educational environments. People with ASD have communication, behavior, and social deficits that make casual learning about sexuality very unlikely. The core deficits associated with autism require specialized sexuality education that is tailored to the unique needs, strengths, and interests of the individual with autism (Realmuto & Ruble, 1999; Travers & Tincani, 2010). Thus, as with any educational intervention, sexuality education for people with ASD requires the use of validated instructional methods, adaptations of and modifications to curriculum, and the integration of concrete stimuli to aid understanding of abstract concepts. Effective and comprehensive sexuality education that is delivered in highly specialized ways helps ensure that the person with ASD achieves satisfactory sexuality-related outcomes (Travers & Tincani, 2010).

Over the past 20 years, special education leaders and government agencies have increasingly promoted the use of evidence-based practices for educating students with disabilities. While the body of empirical evidence demonstrating the efficacy of curricula and methods has accumulated, there remain significant gaps in the research literature and, in some cases, confusion between evidence-based practices, research-based practices, and promising practices (Cook & Cook, 2011). Travers and colleagues (2014) shed light on the paucity of applied research specifically investigating the delivery of sexuality education to people with ASD and other developmental disabilities.

Despite the limited applied research, it is clear that sexuality education is critical for attaining best possible outcomes for people with ASD.

Educators and other support professionals should recognize that specialized sexuality education is warranted not just for sexual and reproductive health because it also is fundamental for healthy development. People with ASD are entitled to instruction that mitigates the risk of sexual abuse, promotes platonic and romantic relationships, enhances self-determination, and supports appropriate engagement in normal and healthy sexual behaviors. Educators and other support professionals need an understanding of what comprehensive sexuality education is and how it can be used to develop specialized lessons for people with ASD.

Components of Comprehensive Sexuality Education

We all are sexual beings (Greenberg, Bruess, & Oswalt, 2013). Almost every aspect of our lives is affected by our sexual development, but when people think about sexuality, the imagery is almost exclusively derived from the physical activity of human bodies (Gagnon & Simon, 2005). Although other methods of sexuality education are used throughout the United States (e.g., abstinence-based, abstinence only), comprehensive sexuality education has many facets and is a lifelong learning process. Comprehensive sexuality education includes age-appropriate and medically accurate information on a range of topics. SIECUS (2004) outlined guidelines for comprehensive sexuality education. The guidelines comprise these six key concepts: (1) human development, (2) relationships, (3) personal skills, (4) sexual behavior, (5) sexual health, and (6) society and culture. Each of these six guidelines contains general "life behaviors," as well as subconcepts with related pieces of specific information. For example, SIECUS Key Concept 2 deals with relationships. One life behavior is to "develop and maintain meaningful relationships" (p. 33). One subconcept is "friendships are important throughout life" and includes several related specific pieces of information, such as "friends can help each other" and "a person can have different types of friends" (p. 35). The guidelines also include information about how to prioritize topics, address gaps in the learner's knowledge, evaluate curricula, and create lessons. Although these guidelines were not developed specifically for people with ASD, they serve as an excellent resource for understanding what to teach a person with ASD about sexuality as well as making decisions about delivering specialized instruction. An overview of each of these areas, as outlined by SIECUS, seems necessary before exploring what and how interventions and supports should be provided to a person with ASD.

Human Development

Human sexual development can be characterized by the ways in which environment affects and is affected by our physical, emotional, social, and cognitive changes (SIECUS, 2004). Teaching people with ASD about human development means facilitating their understanding about human reproduction, anatomy and physiology, puberty, body image, sexual orientation, and gender identity. In the elementary years, children should learn the names and functions of their body parts, how bodies change, aspects of a healthy diet, and how to respect others. During adolescence and young adulthood, young people should be taught biological and physiological information about sperm and menstruation, sexual feelings, intercourse, and contraception, as well as issues related to appearance, attractions, and gender. During adulthood, human development is related to understanding fertility and conception, parenting, menopause, and refined personal understanding of one's own sexual orientation. Given that learning about human development is a lifelong process that people with ASD may not have been afforded, educators and other support professionals will need to consider which of these topics are priorities for their students/clients with ASD, as well as what should be taught later.

Relationships

We all develop relationships that are pivotal to our quality of life. Given that poor or absent social development is a characteristic of ASD, it seems obvious that much effort should be dedicated to facilitating various relationships. However, learning about relationships must be comprehensive. In childhood, we learn about relationships via interactions with our immediate family members. The concept of a family, as well as the different types of families, becomes better understood as relationships begin to extend beyond our own families. Throughout our lives, we learn about different types of friendships, romantic relationships, dating, love, marriage and commitment, and raising children. We also learn about types of love, communication and conflict resolution, peer pressure, rejection, and how love can evolve to grow or dissipate over time. For people with ASD, a fulfilling life will very likely be contingent on the extent to which they are able and allowed to express love and intimacy, develop a variety of meaningful relationships (i.e., relationships beyond their family and network of support professionals), avoid exploitation or harmful relationships, and make choices. Providing comprehensive sexuality education that addresses each of these areas of relationship development will be critical for achieving satisfactory outcomes.

Personal Skills

Personal skills differ from relationship skills in that, when mastered, persons identify and live in accordance with what they value, take responsibility for their behavior, use decision-making and critical thinking skills, negotiate and assert themselves, seek help, and communicate with a variety of people who assume various roles (e.g., acquaintances, coworkers, supervisors, family, friends, romantic partners; SIECUS, 2004). In childhood and adolescence, acquiring good personal skills means using multiple means of communicating, expressing wants and needs, requesting assistance, exercising freedom to choose, listening to others, and setting limits. Adults use their personal skills when consenting to sexual behavior and/or relationships or in understanding the social and legal implications of their decisions or that drugs and alcohol affect decision-making ability. Sexuality is a broad topic composed of many more things than just anatomy and sexual behavior. Teaching these skills, particularly relationship and personal skills, takes an extensive amount of time, planning, and explicit instruction with repeated practice in natural environments. Furthermore, there are other aspects of sexuality education for people with ASD that also require consideration.

Sexual Behavior

Historically shameful and a source of embarrassment, sexual behavior (e.g., exploration of genitalia, masturbation, orgasm) is now recognized as a fundamental and normal part of the human experience (Gagnon & Simon, 2005). Sexually healthy individuals enjoy and express their sexuality throughout life in ways consistent with their values, express their sexual feelings, distinguish between safe and harmful sexual behavior, and engage in safe, consensual, pleasurable sexual relationships (SIECUS, 2004). This means that people with ASD need sexuality education regarding masturbation, abstinence, human sexual response, fantasy, sexual dysfunction, and, when appropriate, shared sexual behavior. Inappropriate sexual behavior, particularly public masturbation, public disrobing, and inappropriately touching others, is perhaps what prompts educators, support professionals, and parents to begin considering sexuality education. This orientation is problematic because sexuality is much more than these few behaviors and inappropriate sexual behavior probably is a reflection of inadequate sexuality education in childhood and early adolescence.

Masturbation is a self-stimulatory behavior and, because of automatic reinforcement, can be difficult to change (Rapp & Vollmer, 2005; Vollmer, 1994). The stigma associated with masturbation often results in use of suppression methods to address it, particularly when it is occurring in public settings (e.g., classroom, place of employment, the community; Koller, 2000; Walsh, 2000). Suppressing masturbation will not likely be effective, especially because it is a healthy and typical part of sexual development. Rather, people with ASD require instruction on where, when, and sometimes how to appropriately and safely masturbate to achieve orgasm (Ruble & Dalrymple, 1993). Thus sexuality education is not a means of preventing inappropriate behavior but a way to support healthy sexual behavior consistent with social norms.

Sexual Health

Sexual health has to do with reproductive health, contraception, pregnancy and prenatal care, abortion, prevention and treatment of sexually transmitted diseases, HIV/AIDS education, sexual abuse, sexual violence, and sexual harassment. Adequate knowledge about and skills in sexual health translate to increased access to preventative treatment, including breast and testes exams, Papanicolaou tests (i.e., Pap smears), prostate cancer exams, and early identification of other problems. Further, sexually healthy individuals use contraception appropriately, recognize when they are pregnant and seek prenatal care, can access emergency contraception, and are better equipped to prevent and report sexual crimes.

Society and Culture

Social and cultural environments influence our behavior and the way we learn about and express sexuality (SIECUS, 2004). Different societies reflect different values about sexuality. These values may be manifested in gender roles, laws pertaining to sexuality, religious beliefs about sexuality, concepts of diversity, and sexuality in the media. Stakeholders should recognize how the concept of sexuality and culture is relevant to people with ASD and may consider categorizing it as a high priority because it is consistent with democratic ideals. People with ASD are a historically marginalized group (Blatt & Kaplan, 1966; Shapiro, 1994). The delivery of comprehensive sexuality education directly and indirectly enhances their ability to influence legislation that affects them. Furthermore, and perhaps more specifically, it empowers people with ASD to confront explicit, implicit, and institutionalized discrimination (e.g., in independent and supported living, sexual relationships, marriage, family planning, sexual health, prenatal care, childrearing). Also, given the frequent objectification of women and use of sexually laden images and messages in American popular media and the widespread availability of legal and illegal pornography on the Internet, people with ASD are entitled to learn how to distinguish between socially acceptable, unacceptable, and criminal sexual behavior (see also Frantz & Zellis, Chapter 14, this volume, on legal issues for people with ASD).

Providing Sexuality Education to People with ASD

Comprehensive sexuality education should begin in early childhood and typically is a lifelong process. However, people with autism (as well as many typically developing children, depending on where they live) often are excluded from comprehensive sexuality education (Konstantareas & Lunsky, 1997; Ludlow, 1991; Stokes & Kaur, 2005). The result can be decades of delay in delivery of instruction to support healthy sexual development and inappropriate behavior that varies in form, intensity, and function (e.g., gaining attention from peers, self-stimulation, gaining access to objects or activities). The delay in sexuality education is perhaps a reflection of sustained perceptions about sexual immaturity, asexuality, and sexuality as a burden for people with ASD (Lesseliers & Van Hove, 2002). Consequently, sexuality education may be delayed until a sexuality-related problem emerges and thus be limited in scope to addressing the problem. Unfortunately, a reactive approach to modifying behavior is less effective than a comprehensive approach that includes prevention components (Wacker, Berg, & Harding, 2006). Thus comprehensive sexuality education should be delivered to people with ASD beginning in early childhood and throughout their lives in order to prevent problems as well as to encourage healthy sexual development (Travers et al., 2014). Despite this philosophy, it remains likely that many educators, support professionals, and family members find themselves in situations in which they are reacting to one or more sexuality-related problems. In such situations, teams need to prioritize components of sexuality instruction, interventions, and behavior supports and to make decisions about what, how, and who should be included in action plans.

Sexuality Education Intervention Research

Travers and colleagues (2014) conducted a systematic review of the sexuality education literature that included participants with ASD and participants with ID. They identified 11 studies that met criteria for inclusion, but, although all reported positive findings, the description of the independent variable (i.e., intervention) was insufficient for replication in most studies. One study included participants who were adolescents, and the remaining 10 included adults. Also, the review indicated that no studies have examined the effects of published curricula on sexuality-related skills of people with ASD. They concluded that, at best, there exists very little empirical information to inform the delivery of sexuality education to people with ASD. However, given that comprehensive sexuality education is critical for attaining the best possible outcomes, educators and other support professionals, as well as parents whenever possible, need to turn to instructional methods, materials, and strategies that are supported by evidence in order to deliver comprehensive sexuality education. To increase the probability of success, stakeholders need to work together and maintain ongoing communication. They also need to become familiar with the guidelines for comprehensive sexuality education developed by SIECUS (2004) and critically evaluate sexuality education curricula. This foundational knowledge can be relied on when selecting general interventions that have empirical support (e.g., task analysis, visual supports, video modeling).

Evaluating Sexuality Curricula

Many commercial curricula for sexuality education exist, but very few are specifically designed for people with ASD. SIECUS (2004) suggests that manuals can be adapted to meet the needs of students with various educational needs but that consumers should critically evaluate curricula for content inclusion and accuracy, as well as the exclusion of fear and shame about sexuality. The most appropriate curricula include content from the six key concepts of comprehensive sexuality education, but there are many other issues to consider. Figure 9.1 is a sexuality education curriculum evaluation tool adapted from SIECUS. Completing a thorough evaluation of curricula being considered for teaching people with ASD can reveal areas of strengths, areas that are lacking, or content that warrants rejection of the entire curriculum.

Evidence-Based Practices with Sexuality Education

People with ASD require specialized instruction and behavioral intervention that considers their unique strengths, weaknesses, preferences, and interests in order to address the priorities of all stakeholders, including the person with ASD. The approach with the largest body of evidence of effectiveness for people with ASD is rooted in applied behavior analysis (National Autism Center, 2009; National Professional Development Center on Autism Spectrum Disorders, n.d.). Behavior analytic interventions include but are not limited to functional communication training, task analysis, time delay, video modeling, prompting and fading prompts, reinforcement, visual supports, shaping, and response interruption. Many of these can be and often are combined to increase the probability of successful behavior change and learning.

EVALUATING FOR APPROPRIATE CONTENT (SIECUS Key Concepts)				
Human Development				
Contains information about reproduction, sexual anatomy, and physiology	0	1	2	3
Contains information about puberty	0	1	2	3
Contains information about reproduction	0	1	2	3
Contains information about body image	0	1	2	3
Contains information about sexual orientation	0	1	2	3
Contains information about gender identity	0	1	2	3
Relationships	0	1	2	3
Contains information about families	0	1	2	3
Contains information about friendship	0	1	2	3
Contains information about love	0	1	2	3
Contains information about romantic relationships	0	1	2	3
Contains information about marriage and lifetime commitments	0	1	2	3
Contains information about raising children	0	1	2	3
Personal Skills	0	1	2	3
Contains information about values	0	1	2	3
Contains information about decision making	0	1	2	3
Contains information about communication	0	1	2	3
Contains information about assertiveness	0	1	2	3
Contains information about negotiation	0	1	2	3
Contains information about looking for help	0	1	2	3
Sexual Behavior	0	1	2	3
Contains information about sexuality throughout life	0	1	2	3
Contains information about masturbation	0	1	2	3
Contains information about shared sexual behavior	0	1	2	3
Contains information about sexual abstinence	0	1	2	3
Contains information about human sexual response	0	1	2	3
Contains information about sexual fantasy	0	1	2	3
Contains information about sexual dysfunction	0	1	2	3

(continued)

FIGURE 9.1. Tool for evaluating sexuality education curricula. Adapted with permission from SIECUS (2004).

Sexual Health	0	1	2	3
Contains information about reproductive health	0	1	2	3
Contains information about contraception	0	1	2	3
Contains information about pregnancy and prenatal care	0	1	2	3
Contains information about abortion	0	1	2	3
Contains information about sexually transmitted diseases	0	1	2	3
Contains information about HIV and AIDS	0	1	2	3
Contains information about sexual abuse, assault, violence, and harassment	0	1	2	3
Society and Culture				
Contains information about sexuality and society	0	1	2	3
Contains information about gender roles	0	1	2	3
Contains information about sexuality and the law	0	1	2	3
Contains information about sexuality and religion	0	1	2	3
Contains information about diversity	0	1	2	3
Contains information about sexuality and the media	0	1	2	3
Contains information about sexuality and the arts	0	1	2	3
EVALUATING FOR CONTENT ACCURACY				
The curriculum only uses scientifically and medically accurate information	0	1	2	3
The curriculum contains information that is not older than 10 years	0	1	2	3
Lessons include various graphics, including line drawings, photographs, and/ or video	0	1	2	3
Curriculum includes or requires concrete materials and examples for lessons	0	1	2	3
Curriculum includes information that is appropriate and accurate for students of different ages	0	1	2	3
Curriculum includes information that accurately represents various racial and ethnic groups	0	1	2	3
Curriculum includes information that accurately represents various sexual orientations	0	1	2	3
Curriculum includes information about people with ASD and other developmental disabilities	0	1	2	3
The curriculum includes information about the benefits of abstinence without relying on fear or shame	0	1	2	3
The curriculum includes accurate information about safe sex	0	1	2	3

(continued)

FIGURE 9.1. *(continued)*

EVALUATING FOR FEAR AND SHAME (Grounds for Exclusion)		
The curriculum uses shame, guilt, or fear to prevent premarital sexual behavior	Y	N
The curriculum uses shame, guilt, or fear to prevent masturbation	Y	N
Curriculum portrays people who engage in premarital sexual behavior as deviant, troubled, or unworthy of respect	Y	N
Curriculum portrays sexuality as a force that young people cannot control	Y	N
Curriculum portrays normal sexual behavior among people with disabilities as devious, dangerous, or criminal	Y	N
Portrays premarital sex as always or almost always causing STDs, unwanted pregnancy, or health problems	Y	N

FIGURE 9.1. *(continued)*

Task analysis is the breaking down of a multistep behavior into smaller steps for teaching a variety of skills to people of various ages (Franzone, 2009). Visual supports (e.g., pictures, words, objects, environmental arrangements, schedules, maps, labels) are ways to support a person's completion of daily activities, tasks related to the activities, and/or behaviors necessary for task completion (Hume, 2008). Video modeling requires the use of video-recorded steps in a behavior performed by another person (i.e., a model) for later review by a person learning the behavior portrayed in the scene (Franzone & Collet-Klingenberg, 2008). Prompting procedures include any assistance given to a person to help him or her respond to natural cues and/or perform a behavior (Neitzel & Wolery, 2009). Time delay is a procedure for eliminating prompts and requires a brief delay between the natural cue and the delivery of a prompt to support learning (Neitzel, 2009). These methods can be combined to effectively teach people with ASD a variety of sexuality-related skills, including dating, safety and reporting, using contraception, reproduction, and hygiene.

How To: Menstrual Care

Women with ASD need explicit instruction to learn to care for their menstrual needs, particularly pain relief and sanitary pad or tampon use. Teaching menstrual care begins in early childhood, with naming and understanding functions of body parts as well as bathing and cleaning the body. As girls grow, they should be taught more skills that are necessary for menstrual care, particularly about reproduction, anatomy, and details about menstruation. Young and mature women should know how to care for their menstrual needs, understand conception and pregnancy, and learn about menopause. Teaching girls and women with ASD about menstrual care likely requires specialized delivery of a comprehensive sexuality education curriculum. Importantly, it is often very difficult to teach menstrual care in the absence of foundational skills achieved with comprehensive sexuality education. For example, without knowledge about, importance of, and skills for cleaning the vagina once a day in the shower, it becomes very difficult to understand why it might need to be cleaned more than once a day outside the shower (i.e., because it is dirty). Girls and women with ASD may not discriminate issues related to "when" (e.g., blood on underwear, lots of blood on a pad, blood on legs) and "why" (e.g., unpleasant odor if pad is not changed; feeling unclean; blood on clothes) menstrual care is important. Thus, women need ongoing and thorough instructions and supports to sufficiently care for their menstrual needs. Table 9.1 outlines how SIECUS (2004) guidelines can be aligned with skills related to menstrual care and effective strategies for educating people with ASD.

Specific skills need to be taught once a young woman begins menstruating. The stakeholders should meet and decide how to teach menstrual care. Professionals should be sensitive to the preferences and cultural beliefs of family members and align interventions and supports accordingly. For example, some cultural or religious beliefs may preclude tampon use if the woman is a virgin (Orgocka, 2004). Once decisions are made about what will be taught, the team should consider evidence-based interventions for implementation. Instruction should result in generalized menstrual care across home, employment, educational, and community settings. To achieve this outcome, menstrual care instruction can be embedded into the daily activities and routines during the week of the month the woman will have her period. Relatedly, interventions and supports should be developed to address setting events, antecedents, behaviors, and maintaining consequences (i.e., the four-term contingency) for various aspects of menstrual care. Figure 9.2 displays how the four-term contingency can be broadly applied to teaching menstrual care to women with ASD.

Setting events for a woman getting her period might include symptoms consistent with premenstrual syndrome. Menstrual care instruction should include recognition of the symptoms in order to prepare for care (e.g., getting/carrying pads or tampons), as well as taking proper doses of pain-relieving medication. Strategies might include social scripts (see Figure 9.3) and visual supports such as concept mapping (see Figure 9.4). Antecedent interventions are necessary for ensuring responding to cues for menstrual care once menstruation begins. Visual supports such as a graphic calendar can help the woman with ASD learn to predict when her

TABLE 9.1. Teaching Menstrual Care across the Lifespan

	Skill taught	Evidence-based strategy
SIECUS Key Concept 1: Human Development		
SIECUS Topic 1: Reproduction and Sexual Anatomy and Physiology		
Ages 5–8 Each body part has a correct name and a specific function.	Correct names of body parts Function of the body part	Direct instruction Visual support: pictures, drawings, etc.
Ages 9–12 A young woman's ability to reproduce starts when she begins to menstruate.	What is menstruation? What happens when a woman menstruates? Why do women menstruate? How long does menstruation last? How often does it happen?	Social scripts Visual support: picture story Visual support: calendar
Ages 15–18 A woman's ability to reproduce ceases after menopause; after puberty, a man can usually reproduce for the rest of his life.	When does a woman stop menstruating? Why does a woman stop menstruating?	Visual support: timeline Social script: when and why women stop menstruating
SIECUS Topic 2: Puberty		
Ages 5–8 Bodies change as children grow older. People are able to have children only after they have reached puberty.	What changes happen to a girl's body? What is the sequence of these changes? When a girl begins to menstruate, she could get pregnant and have a baby.	Visual timeline Visual support: girls/women Venn diagram
Ages 9–12 Puberty begins and ends at different ages for different people. During puberty, girls begin to ovulate and menstruate, and boys begin to produce sperm and ejaculate. Once this occurs girls are physically capable of becoming pregnant and boys of getting a female pregnant.	When does menstruation start? When a girl begins to menstruate, she could get pregnant and have a baby.	Visual support: timeline Social scripts: menstruation, fertility, and pregnancy

(continued)

TABLE 9.1. *(continued)*

	Skill taught	Evidence-based strategy
	SIECUS Key Concept 1: Human Development	
	SIECUS Topic 3: Reproduction	
Ages 13–14 A common sign of pregnancy is a missed menstrual period.	What do I do if I do not get my period? How do I know if I missed my period?	Problem-solving worksheet Visual support: calendar
Ages 15–18 Menopause is the time when a woman's reproductive capacity ceases.	When does a woman stop menstruating? Why does a woman stop menstruating?	Visual support: calendar with timeline
	SIECUS Key Concept 5: Sexual Health	
	SIECUS Topic 1: Reproductive Health	
Ages 9–12 During menstruation, you may need to clean your genitals more frequently.	How do I clean my genitals? How often do I clean my genitals? During menstruation, how often should I clean my vagina? During menstruation, how do I clean my genitals?	Task analysis: how to clean Visual support: steps for cleaning Picture schedule: where and when to clean Prompting: pointing to visual supports Social script: why, how, and where to clean

Setting Events	Antecendent	Teaching Menstrual Care	Consequence
Premenstrual symptoms • Taking over-the-counter medication • Communicating discomfort/pain • Purchasing feminine products	Preparing for menstruation • Visual support—calendar • Social story—how to manage your period • Visual support—concept map of preparation • Checking every 2 hours	• Task analysis • Visual support—steps for menstrual care with task analysis • Video modeling • Backwards chaining with prompts	Positive reinforcement • Reinforce successive approximations • Reinforce behaviors that are part of the entire task

FIGURE 9.2. Four-term contingency plan for premenstrual symptoms.

Once a month, women menstruate, or get their period.

When you menstruate or get your period, blood comes out of your vagina.

I am a young woman and get my period once a month.

It is okay and normal to get my period.

When women get their periods, they wear pads in their underwear to stay clean.

The pads in their underwear need to be changed every 2 hours.

My mom, teacher, and friends are happy when I take care of myself and change my pad.

I know I can change my pad every 2 hours.

I will tell my mom or teacher when I get my period.

I will change my pad and wash up every 2 hours.

I will not talk about my period to my friends in the classroom.

When I talk care of myself by changing my pad, my parents and teacher will be proud of me.

FIGURE 9.3. Social script about getting one's period.

period will start and end. Teaching behaviors associated with menstrual care often requires a task analysis combined with teaching strategies involving backward chaining, prompting and fading, and visual supports. Figure 9.5 provides an example of a task analysis for changing a sanitary pad. The behavior of changing a pad can be maintained by comfort or escape from unpleasant stimuli (e.g., soiled pad, odor, soiled clothing), but additional reinforcing consequences (e.g., rewards for task completion, praise) may be necessary until natural consequences are sufficient to maintain the behavior.

How To: Appropriate Masturbation

The onset of puberty often corresponds with, among other things, an interest in and exploration of one's own genitals. During puberty, young men begin to experience frequent and seemingly random erections. A common reaction is to touch the erect penis, which results in pleasing sensations and, as a result of exploration, usually leads to masturbation. Typically developing young men quickly learn through social interactions that masturbation is something done in private (or, in some cultures, not done at all), but young men with ASD typically do not learn these rules. Young boys with ASD, perhaps because of lack of preparation and the absence of early and ongoing sexuality education, may masturbate in inappropriate

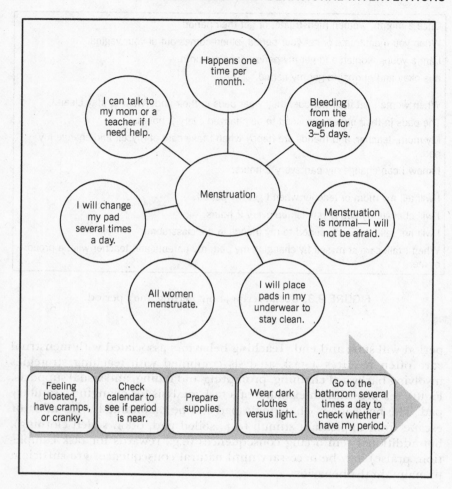

Happens one time per month.

I can talk to my mom or a teacher if I need help.

Bleeding from the vagina for 3–5 days.

Menstruation

I will change my pad several times a day.

Menstruation is normal—I will not be afraid.

All women menstruate.

I will place pads in my underwear to stay clean.

Feeling bloated, have cramps, or cranky.

Check calendar to see if period is near.

Prepare supplies.

Wear dark clothes versus light.

Go to the bathroom several times a day to check whether I have my period.

FIGURE 9.4. Concept maps about menstruation and preparing for your period.

places. As mentioned previously, a common reaction is to try to suppress masturbation entirely. The efforts usually are futile and may backfire because of sexual frustration or for other reasons. Rather than suppressing masturbation, young men and probably many adults with ASD will require specialized instruction to support appropriate masturbation.

As with any topic in sexuality education, support professionals should take steps to ensure that what will be provided is (1) legally allowed, (2) ethically appropriate, and (3) intended to improve quality of life. (Inappropriate masturbation may result in sexual frustration, prevents individuals

1. Go get new pad from _____.
2. Put pad in your pocket or purse.
3. Go to the bathroom.
4. Go into bathroom stall.
5. Shut door.
6. Pull down pants.
7. If pad is red or brown, take pad off underwear.
8. Roll pad and wrap with toilet paper.
9. Put pad in trash can.
10. Take new pad out of your pocket or purse.
11. Take wrapper off new pad.
12. Unfold pad.
13. Pull paper strip off back of pad.
14. Place sticky side of pad on underwear.
15. Throw pad wrapper in trash can.
16. Pull up pants.
17. Leave bathroom stall.
18. Wash hands.

FIGURE 9.5. Sample task analysis for changing a sanitary pad.

from participating in the community or accessing services that enhance independence, and may result in placement in psychiatric hospitals or correctional facilities.) The strategies described in the previous example also may be used to help adult men with ASD learn appropriate masturbation. Figure 9.6 is a four-term contingency plan for appropriate masturbation.

Setting events for masturbation might include a heightened sense of arousal that results from a relatively long period without orgasm, limited or no access to sexual partners, or difficulty achieving orgasm, causing sexual frustration. Antecedents for appropriate masturbation might include visual supports to remind the person where it is okay to masturbate (e.g., the bedroom at home), social scripts about appropriate masturbation, and reminders that vibrating massagers or other sex-related toys are only available at home. Support personnel may also use a highly preferred activity such as a hand-held video game or mobile electronic device to distract the person until he is home and in the bedroom. Supporting appropriate masturbation may require visual supports, such as an instructional video or appropriate pornographic video. The person may be given a vibrating massager or other sex toy specifically and only

Setting Events	Antecedent	Behavior	Consequence
Arousal • Relatively long period since last masturbation • Limited or no access to sexual partners • Inability to achieve orgasm; sexual frustration	Has desire to masturbate; gets erection • Visual support—picture of bedroom where masturbation is appropriate • Social script about appropriate masturbation • Reminder that vibrator or special toy can be used at home • Frequent checks to ensure hands are safe • Use planned distraction (e.g., give portable video game/device)	Teach appropriate masturbation • Visual support—provide instructional or pornographic video • Assistive technology—give vibrating massager or other appropriate sex toy • Task analysis—review steps; teach some steps, if appropriate (e.g., turn on video; plug in vibrating massager, close and lock door) • Video modeling—how to clean up after masturbation	Positive reinforcement • Access to vibrating massager or appropriate sex toy • Rewards and/or praise for safe and private masturbation Negative reinforcement • Escape/avoid hospitals and/or correctional facility

FIGURE 9.6. Four-term contingency plan for appropriate masturbation.

for masturbation. A task analysis of some steps may be helpful, especially for locking the door(s) and turning on a video. Video modeling might be used for teaching the person to clean up after he is done masturbating. Other strategies to support appropriate masturbation might include a social script (see Figure 9.7) or a concept map of masturbation (see Figure 9.8 on page 204). Its worth considering that a person will be more likely to masturbate only in his bedroom if the bedroom affords him the most gratifying experience. Thus, making the bedroom the only location where the man experiences sexual gratification reinforces masturbation in private rather than public places. With comprehensive and appropriate support, men with ASD can experience a better quality of life free of shame, sexual repression, and stigma.

Conclusion

Sexuality affects numerous aspects of our lives, including human development, relationships, personal skills, sexual behavior, and sexual health.

Sometimes I see someone or something that makes me feel excited and my penis gets hard.

This excitement is called sexual arousal.

It is okay to be excited and aroused, but I cannot touch myself unless I am in my bedroom.

When people get aroused, they might masturbate.

Masturbation means touching my penis so that it feels good.

Some people use a vibrator or special toy to masturbate because it feels good.

It is only okay to masturbate in my bedroom.

I will not masturbate if I am not at home in my bedroom.

I will not masturbate anywhere else, even if I am excited, because it is against the law and I will go to jail.

If I am sexually aroused or have an erection, I will quietly tell [*support person's name*].

I will wait until I get to my bedroom to masturbate.

I will close and lock my door so that I am private and safe while I masturbate.

I can masturbate with my hand, vibrator, or special toy.

I will try to be quiet when masturbating because masturbating is a private thing.

I will clean up when I am done masturbating.

When I masturbate in my bedroom, I am safe and private.

FIGURE 9.7. Social script about masturbation.

Sexuality also affects society and culture. Comprehensive sexuality education that begins in early childhood and is delivered throughout adolescence and young adulthood results in better sexuality-related outcomes. People with ASD ought not to be excluded from this human right and should be provided with specialized interventions and supports for sexual development that facilitates relationships, prevents or contributes to reporting of abuse, appropriate sexual behavior, health and hygiene, and increased self-determination. A comprehensive approach requires critical evaluation of curricula, a team approach to making decisions, and application of specialized instruction derived from evidence-based practices. Such an effort will be confronted with numerous barriers, but persistence in the delivery of sexuality education will translate to broad improvements in other domains and, ultimately, improved quality of life for people with ASD.

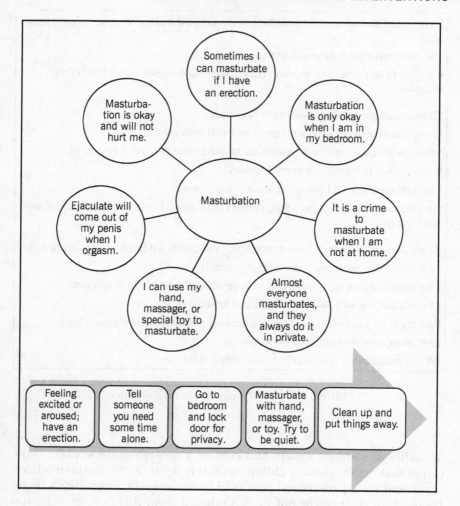

FIGURE 9.8. Concept maps about appropriate masturbation.

REFERENCES

American Academy of Pediatrics. (1999). Sterilization of minors with developmental disabilities. *Pediatrics, 104,* 337–340.

American Psychological Association. (n.d.). Understanding child sexual abuse: Education, prevention, and recovery. Retrieved April 27, 2013, from *www. apa.org/pubs/info/brochures/sex-abuse.aspx?item=4.*

Ashkenazy, E., & Yergeau, M. (2013). Relationships and sexuality: A handbook for and by autistic people. Retrieved on April 27, 2013, from *http://autism-now.org/wp-content/uploads/2013/02/relationships-and-sexuality-tool.pdf.*

Attwood, T. (1998). *Asperger's syndrome: A guide for parents and professionals.* London: Jessica Kingsley.

Blatt, B., & Kaplan, F. (1966). *Christmas in purgatory.* Boston: Allyn & Bacon.

Cook, B. G., & Cook, S. C. (2011). Thinking and communicating clearly about evidence-based practices in special education [White paper]. Retrieved April 27, 2013, from *www.cecdr.org/pdf/thinking_and_communicating_clearly_about_evidence-based_practices_in_special_education.pdf.*

Franzone, E. (2009). *Overview of task analysis.* Madison: National Professional Development Center on Autism Spectrum Disorders, University of Wisconsin, Waisman Center.

Franzone, E., & Collet-Klingenberg, L. (2008). *Overview of video modeling.* Madison: National Professional Development Center on Autism Spectrum Disorders, University of Wisconsin, Waisman Center.

Gagnon, J. H., & Simon, W. (2005). *Sexual conduct: The social sources of human sexuality.* Piscataway, NJ: Transation.

Greenberg, J. S., Bruess, C. E., & Oswalt, S. B. (2013). *Exploring the dimensions of human sexuality.* Burlington, MA: Jones & Bartlett.

Haracopos, D., & Pederson, L. (1992). Sexuality and autism: Danish report. Retrieved April 2, 2013, from *www.autismuk.com/?page_id=1293.*

Harmon, A. (2011, December 26). Navigating love and autism. *New York Times.* Retrieved from *www.nytimes.com/2011/12/26/us/navigating-love-and-autism.html.*

Howlin, P., & Clements, J. (1995). Is it possible to assess the impact of abuse on children with pervasive developmental disorders? *Journal of Autism and Developmental Disorders, 25,* 337–354.

Hume, K. (2008). *Overview of visual supports.* Chapel Hill: National Professional Development Center on Autism Spectrum Disorders, University of North Carolina, Frank Porter Graham Child Development Institute.

Koller, R. (2000). Sexuality and adolescents with autism. *Sexuality and Disability, 18,* 125–135.

Konstantareas, M. M., & Lunsky, Y. J. (1997). Sociosexual knowledge, experience, attitudes, and interests of individuals with autistic disorder and developmental delay. *Journal of Autism and Developmental Disorders, 27,* 397–413.

Krauss, M. W., Gulley, S., Sciegaj, M., & Wells, N. (2003). Access to specialty medical care for children with mental retardation, autism, and other special health care needs. *Mental Retardation, 41,* 329–339.

Lesseliers, J., & Van Hove, G. (2002). Barriers to the development of intimate relationships and the expression of sexuality among people with developmental disabilities: Their perceptions. *Research and Practice for Persons with Severe Disabilities, 27,* 69–81.

Ludlow, B. (1991). Contemporary issues in sexuality and mental retardation. *Advances in Mental Retardation and Developmental Disabilities, 36,* 531–539.

Mandell, D. S., Walrath, C. M., Manteuffel, B., Sgro, G., & Pinto-Martin, J. A. (2005). The prevalence and correlates of abuse among children with autism served in comprehensive community-based mental health settings. *Child Abuse and Neglect, 29*, 1359–1372.

Mansell, S., Sobsey, D., Wilgosh, L., & Zawallich, A. (1996). The sexual abuse of young people with disabilities: Treatment considerations. *International Journal for the Advancement of Counseling, 19*, 293–302.

National Autism Center. (2009). National Standards Report. Retrieved from *www.nationalautismcenter.org.*

National Commission on Adolescent Sexual Health. (1995). *Facing facts: Sexual health for America's adolescents.* New York: Sexuality Information and Education Council of the United States.

National Professional Development Center on Autism Spectrum Disorders. (n.d.). The NPDC on ASD and the National Standards Project. Retrieved April 29, 2013, from *http://autismpdc.fpg.unc.edu/content/national-standards-project#faq2.*

Neitzel, J. (2009). *Overview of time delay.* Chapel Hill: National Professional Development Center on Autism Spectrum Disorders, The University of North Carolina, Frank Porter Graham Child Development Institute.

Neitzel, J., & Wolery, M. (2009). *Overview of prompting.* Chapel Hill: National Professional Development Center on Autism Spectrum Disorders, University of North Carolina, Frank Porter Graham Child Development Institute.

Orgocka, A. (2004). Perceptions of communication and education about sexuality among Muslim immigrant girls in the U.S. *Sex Education, 4*, 255–271.

Ousley, O., & Mesibov, G. (1991). Sexual attitudes and knowledge of high-functioning adolescents and adults with autism. *Journal of Autism and Developmental Disorders, 21*, 471–481.

Putnam, F. W. (2003). Ten-year research update review: Child sexual abuse. *Journal of the American Academy of Child and Adolescent Psychiatry, 42*, 269–278.

Rapp, J. T., & Vollmer, T. R. (2005). Stereotypy: I. A review of behavioral assessment and treatment. *Research in Developmental Disabilities, 26*, 527–547.

Ray, F., Marks, C., & Bray-Garretson, H. (2004). Challenges to treating adolescents with Asperger's syndrome who are sexually abusive. *Sexual Addiction and Compulsivity, 11*, 265–285.

Realmuto, G. M., & Ruble, L. A. (1999). Sexual behaviors in autism: Problems of definition and management. *Journal of Autism and Developmental Disorders, 29*, 121–127.

Rivera Drew, J. A., & Short, S. E. (2010). Disability and Pap smear receipt among U.S. women, 2000 and 2005. *Perspectives on Sexual and Reproductive Health, 42*(4), 258–266.

Ruble, L. A., & Dalrymple, N. J. (1993). Social/ sexual awareness of persons with autism: A parental perspective. *Archives of Sexual Behavior, 22*, 229 –240.

Sexuality Information and Education Council of the United States. (2004). Guidelines for comprehensive sexuality education (3rd ed.). Retrieved from *www.siecus.org.*

Shapiro, J. P. (1994). *No pity: People with disabilities forging a new civil rights movement.* New York: Random House.

Sobsey, D., Randall, W., & Parrila, R. (1997) Gender differences in abused children with and without disabilities. *Child Abuse and Neglect, 21*, 707–720.

Stokes, M. A., & Kaur, A. (2005). High-functioning autism and sexuality: A parental perspective. *Autism, 9,* 266–289.

Taylor, R. L., Richards, S. B., & Brady, M. P. (2005). *Mental retardation: Historical perspectives, current practices, and future directions.* Boston: Allyn & Bacon.

Travers, J., & Tincani, M. (2010). Sexuality education for individuals with autism spectrum disorders: Critical issues and decision making guidelines. *Education and Training in Autism and Developmental Disabilities, 45,* 284–293.

Travers, J. C., Tincani, M., Whitby, P. S., & Boutot, E. A. (2014). Alignment of sexuality education with self-determination for people with significant disabilities: A review of research and future directions. *Education and Training in Autism and Developmental Disabilities, 49,* 232–247.

Vollmer, T. R. (1994). The concept of automatic reinforcement: Implications for behavioral research in developmental disabilities. *Research in Developmental Disabilities, 15,* 187–207.

Wacker, D. P., Berg, W. K., & Harding, J. W. (2006). Evolution of antecedent-based interventions. In J. K. Luiselli (Ed.), *Antecedent assessment and intervention: Supporting children and adults with developmental disabilities in community settings* (pp. 3–28). Baltimore: Brookes.

Walsh, A. (2000). IMPROVE and CARE: Responding to inappropriate masturbation in people with severe intellectual disabilities. *Sexuality and Disability, 18,* 27–39.

Wehmeyer, M. L. (1998). Self-determination and individuals with significant disabilities: Examining meanings and misinterpretations. *Journal of the Association for Severe Handicaps, 22,* 5–16.

Wehmeyer, M. L. (2001). Self-determination and mental retardation. *International Review of Research in Mental Retardation, 24,* 1–48.

Wehmeyer, M. L., & Garner, N. W. (2003). The impact of personal characteristics of people with intellectual and developmental disability on self-determination and autonomous functioning. *Journal of Applied Research in Intellectual Disabilities, 16,* 255–265.

Wehmeyer, M. L., Kelchner, K., & Richards. S. (1996). Essential characteristics of self-determined behaviors of adults with mental retardation and developmental disabilities. *American Journal on Mental Retardation, 100,* 632–642.

Wehmeyer, M. L., & Schwartz, M. (1997). Self-determination and positive adult outcomes: A follow-up study of youth with mental retardation or learning disabilities. *Exceptional Children, 63,* 245–255.

Westcott, H. L., & Jones, D. P. (1999). Annotation: The abuse of disabled children. *Journal of Child Psychology and Psychiatry, 40,* 497–506.

CHAPTER 10

• • • • • • •

Toward a Balanced Leisure Lifestyle for Adults with Autism Spectrum Disorders

• **Phyllis Coyne and Ann Fullerton**

Most adults explore and choose recreation and leisure activities, which, in turn, improve their quality of life. In this chapter, we explore ways to partner with and support adults with autism spectrum disorders (ASD) to create balanced and satisfying leisure lifestyles. Studies suggest that individuals with ASD often have restricted leisure lifestyles and become increasingly isolated in adulthood. However, given the opportunity and appropriate supports, adults with ASD can enjoy a wide range of recreation and leisure activities. The characteristics associated with ASD may present challenges to participation but also strengths for participation that can be incorporated into leisure pursuits. In this chapter, we describe a process to help adults with ASD to develop their leisure lifestyles. This process involves gathering information for use within a person-centered planning process to develop a leisure lifestyle plan, which includes methods to prepare for participation, to support participation, and to teach needed skills to adults with ASD so that they can fully engage in recreation and leisure activities.

The Importance of Leisure and Recreation for Adults with ASD
• • • • • • • • • • • • •

Quality of life for people with ASD consists of the same aspects of quality of life for other people. Leisure provides the milieu in which people may experience positive challenges, social engagement, choice, personal expression, and competence, as well as physical and emotional well-being. Fulfilling and satisfying leisure and recreation opportunities can provide dignity and respect to adults with ASD in a number of ways. Personal freedom, choice, and self-determination are fundamental to recreation and leisure. The opportunity to do things that are fun or relaxing adds meaning to life. Recreation can facilitate the development of affiliations and friendships through mutual interests and shared activities (Godbey, 1999; Howard & Young, 2002). Behaviors that may indicate stress, anxiety, or frustration, such as motoric stereotypies, physical aggression, self-abuse, and property damage, have been found to decrease when individuals are engaged in meaningful recreation activities (Garcia-Villamisar & Dattilo, 2010, 2011; Schleien, Meyer, Heyne, & Brandt, 1995; Schleien, Ray, & Green, 1997; Moon, 1994). Recreation can alleviate unfulfilling idle periods that occur due to unemployment and underemployment. Recreation can bridge the gap between just "being" in the community and actually participating in it.

However, the quality of life related to leisure is less than positive for adults with ASD. Billstedt, Gillberg, and Gillberg (2011) found that the quality of life of adults with ASD was generally positive with the exception of employment and *recreation*. Studies have shown that the leisure lifestyles of individuals with ASD are restricted. Individuals with ASD of all ages tend to engage in leisure activities almost exclusively at home, and they also tend to engage in more passive (e.g., watching television) and solitary activities (e.g., reading) than others both with and without disabilities (Badia, Orgaz, Verdugo, & Ullán, 2013; Buttimer & Tierney, 2005, Hochhauser & Engel-Yeger, 2010; Orsmond, Krauss, & Seltzer, 2004; Reynolds, Bendixen, Lawrence, & Lane, 2011). They participate in leisure pursuits even less often within their limited range of leisure activities (Hochhauser & Engel-Yeger, 2010; Reynolds et al., 2011; Solish, Perry, & Minnes, 2010). The leisure lifestyles of individuals with ASD often become more restricted as they grow older. For instance, Brewster and Coleyshaw (2011) documented that young adults with ASD participated in fewer community pursuits than did children with ASD. Negative experiences in recreation, including bullying and other disrespectful behavior, lack of acceptance, difficulties with relationships and social interaction, safety concerns, and lack of consistency and predictability in the environment may contribute to a gradual retreat into the home and a reluctance to continue or try new pursuits (Brewster & Coleyshaw, 2010; Fullerton & Rake, 2014). Young adults with ASD are often preoccupied with screen-based media, such as television, computers, and video games (Brewster & Coleyshaw, 2011; Hilton, Crouch, & Israel, 2008; Mazurek, Shattuck, Wagner, & Cooper, 2012; Orsmond & Kuo, 2011). Young adults with ASD appear to lack knowledge about available leisure pursuits and a willingness to try other activities (Brewster & Coleyshaw, 2011).

Many adults lack friends with whom to engage in leisure pursuits. According to Orsmond and colleagues (2004), young adults with ASD reported engaging in their leisure activities alone, with members of their immediate or extended families, or with members of their day programs (e.g., classmates). Adults with ASD made no references to friendships outside the school setting (Buttimer & Tierney, 2005). The lack of activity with friends often increases when an adult is not employed or engaged in a structured day program. Without careful planning, the lack of friendships, isolation, and limited leisure opportunities can become a downward spiral as a person ages.

A Satisfying and Balanced Leisure Lifestyle in Adulthood

Leisure is often included in individual support plans (ISPs) and other formal plans for adults with ASD. However, professionals, families, and service providers often have little guidance on how to help an adult with ASD move toward a more satisfying and balanced leisure lifestyle.

Leisure Lifestyle in Adulthood

A satisfying and balanced leisure lifestyle includes choosing and successfully engaging in meaningful recreation activities of sufficient variety to enhance a person's quality of life, including enjoyment, leisure satisfaction, well-being, relationships, and participation in the home and community.

A satisfying and balanced leisure lifestyle encompasses a personal balance of activities at home and in the community, of solitary activities and activities with others, and of active or restful activities. Leisure and recreation encompasses more than community participation or involvement. Important leisure and recreation experiences also take place at home and during breaks at work. Community recreation adds an important dimension to one's leisure lifestyle, but spending discretionary time at home doing enjoyable activities alone or with housemates, family, and friends is equally valuable. Most of us spend the majority of our leisure time at home, so this setting must not be forgotten. To have a balanced leisure lifestyle, an adult with ASD must have a variety of activities that he or she freely chooses to engage in alone and with others at home and in the community.

Balance also implies that an individual has had the opportunity to explore different leisure and recreation options and thus has made an informed choice, based on a variety of prior experiences, regarding how he or she will spend discretionary time. Finally, leisure lifestyle implies that an individual has sufficient skills, knowledge, attitudes, and abilities to participate successfully in and be satisfied with leisure and recreation experiences that are incorporated into his or her individual life pattern.

Individuals express their leisure lifestyles through daily and lifetime choices. During our lifetimes, the activities we enjoy and participate in change. What is most satisfying in leisure often changes as an adult with ASD learns more about leisure options and has new positive leisure experiences. The concept of a balanced and satisfying leisure lifestyle provides a framework for thinking about supporting adults with ASD in this domain of their lives. Moreover, it is useful to both broaden and clarify one's view of what constitutes recreation and leisure.

Leisure and Recreation

In keeping with common usage, the terms *leisure* and *recreation* are used synonymously throughout this chapter and refer to activities or experiences of interest that people choose to participate in for enjoyment, enrichment, and personal expression during their time free from obligations.

A Few Adults with ASD Answer the Question "What Is Leisure for You?"

- Doing things I enjoy.
- An atmosphere where I can be myself; don't have to put on an act.
- Getting together with people I can associate with and sharing ideas and things I like to do.
- I have lots of interests. My first major interest when I was 3 years old was stairways and escalators. Since then, I have intensely studied many other things. At present I consider myself an expert on gear assemblies.
- Being among friends with whom I don't have to explain myself.

Note. From Fullerton and Rake (2014). Reprinted with permission from Sagamore Publishing.

Recreation includes many types of activities, such as hobbies, sports, fitness activities, aquatics and water-related activities, arts and crafts, music, dance, art, drama, nature experiences, and games. In addition to these activities, adults may also participate in a wide range of leisure experiences that are not always considered, such as spectating and appreciating (e.g., sports, museums, and concerts), community service, relaxation and meditation, self-care (e.g., spa visits and massages), religious events or rituals, studying areas of interest, eating, food preparation, shopping, home improvement, caring for pets and plants, computer and Internet activities, travel, sightseeing, vacations, interacting with family and friends, telephone and e-mail conversations, and watching television (Stumbo & Peterson, 2009). Individuals with ASD may desire to engage in any of these categories of activities but may not be given the opportunity because of their diagnosis.

The Impact of Core Characteristics of ASD on Leisure and Recreation

Core characteristics of ASD, such as difficulties with social interaction and communication, unusual responses to sensory information, resistance to change, and restricted interests and obsessions, can influence how an individual participates in recreation both negatively and positively. This section describes a few examples of the challenges that can arise from each characteristic and how they can affect participation in recreation. Then examples of strengths are provided, along with how they can be incorporated into leisure and recreation participation.

Social Communication and Social Interaction

Difficulties with relationships and social interaction during leisure are a concern expressed by individuals with ASD (Brewster & Coleyshaw, 2011; Fullerton & Rake, 2014). Many recreation activities require some form of interaction. For instance, a number of activities are cooperative or competitive, and there may be any number of people involved. However, adults with ASD tend to engage in solitary activities that do not require social interaction (e.g., watching television or going for walks) (Badia et al., 2013; Buttimer & Tierney, 2005; Orsmond et al., 2004), and in fewer casual social activities (e.g., socializing with relatives, friends, neighbors, or work friends) (Orsmond et al., 2004).

The social demands of a recreation activity significantly affect the enjoyment and success of adults with ASD. Depending on the individual and how the activity is structured, an activity can either be a major challenge or a way to meet others and form friendships around mutual interests and shared activities. Too often adults with ASD have difficulty with an activity or refuse to participate because the social skills required are too demanding given their current skills. For instance, the social complexity and pace of interaction in competitive team activities, in which participants must take turns, cooperate as a team, play against another group, and compete, can be particularly confusing for individuals with ASD. Most adults with ASD prefer activities that have fewer social demands. An adult who may not enjoy playing basketball as part of a team may enjoy throwing balls into a basketball hoop on the garage at home, outside or at work alone, or with one or two others. Likewise, an adult with ASD is more apt to enjoy leisure experiences that involve a structured activity with clear rules, such as a table game, rather than an event where the social cues are more complex and vague, such as a cocktail party.

Communication

Challenges in communication often limit the expression of interests and participation in recreation. Chapters 5 and 6 of this volume address how to teach complex communication, including augmentative and alternative communications (AAC) and functional communication, which may be valuable in leisure pursuits.

Verbal instructions, particularly those with multiple steps, can be difficult to understand for many adults with ASD. Moreover, their difficulty understanding nonverbal communication and their literal interpretation of language, including words with double meanings and humor, all contribute to misunderstandings. Providing visual information and structure for an activity both before and during participation can give meaning and encourage independence. Without such support, individuals with ASD may require constant verbal direction from others, forcing them to remain more dependent.

Restricted Interests and Obsessions

Not only do circumscribed interests or intense preoccupations limit leisure pursuits in children with ASD, but also these restricted interests frequently persist into adulthood (Howlin, Goode, Hutton, & Rutter, 2004). Some individuals pursue particular obsessions or narrowly focused interests, such as fixating on train schedules, garage door openers, or a particular DVD, preventing them from doing more traditional leisure activities. Spending hours on end repeatedly engaging in only one or a few activities results in decreased opportunities for both social interaction and leisure skill development. On the other hand, studies have demonstrated that service providers can help individuals with ASD transition from narrow obsessions to new interests and activities (Boyd, Conroy, Mancil, Nakao, & Alter, 2007).

Resistance to Environmental Change or Change in Daily Routine

Adults with ASD like routine, consistency, and predictability in the environment and gravitate toward familiar activities rather than being curious and exploring novel activities. This tendency can limit an individual with ASD from expanding their interests and developing leisure skills. Without preparation before novel leisure experiences and structured, repeated exposure, they are unlikely to explore new leisure options. Yet even with good preparation, difficulty with change itself should be anticipated. Adults with ASD may react strongly to changes such as a new facility, people, or demands, even if they are looking forward to an activity. Even when adults have chosen and desire to participate in a new activity, they may still go through an adjustment period before they begin to enjoy the new activity.

Unusual Response to Sensory Information

The research has shown that atypical sensory processing patterns are associated with lower participation in recreation, especially social, physical, and informal activities (Hochhauser & Engel-Yeger, 2010). Many adults with ASD may avoid recreation settings entirely because of sensory challenges.

Sometimes sensory issues become less obvious as individuals with ASD mature. As a result, sensory issues are often missed, and accommodations are not provided. When not addressed, the sensory issues related to ASD can have even more of a negative impact on adults with ASD and their participation in recreation. Adding something that alleviates the intensity of sensory input, such as headphones for noise, a baseball cap for overhead lights, or a structured arrangement in which individuals with sensory issues can take a break and resume participation when they are ready again, may make their involvement more comfortable.

In addition to being hyper- or hyporeactive to sensory input across sensory modalities, many adults with ASD seek out motor activity, such as running, jumping, spinning, bouncing, pushing, pulling, lifting, and climbing, to meet a variety of sensory needs. Recreation activities that incorporate these actions can also meet these sensory needs.

Using a Person's Strengths in Leisure Activities

Every adult with ASD possesses some strengths associated with ASD that must be carefully considered in the process of developing a balanced leisure lifestyle and facilitating participation. An adult with ASD may have any combination of traits that can be used positively in recreation activities, as shown in the following examples.

• *Hyperattention to detail.* Hyperattention to minute details often results in an adult with ASD being exacting and precise, which is useful in many activities. *Edample*: Ivan may be nonverbal, but he impresses other members of the rock gym with the precise nature of his knot tying.

• *Preference for sameness.* Because of their desire for predictability and routine, adults with ASD often have a tolerance for repetitive activities in leisure. *Example*: Amy makes identical collectible clay figures of a dog that vary only in small details to represent different roles (e.g., Artist Dog, Christmas Dog).

• *Long attention span for activities of significant interest. Example*: Dale spent hours repairing small engines. Those who knew him well had seen the same focus when he was younger while building with Legos.

• *Precise and detailed long-term memory. Example*: Harvey amazes others by giving a play-by-play description of sports games that he has seen. He says, "Autism serves," when others ask him how he remembers all those details.

• *Strong memory for figures and facts they find interesting. Example*: Greg's fellow Sci Fi Film Club members are dismayed if he misses a meeting because they rely on his remarkable ability to recall hundreds of sci-fi movies, down to the last detail.

• *Accuracy in visual perception.* Adults with ASD may replicate exactly from a model. *Example*: Manuel follows the diagram for how to assemble trellises that baffled everyone else in his gardening club, including the leader.

• *Whole-picture learner.* Adults with ASD take in chunks of information quickly, Gestalt processing. *Example*: While the rest of the weaving class is repeating the lesson on how to work the shuttle, Davante demonstrates the skill because he learned it right away.

• *Strong visual–spatial intelligence related to how objects and figures relate in three-dimensional space. Example*: In art class, all watch in wonder as Jerald makes a sculpture from sheets of paper that he tears into a shape and stacks one upon another. The result is a three-dimensional classical bust of a human head.

- *Motor and coordination skills.* Running, jumping, spinning, bouncing, climbing, and the like. *Example*: Noel has stamina and well-developed gross motor skills. He enjoys directing his desire to jump, bounce, and climb into his gymnastics class.

- *Concrete and literal interpretation skills.* Adults with ASD understand and use concrete information and rules. *Example*: When housemates are playing games and there is a lively disagreement about the rules, all turn to José to simply recall and recite the exact language in the rule book.

- *Unusual talents, such as musical or artistic ability. Example*: With his ability to play tunes on the piano after hearing them once, Zack has become an anchor in his community blues band.

- *Persistence in completing tasks with a clear beginning and end. Example*: B. J. stayed after gardening class to complete planting two trays of annuals.

A Framework for Assisting Adults with ASD in Development of a Balanced Leisure Lifestyle

The remainder of this chapter provides a framework for assisting adults with ASD in developing satisfying and balanced leisure lifestyles, which includes choosing and engaging in leisure activities of sufficient variety to enhance their quality of life. This framework involves (1) gathering information, (2) developing a leisure lifestyle plan, and (3) creating and implementing supports and instruction for participation in each activity.

Framework for Developing a Leisure Lifestyle

Gathering information

- Record the person's history related to recreation and leisure.
- Describe the person's current leisure lifestyle.
- Identify the person's interests and features of activities that are of interest.

Developing a leisure lifestyle plan: The four guidelines

- Create a balance of activities.
- Identify opportunities to pursue existing leisure interests.
- Foster and use natural supports.
- Develop new interests through exposure to leisure activities with preferred features.

Creating and implementing supports and instruction for participation

- Determine and create needed supports for participation.
- If necessary, teach the skills needed to participate in the activity.
- If applicable, teach related skills needed so that the person can gain greater independence in leisure/recreation.
- If applicable, prepare staff or others in the setting who may provide formal or informal/natural supports.
- Prepare the adult with ASD for participation.
- Begin participation and adjust supports and teaching as needed.

Gathering Information

Learning as much as possible about the adult with ASD related to his or her past and present leisure is critical to developing a plan that will lead to a satisfying and balanced leisure lifestyle. This plan will also save time and frustration both for adults with ASD and for the people who are concerned about their leisure. There are many methods for gathering this information, such as interviewing the people in his or her life, observing him or her at home and in the community, and using communication strategies that effectively allow the person to express his or her interests and desires. Gathering information involves three steps: (1) Recording the person's history related to leisure; (2) describing his or her current leisure lifestyle; (3) identifying his or her interests and features of activities that are of interest.

Recording the Person's History Related to Recreation and Leisure

First, record a history of his or her past leisure experiences, positive and negative, including former recreation partners and settings. Gather information that is as specific as possible to determine which conditions and/or supports may have contributed to both the positive and negative experiences the person has had.

CASE EXAMPLE

T.J. is a 27-year-old man who lives in a group home. He has a few functional phrases and uses line drawings to make requests and make choices. A case study of T.J. is used to illustrate the process of developing a leisure lifestyle plan, as well as the methods to create and implement the supports and teaching needed to carry out the plan.

T.J.'s History Related to Recreation and Leisure. T.J. lived with his mother and younger sister until he was 22 and then moved into a group home. When he was in elementary school, T.J. spent much of his free time at home in unusual activities, such as spinning and throwing objects at lights. In response to T.J.'s repetitive jumping and spinning, his grandfather made a twirling sit-upon apparatus that T.J. enjoyed for long periods instead of spinning. As T.J. got older, his interest in movement and jumping was partially met by using a mini-trampoline at home.

His mother, who enjoyed bicycling, found that young T.J. enjoyed the movement and wind on his face as he rode behind her in a child trailer. Later in childhood, he learned some bicycling skills riding behind her on a tag-along bike. As an adolescent, T.J. enjoyed cycling local bike trails with his mother on a tandem bike. He did not enjoy riding a stationary bike. Perhaps it did not offer him the same movement and sensations that he enjoyed while bicycling in his community.

Another of T.J.'s unusual activities was to throw objects at lights that were on and, as his aim got better and he succeeded in breaking the light bulbs, laughing uproariously. In an attempt to mimic the tinkling sound of glass breaking and change of lighting, one of his teachers put a glass wind chime and flashing lights on a lowered basketball hoop and taught him to shoot baskets, starting by standing on a rubberized mat with two footprints very close to the hoop. As his interest in throwing the ball into the hoop grew, his teacher removed the chimes and lights from the basket. As his skills and independence developed, his teacher progressively raised the hoop to standard height and moved the footprint mat farther away, placing it at different angles to the hoop. Eventually, at school, T.J. and one of his peers would shoot baskets after lunch. At that point, his family installed a basketball hoop on their garage door, and he stopped throwing objects at the lights.

However, at school he soon found a new noisy object he could activate—the fire alarm. Along with creating loud noises, T.J. would play his favorite song, "Little Drummer Boy" (which he called "Rum Pum"), over and over, and he enjoyed playing pop rock on his cassette recorder. To channel this interest, his teacher worked with the music teacher to teach T.J. how to play a basic rhythm on the bass drum. Eventually, using the aid of a metronome with synchronized visual motion, T.J. could play the bass drum in the school's concert band. He thrived in the structure of the band. T.J. also stopped activating the fire alarms in the school.

To further expand on his leisure lifestyle, and considering the success they had had using lights and sounds, T.J.'s teacher thought T.J. might like the lights and sounds of bowling pins being knocked down. Despite the visual structure that was added to the activity to let him know how many balls to roll down the alley during each turn and to know when his turn was, he did not like bowling because of the random noise, having to wait his turn, wearing shoes that smelled different, and more. His discomfort finally inspired him to initiate his first new phrase in years, "No bowling."

T.J. loved taking hot baths and running through the sprinkler in the yard, so his mother enrolled him in private swimming classes at a pool run by the city's parks and recreation department. He excelled at learning to do the crawl. Although he had good swimming skills, T.J. was asked to leave a specialized swimming program by the volunteer coach, who did not understand his unusual behavior and said he would not follow directions.

In school T.J. was taught to play and cooperated in playing some simple games of chance, such as Sorry! Although he would follow his schedule and the visual structure to play the games, he never showed any particular interest in them or chose them from his choice board. When taught to play a race car game, he appeared to enjoy the lights, the sound of the wheels, and especially the crashing sound whenever a car careened off the track, but T.J. was not interested in the actual progress of the car around the track.

Describe the Person's Current Leisure Lifestyle

To form a picture of the adult's current leisure lifestyle, determine what he or she does during free time alone or with others at home or in the community, the frequency and duration of these activities, and any supports used. Knowing what an individual actually does in an activity is important because it indicates his or her skill levels and interests. If an activity occurs in the community, it is helpful to learn to what degree he or she performs the related skills needed to participate independently (e.g., traveling to and from, taking needed equipment). The places where an individual does activities can indicate knowledge of the community, as well as his or her preferences for certain types of environments. How the person gets involved in activities helps identify self-initiation, motivation, and awareness of resources. Identifying present leisure partners indicates who might be available to help him or her explore new activities.

While exploring his or her current leisure lifestyle, consider the individual's level of understanding of concepts related to use of leisure time. Does the person recognize when he or she has free time? Does he or she know how to make a choice about an activity and then to begin and engage in the activity? What current challenges may be influencing his or her recreation participation, and what kinds of supports are effective to address these challenges? What strengths does he or she have that may be used in leisure activities?

T.J.'s Current Leisure Lifestyle. T.J. is unemployed and spends most of his time alone at home. Although he now has more free time, his leisure pursuits have become more restricted as he has gotten older. He now selects music or basketball from a choice board of pictures. He independently uses his iPod Touch to listen to alternative rock and his enduring favorite song, "Little Drummer Boy," for hours every day. He turns it on and off and chooses the songs he listens to. T.J. retrieves his basketball from a box and throws it at a basketball hoop attached to the garage for about 20 minutes at a time, then puts the basketball away. Two times a week, group home staff take him and two of his housemates to a neighborhood park to shoot baskets. He spends most of his remaining discretionary time lying over a heat vent.

Two to three times a month, his mother and/or sister take him to small music concerts, to family gatherings, clothes shopping, or to small, quiet restaurants. T.J. enjoys the concerts as long as other people listen quietly and as long as he is in the front row or at a table with adequate room so that he is not surrounded by people. At family gatherings, he excitedly responds to seeing all the people he likes by alternating back and forth between being in a room with people, laughing and loudly calling out the name of his favorite person of the moment, and going to his designated break area in a separate room. On shopping trips, T.J. enjoys walking through the racks of clothes and touching the fabric. In restaurants, he loves to order with pictures and eat. He is mostly directed through the steps of these activities by his mother or sister

Identify the Person's Interests and Features of Activities That Are of Interest

It is critical to explore an individual's interests with him or her. However, identifying specific leisure interests may be challenging. Their responses are often limited by their lack of experiences or opportunities for leisure pursuits. If adults lack experiences or knowledge of leisure activities, then identify the person's interests and preferred activities, including obsessions. Often idiosyncratic interests can be utilized in leisure activities.

Because answering questions is generally difficult even for the most verbal person with ASD, interviews need to be carefully structured and conducted by someone the individual with ASD knows well. Pictures of activities may help generate responses, but because of the nature of ASD, the individual's answers may focus on irrelevant detail(s) within the visual representation of the leisure activity.

T.J.'s Interests and Features of Activities That Are of Interest. When T.J. is shown photos of a variety of leisure activities, he does not have the experience to know what most of them are. However, he chooses some activities from pictures that depict activities he has experienced, including listening to music, playing drums, tandem bicycling, shooting baskets, and swimming. His past and present activities during free time indicate that he has a preference for activities involving movement (particularly vestibular), creating loud sounds, controlling lighting, moving air—particularly warm air—being in hot or cool water, and touching material of different textures.

Developing a Leisure Lifestyle Plan

A leisure lifestyle plan serves as a working document that evolves as the adult's needs, interests, and opportunities change. It reflects his or her current interests and preferences but may also include expanding existing activities to additional settings or people and trying new activities with a high probability of interest. Without an individual leisure lifestyle plan, activities are often based on staff skills or interests, available facilities, and limitations of the budget and therefore reflect staff or agency priorities rather than the interests of the adult with ASD.

It is highly recommended that person-centered planning, such as Personal Futures Planning (Mount & Zwernik, 1994), be used so that the adult creates a plan with persons concerned about his or her leisure. Person-centered planning, with its structured process and roles and use of visuals, helps an adult with ASD share his or her interests, choices, and needs and can strengthen naturally occurring opportunities for support at home and in the community.

Developing a leisure lifestyle plan begins with examining the information gathered regarding how the adult historically and presently has spent his or her free time. The balance and variety of activities at home and in the community, alone and with others, active and passive, and the degree of participation in desired activities are reviewed.

T.J.'s Current Leisure Lifestyle. T.J. presently has a restricted leisure lifestyle, with two activities he does alone at home—listening to music, a passive activity, and shooting baskets, an active activity—and one regularly scheduled, active pursuit in the community that he does with paid staff, shooting baskets. However, he has additional leisure interests that he could pursue both at home and in the community, as well as preferences that could be matched to activities.

Each adult's plan is individualized, but the following four guidelines are useful in determining which activities will be prioritized, where they will be pursued, and with whom.

Create a Balance of Activities

There is no rule for how many or what kinds of leisure activities make up a balanced leisure lifestyle. Reality dictates that any of us can learn and participate in only a finite number of activities, so it is judicious to choose carefully. This decision process includes prioritizing activities that are likely to be engaged in regularly and can be done in more than one place. The plan should include activities that occur at home and in the community. If the adult has little or no satisfying leisure activity at home, this should be the first priority because the majority of all of our free time is spent at home. Both activities alone and with others should be considered, keeping in mind that many or all of our leisure activities at home are done alone and that many adults with ASD are more inter-ested in an activity itself than in any social interaction associated with it. Additionally, both active and passive activities should be considered. Finally, consider how independent an individual is in doing each activity, including traveling to and from an activity, getting and putting away nec-essary equipment, initiating the activity, and more. Having a few leisure activities that an adult can do independently or semi-independently given visual or other supports can outweigh having a dozen activities that will require intense staff support.

Identify Opportunities to Pursue Existing Leisure Interests

Clearly, the activities selected need to reflect the adult's current or observed interests, so that he or she will enjoy and continue to pursue them. Activities that can be pursued in more than one setting should be prioritized.

  Opportunities for T.J. to Pursue Current Interests. T.J. expressed interest in drumming, an activity he has not done since high school, and listening to music. One of the members of his planning team knows of a drumming circle that meets weekly in a community center that she thinks would be a good fit for T.J. Another member of T.J.'s planning team thinks that he would enjoy the variety of rock music in Wii's Rock Band and that it could help him expand his drum skills at home. Both of these become part of the plan.

Foster and Use Natural Supports

Interests of people with whom the focus person lives, such as family mem-bers, partners, friends, coworkers, or service providers, need to be iden-tified because these people are potential leisure companions who can expand the focus person's repertoire of leisure possibilities.

Natural Supports for T.J.'s Leisure Interests T.J.'s sister, Shanna, enjoys bicycling and wants to ride local bike trails with him two Saturdays a month on the tandem bicycle that T.J. and their mother had used together. She is a social person, so she goes online to find a relaxed recreational bicycle club that they can join. She thinks other club members will be intrigued by the tandem bike and T.J.'s contagious laughter when he bicycles, and that they will ask if they can trade off with Shanna. She is looking forward to this new experience, meeting new people, and getting fitter. Meanwhile, T.J. excitedly expresses his interest by flapping his hands and saying "Bike! Shanna!"

T.J. wants to start swimming again. He has the opportunity for a membership at the YMCA and can bring a leisure companion as an Americans with Disabilities Act (ADA) accommodation. He is particularly fond of Tyrone, one of Shanna's lifelong friends, who is a regular at family gatherings, and the feeling is mutual. Tyrone wants to support T.J.'s return to swimming, while also enjoying swimming laps himself. The fact that the Y has a hot tub makes going there additionally appealing to both of them. They schedule time to go to the Y at the least busy time on Wednesdays.

Develop New Interests through Exposure to Leisure Activities with Preferred Features

If an adult's leisure interests are underdeveloped or unclear due to limited experience, then exposure to new activities will be an important component of the leisure lifestyle plan. Ultimately, the goal is to offer sufficient exposure to a variety of leisure pursuits so that the adult with ASD can make informed choices based on personal experience.

A new activity has a greater chance of being successful and becoming a preferred activity if it contains features important to the individual. We cannot always predict what activities an adult with ASD will prefer and enjoy, but given the characteristics of persons with ASD, there are some properties within leisure activities that increase the possibility that they will be meaningful and enjoyed by the person with ASD. For instance, clear, static rules, a well-defined beginning and end, a predictable or repetitive quality, minimal verbal direction, structure, a predictable and discernible routine, and a slow to moderate pace are all features that may be beneficial. See Coyne, Nyberg, and Vandenburg (2011) and Coyne and Fullerton (2014) for information on assessing features of an activity.

For many adults with ASD, particular features of an activity are more important than the leisure activity itself. Therefore, knowing what an adult with ASD is attracted to in activities or his or her preferences in general will lead to the best match of activities. Carefully choosing activities with preferred features ensures more enjoyable and meaningful participation and reduces the time spent trying new activities. For instance, a person may prefer activities that are outdoors, solitary, and involve water. The planning team should translate preferences such as these into activities.

Trying a New Activity That Includes Features T.J. Enjoys. As an unemployed person, T.J. has a good deal of free time and limited leisure activities at home. T.J. spends a lot of time lying over heat vents, and the team would like to introduce T.J. to a different activity that involves warm, moving air. His planning team brainstorms what activity might include his preferences for touching material with different textures, water, moving air, and a tinkling sound. The team decides on the craft of making cat and dog toys by hand felting around balls with tinkling bells inside. The process involves rubbing wet fibers and use of a dryer. T. J. can learn this activity at the recreation center and then, if he sufficiently likes it, he can continue to pursue the activity at home. Although the team is not sure at this point, T.J. might enjoy making the pet toys as something that he can give as presents to his extended family.

As described earlier, considerable thought goes into developing a leisure lifestyle plan, including the nature of the activities, where they will occur, and who will accompany the adult.

Creating and Implementing Supports and Instruction for Participation

Careful preparation is often critical to successfully supporting an adult's participation in an activity and is accomplished through six steps that are described in this section. First, determine and create needed supports for participation. Second, depending on the activity and the individual, determine whether the individual will need to be taught particular skills in order to participate in the activity. Third, determine whether the individual will be taught related skills (such as transportation or interacting with leisure partners in a setting) in order to be independent or semi-independent in the activity. Fourth, if applicable, prepare staff or others in the setting who may provide formal or informal/natural supports. Fifth, it is critical to prepare the adult with ASD for participation. Sixth, as actual participation begins, the supports and teaching are implemented, observed, and adjusted as needed.

Determine and Create Needed Supports for Participation

The autism spectrum is very broad and includes adults with a wide range of skills and needs. However, because of the nature of ASD, many individuals, regardless of their intellectual level or severity of ASD, will need some type of the following:

- Visual supports to convey instructions, meanings, routines, schedules, changes, and expectations (e.g., tangible, pictorial or written daily schedule; visual directions, templates, finished examples, mini-schedules, reminder cards for rules and expectations).
- Visual organization of the environment and materials to provide structure and predictability, while conveying boundaries, expectations, routines, and schedules (e.g., clear physical boundaries in the environment, such as lines on floor, carpet squares, color-coding objects, clear beginning and ending to activities/tasks).
- Environmental modifications and/or accommodations for sensory regulation (e.g., relaxation protocol, break areas, headphones to reduce noise, fidget toys for waiting times, personal space for breaks).
- Communication supports to help the participant to communicate and understand communication, ask for help, indicate needs and choices, and respond to requests (e.g., augmentative or backup communication systems, allowance for delayed processing time, use of gestures, models, visual supports, demonstration with verbalizations, concrete language).
- Social information about the social context, including roles, norms, standards of behavior, and expectations of others in a setting or activity (e.g., social narratives on roles and social conventions, reminder cards for rules and expectations).

Supports are needed not only for the actual leisure activity but also for other aspects of the situation. It may be necessary to support the individual in knowing what to do during breaks, how to use the bathrooms, how to handle anxiety, who to go to if he or she has a problem at the site, or other issues.

In order to determine what supports are necessary, the leisure activity, procedures, and the environment are observed and analyzed in relation to the needs of the individual. Observe typical adults doing the activity to identify the leisure activity skills (e.g., yoga postures) and related skills (e.g., bringing a mat to class, knowing when to be quiet in yoga class) that are needed to independently participate in the activity. In addition, identify the procedures involved in the activity. Many behavioral challenges of individuals with ASD are the result of misunderstood procedures, so the procedures need to be identified and taught.

The environment can have a major impact on the ability of a person with ASD to participate in recreation activities. The behavior of a participant with ASD will vary depending on aspects of the setting, such as novelty, degree of structure provided, and complexity of the environment, so observation of the environment is vital. Surveying the recreation environment for factors that may lower a participant's ability to function in activities can help determine whether there is a good match between the participant and the inherent demands of the activity. An environmental inventory can help determine what accommodations and/or modifications are needed. See Coyne and colleagues (2011) and Coyne and Fullerton (2014) for methods of observing and analyzing leisure environments and procedures for selecting activities in light of the needs of an individual with ASD. Then determine what leisure activity or related skills will require instruction and/or supports.

Involving the adult with ASD in planning supports as much as possible usually results in the best fit and provision of supports that he or she will be more motivated to use. Adults with ASD do not necessarily know how to use supports when they are first presented. Therefore, they should be explicitly taught how to use supports with lots of opportunity to practice until they independently use the support structure. For instance, if an adult is given a pictorial sequence for making tie-dyed T-shirts, he or she will need to be taught to follow each picture and proceed to the next picture.

Supports, such as visual schedules and reminder cards, can help an individual with ASD perform more independently and do so without the constant verbal direction of others. Once an adult with ASD is competent in the use of needed supports, the supports are not faded or removed. Instead, a system to reinforce and monitor the adult's continued use of the supports must be implemented. Many individuals with ASD will always need others to develop and maintain supports for them. They are likely to need accommodations in community activities. These adults also need to learn to ask for the supports that they need at home and in community activities.

A number of supports have been designed to utilize the underlying strengths and accommodate the needs of individuals with ASD. Most of these supports are evidence-based or promising practices for children with ASD, but given the similar characteristics of ASD throughout the lifespan, they are also likely to be effective with adults. Coyne and Fullerton (2014) give many examples of support strategies and how they have been used in a variety of recreation activities and settings for people with ASD.

Supports for T.J. One of T.J.'s service providers observed and analyzed the activity, procedures, and environment at the YMCA pool to address T.J.'s support needs. She determined that the following supports were needed: (1) a video to prepare him for the environment, including entering the building, going to the reception area, going to the locker room and bathroom, and entering the pool area; (2) a visual schedule of line drawings for the routine, including presenting his membership card to the receptionist, changing into a swimsuit, putting his clothes in a locker, and so forth; (3) a prepacked athletic bag with materials always in designated compartments; (4) a membership card on a cord attached to the athletic bag; and (5) a waterproof MP3 player with a playlist that ended in 20 minutes, the length of time he would swim.

If Applicable, Teach the Skills Needed to Participate in the Activity

In some cases, explicit instruction is required to enable an adult with ASD to engage in an activity. Evidence-based practices (EBPs) are available to teach individuals with ASD leisure skills. Of the 24 EBPs identified by the National Professional Development Center (NPDC) on Autism Spectrum Disorders (2008) for people between the ages of birth and 22 years, 6 met the criteria specifically for leisure and recreation. These include prompting, reinforcement, self-management, structured work systems, task analysis, and visual supports. These strategies are often used in conjunction with each other. For instance, prompting, reinforcement, and visual supports are frequently used with other strategies. Additional EBPs were added in 2014. Service providers can learn how to implement these and other EBPs in the NPDC Briefs (*http://autismpdc.fpg.unc.edu/content/briefs*) and the Autism Internet Modules (*www.autisminternetmodules.org/user_mod.php*). Because two of these practices, structured work systems and visual supports, are frequently used both as supports and in teaching skills in recreation, they are described here.

STRUCTURED WORK SYSTEMS

A structured work system is a visually structured intervention used to organize a series of activities for individuals with ASD (Hume & Carnahan, 2008; Mesibov, Shea, & Schopler, 2005).

VISUAL SUPPORTS

Visual supports for individuals with ASD include but are not limited to visual schedules to increase task engagement, visual scripts to encourage social interaction, and picture cues to support play skill development (Massey & Wheeler, 2000; Morrison, Sainato, Benchaaban, & Endo, 2002).

Visual schedules, also referred to as activity schedules, are one of the most commonly used visual supports. They involve a display of objects, pictures, or written words in the desired sequence of activities. Activity schedules have repeatedly been shown to be effective in promoting leisure and interactive play skill acquisition for children with ASD (Betz, Higbee, & Reagon, 2008; Cuhadar & Diken, 2011; Machalicek et al., 2009). Coyne and colleagues (2011) used activity schedules within their activity cards for over 40 leisure activities in the home, school, and community. Many examples of structured work systems and of visual supports developed for use in recreation are found in Coyne and Fullerton (2014).

VIDEO MODELING

Video modeling involves the viewing of a video clip that provides a model for an individual to imitate (McCoy & Hermansen, 2007). Video modeling is emerging as a promising EBP and has been used to teach children with ASD play skills (Blum-Dimaya, Reeve, Reeve, & Hoch, 2010; Dauphin, Kinney, & Stromer, 2004; Paterson & Arco, 2008; Yanardag, Akmanoglu, & Yilmaz, 2013). In addition, it has been used to teach children with ASD to play the video game Guitar Hero II (Blum-Dimaya et al., 2010).

Instruction for T.J. T.J. needed instruction in how to play Wii's Rock Band drum game. He learned it quickly through the combined use of an activity schedule and video modeling. An activity schedule of the steps for turning on and off the game and system was developed, and as T.J. learned to use the schedule to cue him to perform each step, prompting was faded. Video modeling was embedded in the game itself, providing demonstration and practice in using the game controller to manipulate the drum set. Selection of different rhythms was demonstrated and then practiced until T.J could select from the array of options. Once T.J. mastered the steps involved, he selected new songs and rhythms that were not used during training.

If Applicable, Teach Related Skills Needed to Gain Greater Independence in Leisure/Recreation

In order to engage in most leisure activities as independently as possible, an adult may need to learn and perform many related skills, such as using transportation, making purchases, remembering and packing needed equipment and clothing, keeping track of the time, and so on. (Independent living skills are discussed by Myles et al., Chapter 12, this volume.) Semi-independent or independent participation may also require an awareness of free time, the identification of resources, choice making, initiation, social interaction, and problem-solving skills related to the activity. The service provider considers what related skills may need to be taught for optimal independence. When an adult is highly interested in an activity, he or she is more likely to be motivated to develop and practice related skills.

If Applicable, Prepare Staff or Others in the Setting Who May Provide Formal or Informal/Natural Supports

Staff in organized recreation programs often need to be prepared to support a participant with ASD. Organized recreation programs often have a process for providing accommodations to persons with disabilities, but the staff will need to know what are the most effective supports for the individual with ASD. The adult with ASD may be assisted to request ADA accommodations, and adult service providers who know the individual can assist recreation staff to provide adequate supports. For example, the adult service provider may help the recreation staff develop a visual schedule for the activity time period and use it to signal all participants when transitions will occur. Other participants may interact with their fellow participant with ASD and become natural supports. See Coyne and Fullerton (2014) for examples of supports provided by recreation staff.

A Few Suggestions for Recreation Leaders from Adults with ASD

- Give the person with ASD complete information and all the details in sequence. Make things clear and don't leave steps out.
- Don't leave people out or force them into things.
- Be creative; use their interests.
- Some may need one-on-one time. Don't get mad if they do not "get it" at first.

Note. From Fullerton and Rake (2014). Reprinted with permission from Sagamore Publishing.

Prepare the Adult with ASD for Participation

Preparing the adult for a new activity is often critical to successful participation. It is important to provide the adult with information about what to expect, what will happen, what the activity entails from start to finish, and any possible sensory challenges (e.g., unexpected sounds, ambient noise level, lighting). For many, a visual schedule and social narrative that are reviewed several times before going to the setting to participate for the first time are critical. For example, Coyne and colleagues (2011) used written and pictorial information on activity cards to help persons with ASD get ready for an activity. Other methods are described in Coyne and

Fullerton (2014). Sometimes it is helpful to have the adult visit the site and meet staff prior to beginning participation, but this is not advised if the person will have difficulty unlearning the "visiting" routine and learning the "participating" routine. For some individuals, providing a map of the building, including the bathrooms and other areas the person will access, is helpful. An alternative is creating digital video walkthroughs of the site and the routine with locations of restrooms and water fountains, as well as introduction of instructor and activity.

Begin Participation and Adjust Supports and Teaching as Needed

As the adult with ASD begins participation in the activity, the service provider needs to provide planned supports and instruction. Once the adult is participating, the areas in which supports or instruction need to be adjusted will become clear and then be addressed.

Conclusion

An important aspect of adulthood is the ongoing development of a leisure lifestyle that enhances our quality of life. This chapter describes a process for affording adults with ASD the same opportunity. Many examples exist of individuals with ASD participating in a wide range of leisure and recreation activites (Coyne & Fullerton, 2014), attesting to the potential and capability of all adults with ASD to expand this important aspect of life.

REFERENCES

Badia, M., Orgaz, M. B., Verdugo, M. Á., & Ullán, A. M. (2013). Patterns and determinants of leisure participation of youth and adults with developmental disabilities. *Journal of Intellectual Disability Research, 57*(4), 319–332.

Betz, A., Higbee, T. S., & Reagon, K. A. (2008). Using joint activity schedules to promote peer engagement in preschoolers with autism. *Journal of Applied Behavior Analysis, 41,* 237–241.

Billstedt, E., Gillberg, I. C., & Gillberg, C. (2011). Aspects of quality of life in adults diagnosed with autism in childhood. *Autism: The International Journal of Research and Practice, 15*(1), 7–20.

Blum-Dimaya, A., Reeve, S. A., Reeve, K. F., & Hoch, H. (2010). Teaching children with autism to play a video game using activity schedules and game-embedded simultaneous video modeling. *Education and Treatment of Children, 33*(3), 351–370.

Boyd, B. A., Conroy, M. A., Mancil, G. R., Nakao, T., & Alter, P. J. (2007). Effects of circumscribed interests on the social behaviors of children with autism spectrum disorders. *Journal of Autism and Developmental Disorders, 37*, 1550–1561.

Brewster, S., & Coleyshaw, L. (2011). Participation or exclusion?: Perspectives of pupils with autistic spectrum disorders on their participation in leisure activities. *British Journal of Learning Disabilities, 39*(4), 284–291.

Buttimer, J., & Tierney, E. (2005). Patterns of leisure participation among adolescents with a mild intellectual disability. *Journal of Intellectual Disabilities, 9*(1), 25–42.

Coyne P., & Fullerton, A. (2014). *Supporting individuals with autism spectrum disorder in recreation*. Urbana, IL: Sagamore.

Coyne, P., Nyberg, C., & Vandenburg, M. L. (2011). *Developing leisure time skills in persons with autism* (2nd ed.). Arlington, TX: Future Horizons.

Cuhadar, S., & Diken, H. (2011). Effectiveness of instruction performed through activity schedules on leisure skills of children with autism. *Education and Training in Autism and Developmental Disabilities, 46*(3), 386–398.

Dauphin, M., Kinney, E. M., & Stromer, R. (2004). Using video-enhanced activity schedules and matrix training to teach sociodramatic play to a child with autism. *Journal of Positive Behavior Interventions, 6*, 238–250.

Fullerton, A., & Rake, J. (2014). A few perspectives and experiences of individuals with autism spectrum disorder related to recreation. In P. Coyne & A. Fullerton (Eds.), *Supporting individuals with autism spectrum disorder in recreation* (2nd ed.). Urbana, IL: Sagamore.

Garcia-Villamisar, D. A., & Dattilo, J. (2010). Effects of a leisure programme on quality of life and stress of individuals with ASD. *Journal of Intellectual Disability Research. 54*(7), 611–619.

Garcia-Villamisar, D., & Dattilo, J. (2011). Social and clinical effects of a leisure program on adults with autism spectrum disorder. *Research in Autism Spectrum Disorders, 5*(1), 246–253.

Godbey, G. (1999). *Leisure in your life: An exploration* (3rd ed.). State College, PA: Venture.

Hilton, C. L., Crouch, M. C., & Israel, H. (2008). Out-of-school participation patterns in children with high-functioning autism spectrum disorders. *American Journal of Occupational Therapy, 62*(5), 554–563.

Hochhauser, M., & Engel-Yeger, B. (2010). Sensory processing abilities and their relation to participation in leisure activities among children with high-functioning autism spectrum disorder (HFASD). *Research in Autism Spectrum Disorders, 4*(4), 746–754.

Howard, K., & Young, M. E. (2002). Leisure: A pathway to love and intimacy. *Disability Studies Quarterly, 22*(4), 101–120.

Howlin, P., Goode, S., Hutton, J., & Rutter, M. (2004). Adult outcomes for children with autism. *Journal of Child Psychology and Psychiatry, 45*, 212–229.

Hume, K., & Carnahan, C. (2008). *Overview of structured work systems*. Chapel Hill: National Professional Development Center on Autism Spectrum Disorders, University of North Carolina, Frank Porter Graham Child Development

Institute. Retrieved January 4, 2013, from *http://autismpdc.fpg.unc.edu/content/structured-work-systems.*

Machalicek, W., Shogren, K., Lang, R., Rispoli, M. J., O'Reilly, M. F., Sigafoos, J., et al. (2009). Increasing play and decreasing the challenging behavior of children with autism during recess with activity schedules and task correspondence training. *Research in Autism Spectrum Disorders, 3,* 547–555.

Massey, N. G., & Wheeler, J. J. (2000). Acquisition and generalization of activity schedules and their effects on task engagement in a young child with autism in an inclusive pre-school classroom. *Education and Training in Mental Retardation and Developmental Disabilities, 35*(3), 326–335.

Mazurek, M. O., Shattuck, P. T., Wagner, M., & Cooper, B. P. (2012). Prevalence and correlates of screen-based media use among youths with autism spectrum disorders. *Journal of Autism and Developmental Disorders, 42*(8), 1757–1767.

McCoy, K., & Hermansen, E. (2007). Video modeling for individuals with autism: A review of model types and effects. *Education and Treatment of Children, 30,* 183–213.

Mesibov, G., Shea, V., & Schopler, E. (2005). *The TEACCH approach to autism spectrum disorders.* New York: Springer.

Morrison, R. S., Sainato, D. M., Benchaaban, D., & Endo, S. (2002). Increasing play skills of children with autism using activity schedules and correspondence training. *Journal of Early Intervention, 25*(1), 58–72.

Moon, M. S. (1994). *Making schools and community recreation fun for everyone: Places and ways to integrate.* Baltimore: Brookes.

Mount, B., & Zwernik, K. (1994). Making futures happen: A manual for facilitators of personal futures planning. Retrieved from *www.mncdd.org/extra/publications/making_futures_happen.pdf.*

National Professional Development Center on Autism Spectrum Disorders. (n.d.). Briefs. Retrieved from *http://autismpdc.fpg.unc.edu/content/briefs.*

Orsmond, G., Krauss, M., & Seltzer, M. (2004). Peer relationships and social and recreational activities among adolescents and adults with autism. *Journal of Autism and Developmental Disorders, 34,* 245–256.

Orsmond, G. I., & Kuo, H.-Y. (2011). The daily lives of adolescents with an autism spectrum disorder: Discretionary time use and activity partners. *Autism: International Journal of Research and Practice, 15*(5), 579–599.

Paterson, C. R., & Arco, L. (2008). Using video modeling for generalizing toy play in children with autism. *Behavior Modification, 31,* 660–681.

Reynolds, S., Bendixen, R. M., Lawrence, T., & Lane, S. J. (2011). A pilot study examining activity participation, sensory responsiveness, and competence in children with high-functioning autism spectrum disorder. *Journal of Autism and Developmental Disorders, 41,* 1496–1508.

Schleien, S. J., Meyer, L. H., Heyne, L. A., & Brandt, B. B. (1995). *Lifelong leisure skills and lifestyles for persons with developmental disabilities.* Baltimore: Brookes.

Schleien, S. J., Ray, M. T., & Green, F. P. (1997). *Community recreation and people with dusabilities: Strategies for inclusion.* Baltimore: Brookes.

Solish, A., Perry, A., & Minnes, P. (2010). Participation of children with and without disabilities in social, recreational and leisure activities. *Journal of Applied Research in Intellectual Disabilities, 23*(3), 226–236.

Stumbo, N. J., & Peterson, C. A. (2009). *Therapeutic recreation program design: Principles and procedures* (5th ed.). San Francisco: Pearson Benjamin Cummings.

Yanardag, M., Akmanoglu, N., & Yilmaz, I. (2013). The effectiveness of video prompting on teaching aquatic play skills for children with autism. *Disability Rehabilitation, 35*(1), 47–56.

PART IV

• • • • • •

Employment, Independence, Aging, and Policy

CHAPTER 11

• • • • • • •

Meaningful Employment for Individuals with Autism Spectrum Disorders

• **Paul Wehman, Pamela Sherron Targett, Carol Schall, and Staci Carr**

Autism spectrum disorders (ASD) comprise the fastest-growing developmental disability (Centers for Disease Control and Prevention, 2012), with 1 in 88 children in the United States being diagnosed. Functional limitations from ASD continue into adulthood and often create barriers to employment (Schall, Targett, &Wehman, 2013). As the number of children diagnosed with ASD increases, so does the need to focus on the knowledge, skills, abilities, and connections that enable youth with ASD to gain and maintain employment in their communities (Schall et al., 2013).

Youth Transition from School to Work
• •

The majority of individuals diagnosed with ASD are rapidly approaching adolescence and adulthood. Yet recent research shows that transition planning is inadequate. Shattuck and colleagues (2012) found that more than 50% of young adults with ASD were neither working nor in school 2 years after leaving high school. Notably, the rate of of employment participation among persons with ASD was the lowest of all disability categories studied. In an earlier study, Newman, Wagner, Cameto, and Knokey (2009) found that only about 37% of individuals with ASD had been employed for 12 months or more 4 years after exiting high school. The National Longitudinal Transition Study–2, a primary source of information about outcomes for students with disabilities, followed a large sample of youth with ASD as they transitioned from school to adulthood from 2001 to 2009. Among the overall sample of 11,000 individuals with disabilities, 922 were people with ASD. Shattuck, Wagner, Narendorf, Sterzing, and Hensley (2011) examined patterns of service for this sample. They found that 6% of those youth had competitive jobs. This is among the lowest employment rates for individuals with disabilities (Wehman, Schall, Carr, et al., 2014). This rate is most disappointing in light of recent efforts to develop "Employment First" initiatives nationally. According to the Office of Disability Employment Policy:

> Employment First is a concept to facilitate the full inclusion of people with the most significant disabilities in the workplace and community. Under the Employment First approach, community-based, integrated employment is the first option for employment services for youth and adults with significant disabilities. (U.S. Department of Labor, Office of Disability and Employment Policy, n.d.)

At the same time, however, this low rate of employment should come as no surprise, given that a review of the extant literature on interventions for individuals with ASD reveals a paucity of research regarding transition practices and models that would change this pattern of significant underperformance in the transition to adulthood by incorporating autism-specific interventions (e.g., Schall et al., 2013; Shattuck et al., 2012; Wehman, Schall, Brooke, & McDonough, 2012). The International Autism Coordinating Committee notes that only 4% of all studies on ASD in 2010 were "lifespan studies" (Office of Autism Research Coordination, 2012). However, none of these studies comprises a complete model of intervention for transition-age youth with ASD. One model that has been utilized nationally is Project SEARCH, an intensive internship program (Daston, Riehle, & Rutkowski, 2012). Most of the existing literature has described the characteristics of the transition-age young adult population of individuals with ASD, the services or lack thereof that young adults with ASD can access, or the poor outcomes achieved by this group of individuals (e.g., Barker et al., 2011; Cimera & Cowan, 2009; Henninger & Taylor, 2012; Shattuck et al., 2011, 2012). The findings from this literature indicate that, despite a slight lessening of the original symptoms, individuals with ASD continue to have significant challenges in all environments related to social interaction and communication into adolescence and adulthood.

Adults and Employment

• • • • • • • • • • • • • • • •

Adults with ASD experience high rates of unemployment and underemployment, frequently change jobs, earn less money, and are less likely to be employed than their typically developing peers (Howlin, 2000; Hurlbutt & Chalmers, 2004; Jennes-Coussens, Magill-Evans, & Koning, 2006; Müller, Schuler, Burton, & Yates, 2003, Wehman, Schall, Carr, et al., in press). Even individuals with postsecondary education degrees and experiences commonly have challenges in acquiring and maintaining employment commensurate with their abilities (Howlin, 2000). The reasons for the challenges that individuals with ASD face in achieving employment have been explored. Recently, Holwerda, van der Klink, Groothoff, and Brouwer (2012) completed a systematic literature review on factors hindering work for individuals with ASD. They identified one factor that was consistently associated with hindering work participation: limited cognitive ability. In addition, they found two factors that had a positive impact on job participation; higher educational attainment and family support for work.

Several researchers have focused on interventions designed to improve job retention by using strategies to match a job seeker with ASD to the workplace. For example, assessments have been used to determine the job seeker's task preferences (Lattimore, Parsons, & Reid, 2006; Nuehring & Sitlington, 2003). Social and communication needs have been evaluated (Müller et al., 2003). Hagner and Cooney (2005) looked at improving outcomes by adding necessary modifications and adaptations to the workplace.

It appears that functional limitations related to impairment in social functioning, communication, and repetitive and unusual patterns of behavior often create barriers to ongoing employment for adults with ASD (Cameto, Marder, Wagner, & Cardoso, 2003; Dew & Alan, 2007). Research shows that individuals are more likely to lose their employment because of communication and social difficulties rather than because of inability to perform the job (Bolman, 2008; Camarena, & Sarigiani, 2009; Dew & Alan, 2007; Hurlbutt & Chalmers, 2004; Müller et al., 2003; Ruef & Turnbull, 2002; Sperry & Mesibov, 2005). Notably, Schaller and Yang (2005) found that employment outcomes can be improved with effective behavior support and social interventions.

In addition to the descriptive literature, there are a number of single-subject and small studies that research the efficacy of discrete interventions designed to strengthen adaptive or weaken maladaptive behaviors associated with ASD for young adults (e.g., Dogoe, Banda, Lock, & Feinstein, 2011; Gentry, Lau, Molinelli, Fallen, & Kriner, 2012; Gentry,

Wallace, Kvarfordt, & Lynch, 2010; Hillier et al., 2007; Hillier, Fish, Siegel, & Beversdorf, 2011; Kandalaft, Dibehbani, Krawczyk, Allen, & Chapman, 2013; Lattimore et al., 2006; Mechling, Gast, & Seid, 2009; Mechling & Seid, 2011; Southall & Gast, 2011). These studies indicate that there is a growing collection of individual interventions that support adults with ASD in achieving improved independence, employment, communication, and social interaction. These interventions include supported employment, the use of augmentative and alternative communication, social skills instruction, and the use of personal digital devices for communication and cognitive organization (Schall et al., 2013). Despite this work, there continues to be a paucity of research on interventions for adults with ASD.

Perhaps the most promising studies to date, though, involve supported employment and the use of the Project SEARCH model adapted for transition-age youth with ASD (Wehman et al., 2012; Wehman, Schall, McDonough, et al., 2014). For example, Wehman and colleagues (2012) studied the effect of supported employment for young adults with ASD. In this study, 27 of 33 adults with ASD achieved competitive employment at the prevailing wage. This study demonstrated that, with intensive initial supports, individuals with ASD achieved a reasonable level of workplace independence within a year of intervention. Wehman, Schall, McDonough, and colleagues (2014) also presented the effect of Project SEARCH with supports for individuals with ASD in a randomized clinical trial. In this study, youth with ASD were placed in an intensive internship model in a community business during their final year of high school. The treatment group achieved competitive employment at 87.5%, whereas the control group only reached 6.25%. Finally, the employment outcomes of the treatment group were notably in "nontraditional" jobs such as hospital pharmacy assistant and surgical care technician (Wehman, Schall, McDonough, et al., 2014). In both studies, the researchers used supported employment and customized employment strategies, applied behavior analysis, and positive behavior support for skill acquisition and self-management strategies (Wehman et al., 2012, 2013; Wehman, Schall, McDonough, et al., 2014). Although there is emerging literature establishing evidence-based practices related to supported employment, there is not yet enough evidence to make strong conclusions regarding the validity of these interventions across settings. This chapter examines promising practices to help improve work outcomes. It begins with an overview of two Employment First strategies, supported employment and customized employment. Next, some basic guidelines to effectively implement these Employment First options are provided. This includes information on working with businesses. Finally, the chapter concludes with a case study.

Promising Practices
• • • • • • • • • • •

As noted earlier, more empirical research is needed to identify strategies and models that will improve employment outcomes for individuals with ASD (Hendricks, 2010; Hendricks & Wehman, 2009; Wehman, Datlow, Smith, & Schall, 2009; Wehman, Schall, Carr, et al., 2014; Westbrook et al., 2012). Nevertheless, attention is on the growing body of emerging literature that documents promising practices to enhance employment outcomes, such as supported employment and customized employment (Barnhill, 2007; Cimera & Cowan, 2009; Gerhardt & Holmes, 2005; Hillier et al., 2007; Hurlbutt & Chalmers, 2002, 2004; Lawer, Brusilovsky, Salzer, & Mandell, 2009; O'Brien & Daggett, 2006; Schall, 2010; Schall, Wehman, & McDonough, 2012; Schaller & Yang, 2005; Smith & Philippen, 1999; Taylor & Seltzer, 2011; Wehman et al., 2012, 2013; Wehman, Schall, Carr, et al., 2014). Prior to examining these two promising practices in more detail, a brief look at state vocational rehabilitation services, a primary provider and funder for employment support services, is provided.

State Vocational Rehabilitation

The Rehabilitation Act of 1973 (Public Law 93-112), as amended in 1998 (Public Law 105-220) (35), provides federal grants to states to operate comprehensive programs of vocational rehabilitation (VR) services to individuals with disabilities. It is a cooperative program between state and federal governments and should be considered a core resource for individuals with ASD. State VR services employ counselors who provide an array of services and supports focused on assisting a person with a disability in finding employment. Services can include, but are not limited to, the following: assessment for determining eligibility for services; vocational counseling, guidance, and referral services; vocational training, including on-the-job training; personal assistance services; rehabilitation technology services; job placement services; and supported employment services. Once eligibility is determined, an individualized plan of employment is developed with the job seeker by the counselor. The plan includes an employment goal and services needed to obtain it. VR counselors have access to case service funds that can be used to purchase services from authorized vendors, such as postsecondary education and training, supported employment, transportation, assistive technology, and uniforms. It is also important to note that state VR services are time-limited.

There is little doubt that state VR programs will see a substantial increase in the number of youth with ASD seeking services in the near future (Migliore & Zalewska, 2012a). However, relatively few vocational support service providers, including state VR counselors, have the knowledge, skills, or resources necessary to successfully serve them (Cimera & Cowan, 2009; Dew & Alan, 2007; Lawer et al., 2009; Schall et al., 2013). In addition, the services provided by VR are less than optimal and do not provide sufficient support (Cimera & Cowan, 2009; Lawer et al., 2009). For example, Cimera, Wehman, West, and Burgess (2012) found that the most common approach to employment for individuals with ASD who were served through the Rehabilitation Services Administration was sheltered workshops. This outcome ignores the fact that sheltered work does not increase the probability of employment in the community. It has long been known that individuals who attend sheltered workshops typically do not transition to competitive employment—and the costs are high (Wehman et al., 2013). Therefore, after decades of research for individuals with intellectual and other severe disabilities, as well as advocacy on the effectiveness of Employment First approaches, such as supported employment and customized employment, it is difficult to understand why this option even exists. Unfortunately, this distressing truth, paired with inconsistencies in employment policies, practices, and procedures, may mean that individuals with ASD, their families, educators, vocational support specialists, policymakers, and other stakeholders may be destined to repeat the past—that is, unless a loud and clear message that competitive employment must be a priority is adopted and effective individualized support services are readily available.

Supported Employment

Supported employment is an individualized approach to assist a person with a severe disability in gaining and maintaining competitive employment in the community. Supported employment, initially viewed as a concept in the 1970s, was devised to assist a person with the most severe disabilities to exit from or avoid enrollment in a sheltered workshop, and instead go to work in the community. It should be noted that this approach is not for someone with ASD who would benefit from a less intensive vocational service, such as career guidance and counseling, job clubs, or placement services, to gain and maintain work. Supported employment is an intensive service. Readers should also be familiar with the federal legislation that defines for whom the service is intended. Supported employment is for individuals with the most significant disabilities who (1) are in need of ongoing supports, (2) have interrupted or no work histories, or (3) have intermittent employment records. Over the years, there has been some confusion over the meaning of the term *significant disability*.

This is most likely due to various interpretations by service providers. For instance, a "high-functioning" adult with ASD who has a college degree may qualify for supported employment. Too often, referral agencies such as state VR services have accepted proof of significant disability from the U.S. Social Security Administration's Disability Determination or Special Education Services and do not consider other parts of the definition. For instance, it is very possible that a woman with high-functioning ASD could gain employment on her own. She may be able to conduct a job search, locate job openings, apply for jobs, sell herself at an interview, get an offer, negotiate any terms, and accept a suitable position. However, once employed, she may begin to experience problems at work. She may remain employed for a few months and then be terminated or quit her job. If this work history becomes a pattern, such an individual would likely qualify for supported employment services. In a supported employment approach, a woman would get assistance with analyzing what went wrong in the past, developing an employment plan, and choosing a "better" job. Then, once employed, she would receive on-the-job support specifically designed to help improve retention at her new place of employment.

Supported employment can be ideal for adults with ASD. One of the learning characteristics of individuals with ASD is difficulty in generalizing skills from one environment to another. Consequently, skills learned in a "prevocational" environment do not necessarily result in the acquisition of employment, as is the case in sheltered workshops. With supported employment, individuals do not have to spend time "getting ready" to work in contrived environments. Instead, with supported employment, a job coach gets to know the job seeker, then works with employers to develop a job with that person in mind. After the person is hired, the job coach is available to provide on-the-job training and support to the new employee *and* the business. Once the employee learns to perform the job, the coach fades from full-time support to provide long-term follow-up services for the duration of the person's job tenure. Individuals who access supported employment will need sources of funding for this ongoing long-term follow-up. Notably, over the decades, supported employment has evolved into an effective, yet often underutilized, VR service and transition to work intervention for individuals with severe disabilities (Wehman et al., 2013).

Supported employment increases employment rates, earnings (Howlin, Alcock, & Burkin 2005), and quality of life for individuals with ASD (Garcia-Villamisar, Wehman, & Navarro, 2002). Garcia-Villamisar and Hughes (2007) found that cognitive performance also improved among individuals with ASD who accessed supported employment. Reviews of literature on transition from schoolwork (Hendricks & Wehman, 2009) to adult employment (Hendricks, 2010; Holwerda et al., 2012) reveal examples of successful supported employment programs and case studies that offer guidance for developing recommendations for vocational supports. For example, Hendricks (2010) grouped vocational supports into five major themes: job placement, supervisors and coworkers, on-the-job provisions, workplace modifications, and long-term support. In addition, she warned that although the literature gives shape to the topic, many limitations remain. For example, there are few peer-reviewed articles, and those that do exist are based on limited sample sizes and restricted population ranges. Although much can be learned from vocational support programs for individuals with ASD, descriptions to date are sparse, except for information about the Project SEARCH Model plus ASD supports (Wehman et al., 2013; Wehman, Schall, McDonough, et al., 2014).

In an exhaustive review of the literature on supported employment for adults with ASD, Westbrook and colleagues (2012) examined 8,528 citations for the first stage of review. Of these, a total of 77 citations were selected for second-stage full-text review of each study. Upon review of the full text for each of the 77 studies, only two studies—by Mawhood and Howlin (1999) and Garcia-Villamisar, Ross, and Wehman (2000)—were retained, having met the inclusion criteria, and both were quasi-experimental research designs. The studies described the effects of a supported employment intervention for adults with ASD on either employment outcomes or aspects of cognitive functioning. The nature of the data provided did not lend itself to a traditional meta-analysis. Given the number of studies, study designs, and the diversity of outcomes across the two studies, it was not possible to aggregate results across studies. Qualitative and other relevant research studies connected to the employment of persons with ASD were also reviewed by Westbrook and colleagues. This revealed some elements that may promote successful employment of individuals with ASD, including identification of the most appropriate work settings and positions and providing on-the-job supports and ongoing long-term support to the employer and the employee with ASD. Westbrook and colleagues also indicated that the costs for community-based employment interventions are greater than for other employment alternatives, such as sheltered, nonintegrated workshops. However, as Howlin, Alcock, and Burkin (2005) and others (e.g., Cimera & Cowan, 2009) reported, supported employment service interventions are becoming less expensive to deliver. These researchers also stressed that community-based integrated employment interventions such as supported employment, although expensive, expand options for mainstream social integration, competitive wages, and community involvement.

Since the publication of that review, Wehman and his colleagues have published more research on the transition to competitive employment and supported employment for individuals with ASD. As cited earlier, Wehman and colleagues (2012) reported on the effect of supported employment for 33 adults with ASD. Of those 33 participants, 27 achieved competitive employment. The authors emphasize the importance of an individualized approach in the implementation of a four-step supported employment model: (1) job seeker assessment and profile development, (2) career search and job development, (3) job site training, and (4) job retention. On the job the employee with ASD received individualized interventions. For example, the provision of behavior supports, intensive job training, planned fading, environmental modification, and the use of personal digital assistants to provide visual supports (Wehman et al., 2012).

In addition, Wehman and colleagues (2013) provided two quasi-experimental case studies in a description of their modification of Project SEARCH. This paper described the supports and services provided to two young people with ASD who were employed in a hospital setting upon the completion of an intensive school-to-work transition program. This study described additional supports added to the Project SEARCH model that resulted in successful competitive employment outcomes. Those supports included (1) weekly consultation with a behavior analyst, (2) consistent structure, (3) defining social expectations, (4) providing visual supports, (5) implementing self-management behavior interventions, (6) teaching social skills, and (7) monitoring student success through data collection (Wehman et al., 2013) These studies point to an emerging literature indicating that individuals with ASD can be competitively employed.

Customized Employment

Customized employment describes a myriad of strategies used to successfully facilitate employment. The *Federal Register* defines it as "individualizing the employment relationship between employees and employers in ways that meet the needs of both. It identifies the strengths, needs, and interests of people with disabilities, addresses the specific needs of employers, and is a process of negotiation." Essentially, it is often viewed as an umbrella term that consists of a variety of services and strategies that consider both the unmet needs of an employer and the goal of employment for the job seeker, based on her or his own preferences. In order to implement the service, funds are typically blended or braided from a variety of resources (e.g., state VR, individual training account funds from one-stop career centers, social security work incentives) The term was coined around 2001, when the Office of Disability Employment Policy, with the Department of Labor, funded several customized employment grants to help One-Stop Career Centers provide employment services to individuals with disabilities. Notably, customized employment embraces the very same values and practices as supported employment. It is a comprehensive, inclusive term to describe the services and techniques that have been developed to enhance the employment of all people who face challenges to work, including those with disabilities. Supported employment is an employment model exclusively for individuals with significant disabilities who are unemployed or underemployed.

Many of the strategies and services that make up customized employment have been in existence for years. Support strategies are based on each person's specific needs. For example, one individual with ASD may benefit from assistance in developing a resume or from role-playing interviews and select job placement assistance; another may benefit from more intensive job negotiations and on-the-job training to learn how to communicate with coworkers and use assistive technology, such as an iPad or smartphone application, to self-manage at work. The range and intensity of support the person receives will vary. In fact, in this approach, the person with the disability may not choose to disclose his or her disability to an employer, especially if no on-the-job support is needed. In other instances a vocational support professional, sometimes referred to as a personal representative, may be required to help the person develop a job and support the person at work once hired.

One of the primary tenets of customized employment is working closely with an employer in order to negotiate a job design for a specific person. This strategy is useful for many job seekers with ASD and is often used in supported employment, too. Jobs that are created should solve a problem for the employer and offer satisfaction to the employee. Using this strategy, any aspect of employment may be negotiated, such as the job duties, the work setting, the type of supervision or expectations, or more. Essentially, the employer and job seeker strike a deal to meet the need of both parties. How a job is designed can play a major role in determining whether a new hire with ASD is successful on the job and socially included. Often, newly negotiated jobs can help employers save money or enhance efficiency by improving productivity of others.

Customized employment may also include supporting an individual in developing his or her own business, working either in or outside the home. Some of these ventures have been referred to as microenterprises and may include a business within a business. Some examples of new start-ups include raising and selling meal worms to bird rescuers, laundering towels for a number of hair salons, delivering sandwiches from local shops to employees in area businesses, and selling magazines and newspapers in a coffee shop. Check out some other examples under "Training" at *worksupport.com* (Virginia Commonwealth University's Rehabilitation Research and Training Center [RRTC] website).

Natural Supports

Both supported employment and customized employment promote the use of natural supports at work. A mentor is one valuable resource in most companies who can guide and train new employees. Although some companies have formal programs, often mentoring is informal. Among other things, a mentor may make introductions to others, offer up tricks of the trade give insights into office politics, and provide support the new hire beyond initial training. Identifying a mentor, arranging a training schedule, and working as a consultant to train the mentor on how the new employee best learns and communicates are roles often assumed by the person's vocational support services professional such as a job coach or personal representative.

Meeting Individual Needs

Many individuals with ASD benefit from comprehensive, individualized services such as those offered in supported or customized employment approaches. Although understanding the requirements laid out in federal legislation for each practice is helpful, these policies do not ensure that individuals with ASD will receive high-quality services. Assisting each individual to make informed choices and achieve desired outcomes requires a structured and well-defined process. Neither supported nor customized employment services are ends unto themselves—both are dynamic and flexible processes.

Because many individuals with ASD have a complex set of needs, untapped talents, and variable skills, they often need a job developed to best suit these. In addition, once the person is hired, an individualized plan may be needed to teach him or her the necessary job skills and personal qualities, habits, and attitudes associated with a good employee such as time management, social communication skills, and teamwork. Furthermore, some will also require ongoing support throughout their employment. As a matter of fact, the provision of long-term follow-up is a key feature that distinguishes supported employment from other options (e.g., customized employment, job coaching services, job placement services). This section provides an overview of the best practices associated with career planning, as well as considerations for supporting an individual with ASD once he or she is hired. These practices are typically associated with high-quality vocational support services (i.e., supported and customized employment).

Career Planning

Many individuals with ASD who access vocational support service such as supported or customized employment may have limited experiences. Some individuals may arrive having previously been deemed as unemployable. Lacking experiences and being uncertain about interests and abilities may make it difficult to choose a career direction. Therefore, a first step is to find out where the person stands in terms of career awareness or exploration. Then, as indicated, time must be dedicated to getting to know the person and identifying his or her interests, strengths, and support needs. This step typically involves talking with the person and those who know him or her best, observing the person's abilities, and gauging his or her interest in various work and community settings. Sometimes a report may be reviewed. However, to be effective it must be recent and support an individual's career planning. For example, any report citing reasons a particular person with ASD cannot work or might be "better" suited for nonintegrated work options, such as sheltered work, would not be useful because supported employment is a service specifically designed to meet the needs of individuals with the most severe disabilities who are in need of ongoing supports, who have interrupted or no work histories, or who have intermittent employment records. On the other hand, functional vocational reports that list interests, abilities, and potential support leads from internships in high school or person-centered planning documents that state future dreams, strengths, and support needs could be extremely helpful. No matter what vocational support service (supported vs. customized) is used by a person with ASD, the goals of career exploration and assessment should relate to those in Table 11.1.

Some individuals may have interfering behavior, including agression or self-injurious behavior. A structured approach to addressing this issue while on the job should be developed and may require the expertise of a trained behavior analyst, positive behavior support facilitator, or psychologist. The implementation of effective behavior support plans can enable individuals with such challenges to work in their communities. Therefore, job coaches or others who support the person on the job will need to be skilled at developing and implementing effective behavior support plans or to have access to other professionals in this area (see also Tincani & Crozier, Chapter 7, this volume). Wehman and colleagues (2013)

TABLE 11.1. Career Exploration and Vocational Assessment Activities

- Expose the job seeker to a variety of work settings and activities to facilitate discovery of personal talents and strengths to help determine what an optimal job may look like (e.g., what should the setting, job tasks, supervision be?).
- Develop practical ideas about potential work supports that will help the job seeker learn to perform the job tasks and avoid or adapt to any environmental considerations.
- Empower the job seeker and/or his or her family and vocational support services professional (e.g., job coach or personal representative) to consider and establish a direction for job development (e.g., businesses to contact, how to present the job seeker, what to look for and avoid when developing a work opportunity).

described the implementation of positive behavior supports at work in their presentation of case studies for two young people who achieved competitive employment in a hospital.

Gathering career planning information during assessment should help the service provider, job seeker, and others begin to develop criteria (preferences, interests, abilities, environmental factors, support needs, etc.) about what would constitute a good job and work environment. With this information in mind, the next step is contacting employers to discuss their needs and possible opportunities to develop a job. Most employment service providers use a tool such as a vocational profile to guide them in collecting appropriate career planning information. The profile provides essential information in job development and can also be useful when developing a work support plan once the person is hired.

Career Search

Once support providers understand the characteristics of an optimal job match, they can contact businesses and talk with potential employers. It is important to note that jobs are *developed*. In other words, this is not a typical job search in which openings for positions are pursued and applications are then submitted. Instead, time is spent with an employer to look for ways the job seeker's strengths can meet a business's needs. Because relating to businesses is so important, the next section of the chapter is dedicated to this topic. Some important considerations for developing a suitable job match are offered in Table 11.2.

When a job seeker is hired, sometimes on-the-job support will be required from day 1 of employment (i.e., a supported employment approach). For example, the new hire may need specialized training and other work supports to learn the job and meet performance standards.

TABLE 11.2. Important Considerations for Job Matching

- Which job tasks would the job seeker prefer (Hagner & Cooney, 2005; Lattimore, Parsons, & Reid, 2006)?
- What settings would the job seeker prefer?
- What types of changes in tasks are required throughout the day? How will these affect the job seeker? What supports (including environmental or job description) may be needed?
- What supports will be needed to assist the new hire with learning to perform the job to meet expectations (Targett & Smith, 2009)?
- What are the social demands? Is there a high degree of interaction with others? How will these affect the job seeker? What supports may be needed (Wehman et al., 2009)?
- What are the communication demands? How will these affect the job seeker? What supports may be needed (Müller et al., 2003; Wehman et al., 2009)?
- How supportive is the workplace (e.g., interactions with supervisors and coworkers are friendly; personnel seem open, accepting, and supportive of one another; management open to modifications or adaptations to the environment or on-the-job support via job coach)?

Obviously, what support is needed will vary from person to person. Some examples of possible work supports for individuals with ASD are listed in Table 11.3. It is also important to note that the success of an employee with ASD may be contingent upon supervisors and coworkers who are willing to allow support from a vocational professional, and perhaps themselves. Under these circumstances, worksite personnel may need training in effective ways to communicate with and support the employee.

TABLE 11.3. Work Supports

- Systematic approach to instruction using specific prompting procedures; may include use of least prompts or time delay.
- Social and communication skills development and coaching by determining social and communication skills needed in various environments (e.g., how do people communicate, what are typical interactions, how do people get what is needed?) or analyzing problem behavior to identify social skills needed.
- Introducing structure into basic routines.
- Providing information for coworkers about ways to offer supports.
- Training individual to use personal calendar, appointment book, or a PDA/smartphone with scheduling and prompting applications.
- Creating a work station with minimal distractions or providing accommodations to minimize such distractions (e.g., closing a door, wearing headphones or sunglasses, turning off lights, wearing gloves).
- Implementing task checklists (with symbols or color coding).

Supporting Business

There is little doubt that employment will advance the well-being of individuals with ASD, their families, and their communities (Wehman et al., 2009). To make this happen, service delivery systems must adhere to best practices and, as needed, adopt new strategies to ensure integrated competitive employment for those served. Furthermore, employers must embrace the principle that all people, including those with significant disabilities, can and should work in their communities. For some employers, this concept will come naturally and essentially fit into the way they currently do business. On the other hand, some companies may need to develop a series of policies, practices, procedures, and guiding principles to support the employment of individuals with ASD within their workforce.

Regardless of the company's approach, one thing will remain consistent: Employers will want to see value. The employer will need to understand how hiring a specific job seeker in an existing, restructured, or created job will benefit the business. In situations in which the job seeker is receiving advocacy services, as in a supported employment approach, the employer will also need to understand the nature and benefit of the recommended vocational support services.

This means vocational support services must align practices, policies, and procedures, and fund services and supports that meet the needs of both the individual with ASD and the employer. In some instances, this may require organizations to close segregated day activity programs and sheltered workshops and start Employment First initiatives. It has been known for decades now that people with significant disabilities can succeed in the workforce when the right type, level, and intensity of support is available to them and the employers who choose to hire them (Wehman et al., 2013). Individuals with disabilities do not have to settle for performing piecemeal or contact work. They can and should look forward to the norm—real work for real pay in their communities (Rogan & Rinne, 2011). Again, vocational service providers must recognize both individuals with disabilities and employers as their customers. This is a necessary first step in promoting integrated, competitive employment for individuals with ASD.

Relating to Employers as Customers

If an individual with ASD is represented by a vocational support professional (e.g., employment specialist or job coach), employers must be viewed as a customer for his or her services. Thus it is critical to develop relationships with community employers. Often, when providers and employers do make contact, their attempts may be superficial at best. They simply accept the businesses practices for what they are (e.g., hiring individuals in accordance with the Americans with Disabilities Act) rather than addressing employer concerns and developing a relationship to adopt new and creative business practices that would bring value to the business while welcoming individuals with more significant disabilities in their workforce. Vocational professionals must have ongoing outreach, education, and follow-up with businesses to begin to develop relationships (Luecking, Fabian, & Tilson, 2004). They must also be prepared to learn about a business and its needs—by listening to one employer at a time.

To accomplish these goals, service providers must have skilled and talented vocational professionals leading the way. These staff members will understand how to relate to business and, as indicated, to convince an employer how hiring a particular individual with a disability can bring value to the workplace. They will also be skilled at providing support to an employer once the job seeker is hired. A study by Luecking, Cuozzo, and Buchanan (2006) supports the arguments for why it is essential for rehabilitation professionals to understand employer needs, circumstances, and perspectives. They found that employers cited the value of competent disability employment professionals who help identify operational improvements as a key reason for hiring and retaining individuals with intellectual and multiple disabilities, despite the fact that their employment was contingent on significant customization of job duties and conditions of work. Some other important employer views that professionals need to be aware of are cited in Table 11.4.

Representatives of individuals with disabilities must understand these views and other business perspectives, including how to address their concerns. They must also know how to make employers aware of the contributions a job seeker with ASD can make to their workforce. A brief discussion of each of these areas follows.

Addressing Employer Concerns

Service providers should be prepared to change a potential employer's perceptions about hiring someone with ASD by anticipating some likely concerns in advance. They should also recognize the fact that businesses will rarely admit the real reasons that keep them from hiring individuals with disabilities. "We are not hiring right now . . . we are not set up to train a person with a disability . . . we cannot create a job because it is not fair to our other employees . . . have the person apply for the position and if he is qualified we will call him . . . "—this list of possible employer objections to hiring someone with ASD could go on. In addition to these

TABLE 11.4. Employer Views

- There is a growing group of employers (e.g., Walmart, Walgreen's, Lowe's) that have made it part of their mission to hire individuals with disabilities (Nicholas, Krepcio, & Kauder, 2011). This is prompted by business-to-business initiatives such as the U.S. Business Leadership Network.
- Companies that have diversity programs do not include disability as an element of diversity. This indicates that, in spite of growing awareness, employers still do not attend to employing individuals with disabilities (Kessler Foundation/National Organization on Disability, 2010).
- Employers report that partnering with organizations experienced in disability issues and the ability of those organizations to positively contribute to the businesses' operations improve their success with workers with disabilities (Luecking, 2004).
- Employers are more positive about workers with intellectual disabilities when appropriate supports are provided (Morgan & Alexander, 2005).
- Employers report that disability employment personnel are not familiar with business practices (Luecking, 2008).
- Employers have difficulty making the connection between the mission of employment service providers and their business protocol and demands (Katz & Luecking, 2009).
- Employers indicate that the jargon that is characteristic of the disability employment field is mostly foreign to them (Luecking, Fabian, & Tilson, 2004).

reasons that circumvent moving forward with employment, the employer may have concerns or fears regarding hiring a person with a significant disability (Targett & Griffin, 2013). Individuals with ASD who choose to self-represent or vocational professionals representing them must be prepared to address these often present but typically unspoken fears. Table 11.5 briefly highlights some employer concerns and offers possible strategies to help overcome each. Fortunately, such attitudes are typically amenable to change. Professionals must understand these and other employer attitudes and perspectives in order to begin the transformation.

Presenting Job Seeker Assets

It is also important to project the job seeker's assets. Being open and honest about this and his or her needs for support are necessary for success. Hiding concerns or overestimating performance can lead to disaster. Full and open communication with potential employers is vital. Furthermore, employers and work environments that hold the promise of being a good fit must be targeted.

TABLE 11.5. Strategies to Address Employer Concerns

Possible concern	Strategy to address concern
How much will this cost? This question is associated with concerns related to cost associated with training the person and/or lost productivity and/or quality of work due to the new hire's inability to get the job done to standard. Employers may be stereotyping or misunderstanding the possibilities,	Assure the employer that doing a good job is of utmost importance; describe how the job tasks will get done by emphasizing personal assets and support; if a job coach is involved, emphasize his or her role related to providing on-the-job skills training and/or facilitating supports and long-term support at no cost to the employer. Provide examples of past successes; to move ahead, find a way to make sure connections are made with the job applicant(s).
What will happen if this does not work out? This question is associated with concerns related to repercussions for letting go an individual with a disability if he or she does not meet expectations.	Let the employer know that an opportunity is desired and if the position does not work out the person will look for a more suitable job. Explain how this would be handled in the same way as with other employees who do not work out. Reemphasize assets and the vocational support professional's role (i.e., job coach or personal representative).

Relaying information about a job seeker's abilities and interest to an employer becomes easy with proper planning. However, presenting the person's support needs may present more of a challenge. Before an employer is contacted on behalf of a job seeker with ASD, a discussion about disability and how this will be addressed should take place. Time should also be spent considering the factors listed in Table 11.6. Perhaps the most important thing for a vocational support provider to keep in mind is that talks with potential employers should focus on job performance and how the new hire will bring value to the business. Naturally, in order to have such discussions, the job seeker or vocational support

TABLE 11.6. Tips on Describing Job Seeker

- Avoid labels and describe disability in terms of support needs. *For Susan to do well on the job, she will need a job coach to help her learn the job.*
- Describe abilities in functional terms. *Susan is very reliable and pays attention to detail.* Rather than *Susan is autistic and does not like change. She needs a routine and a place to take a timeout if she gets overwhelmed.*
- Describe services offered. *We are available to work with you and Susan as much as you need.* Then go on to describe the service and state that it is at no cost to the employer.

professional will have to learn about a specific business's operations and needs in advance. This requirement means spending time with the employer and is applicable whether the job being investigated happens to be an existing position or a job creation.

After describing a job seeker, the vocational support professional will have to ask the employer about next steps. Sometimes, an interview will be necessary. However, it may take an alternative format. For instance, for a job seeker receiving advocacy-level services such as supported employment, he or she might be introduced to the employer and tour the workplace. The introduction may also be paired with video resumes or other tools that highlight the job seeker's assets. These alternative-format interviews can be very helpful to individuals with ASD, who frequently have social communication challenges that may impede their ability to "sell themselves."

Developing Knowledge and Skills to Foster Relationships

As mentioned earlier, employers are interested in meeting their needs. We end this section with some advice on what vocational professionals must know prior to connecting with employers is offered in Table 11.7. These tips have been derived from the limited literature on this important topic and our personal experiences.

TABLE 11.7. Tips for Making Employer Connections

Be prepared by gaining the knowledge and developing the skills needed to . . .

- Address general employer concerns about hiring individuals with ASD.
- Relate job seeker's assets and how they bring value to business.
- Relate potential supports needed to help job seeker succeed in a workplace.
- Explore business needs with an eye toward recommending a "customized" job by looking for opportunities for a new hire to save the employer money, or help the employer make money, help the employer's operation run more smoothly or efficiently.
- Listen to an employer and probe for information about needs.
- Explain support services available to the employer in a simple and straightforward way that makes sense to business and is void of any disability service provider jargon.
- Get familiar with business terminology and use it during talks with employers.
- Influence workplace operations to create a demand for job seekers and employment services by emphasizing value and mutual benefit.
- Build lasting relationships by participating in business events and staying in touch with contacts even when they have not hired.
- Offer something (training, resources, job analysis, etc.) to the employer prior to asking for something in return (meeting a job seeker).

Above all, the reader should note that preparation, flexibility, and professionalism are critical when developing relationships with businesses and assisting them in their pursuit to hire and support individuals with ASD. Taking the necessary time to further investigate the best practices associated with supported employment and customized employment, should also help vocational professionals get ready to do business with business. Then calling on businesses will be the next step forward in the process of assisting individuals with ASD with gaining and maintaining a real job for real pay!

To further illustrate the concepts presented in this chapter, the following case study highlights implementation of supported employment services.

Case Example: James

James is a 22-year-old male who has a diagnosis of ASD. He received his diagnosis when he was 3 years old and has been in self-contained special education classes throughout his educational career. James lives at home with his mother, father, and younger sister (16 years old). James had significant deficits in many adaptive skill areas and in his social-emotional development and was significantly behind his peers. James was described by his parents as a sweet young man who was very sensitive to the environment around him. If their home was calm, he was calm, but if anyone in the family was anxious or loud he became very agitated. This agitation, his parents explained, was never directed toward others; rather, he exhibited self-stimulatory behaviors, such as rocking back and forth while sitting or twisting his torso when standing. When he was extremely agitated or anxious, he would become self-injurious and bite his hands and arms. He would often bite hard enough to draw blood. Other times he would screech or scream hysterically. Calming him down was difficult and generally necessitated removing him from the environment or taking him for a walk outside. James is able to speak in full sentences; however, he struggles with social interactions and has difficulty maintaining a conversation. He rarely asks for help and mostly replies with a very brief "yes" or "no" response.

Job Seeker Profile and Assessment

Each individual with ASD has strengths and skills that can benefit an employer. The key to unveiling those strengths is completing a comprehensive profile on the individual. These profiles can be developed through a variety of informal and formal measures, including interviews, observations, situational assessments, and interest inventories. Compiling this information can establish the groundwork needed for job exploration, development, and supports.

Through situational assessments, interviews, and observations, the job coach found James to be most calm in smaller stores, restaurants, and places that played soothing music. He could lift a fair amount of weight, and when given the task of organizing plants and planting materials in a large home improvement store, he worked consistently for over 2 hours with minimal redirection. He removed dead leaves, watered plants, and replenished 40-pound bags of soil and fertilizer. He took a break to sit every 20 minutes for 5 minutes. He followed directions on a visual schedule with intermittent prompting and supervision. When he was greeted by other employees or customers, he waved and said "hi." When an announcement was given over the public address system, he screeched, plugged his ears, and began rocking until it was over and he was redirected to the task.

Job Development and Career Search

The career search phase consists of the job coach and the individual working together to identify employment options based on the results of the assessments and the strengths and desires of the individual.

James excelled at his situational assessment in the garden department at a large home improvement store. He enjoyed being outside and completing the tasks associated with that department. He did not like going into the larger part of the store and was agitated by the noise of the loudspeaker.

Currently, that store was not hiring; however, through careful observation, the job coach found that many of the plants were not being cared for and that several of the shelves were running low on stock. When the job coach asked whose responsibility it was to take care of the plants, the response was, "whoever has time." Additionally, restocking only happened at the end of the day or if a customer needed an item that was not on the shelf.

Seeing a need, the job coach asked the store manager to perhaps create a position to take care of plants and alert the garden manager of low inventory. The manager liked this idea.

Job Site Training and Support

After a job has been secured, the training and support phase begins. The job coach helped James learn the skills, routines, expectations, and responsibilities of his new job. This included identifying what supports were needed, such as visual schedules, reinforcement, prompting, and fading support strategies.

James worked 4 days a week for 3 hours each day. During this time, he would water plants, remove dead leaves, and check inventory. To alert the manager that inventory was low, he would circle the picture of the item on his list. Once he completed this, the list would be put in the garden manager's box.

Because James had the potential to engage in self-injurious behaviors, a positive behavior support plan was developed so those involved would know what needed to be done if this behavior were to occur. It was also noted that James had minimal sight word recognition; because of this a visual schedule was implemented with pictures of the tasks that needed to be completed, embedded breaks, and other needed routines. In addition to pictures, James was trained to use an iPod Touch to support independence. Until he became fluent with this device, the pictures were the support.

Long-Term Supports to Aid Job Retention

Planning for ongoing long-term support services is essential for some individuals with ASD to maintain and advance in their jobs. The types of supports needed range in intensity based on the needs of the individual and the business. For example, if a person is successful with current job duties, additional tasks may be added to his or her routine that may require adjustments to supports. Additionally, changes in an individual's life may require community or targeted supports away from the job, such as housing or development of leisure activities.

James used the iPod and other supports to get his job done. His supervisor and colleagues reported that he was pleasant to work with. Due to his success, James was asked to take on additional responsibilities like helping customers load their cars. This required the job coach to make changes to his iPod schedule and provide specific customer interaction/social skill instruction that included role playing.

Conclusion

In summary, although promising practices are emerging, current research overwhelmingly demonstrates disappointing employment outcomes for adults with ASD. The vast majority are unemployed and, for those who do have gainful employment, underemployment is common.

The increased prevalence of ASD coupled with unique social, communication, and behavioral characteristics translate into the need for individualized support services to help them achieve success at work. For now, we do know that consideration of individual characteristics, including strengths, needs, and specific interests, coupled with implementation of proper supports, can result in successful and ongoing employment. We also know that employers must also be supported in employing individuals with ASD. Finally, we know that Employment First approaches such as supported employment and customized employment hold much promise to improve outcomes for individuals with ASD.

ACKNOWLEGMENTS

Preparation of this chapter was supported in part by Cooperative Agreement No. H133A100007 from TransCen, Inc., and by the National Institute on Disability and Rehabilitation Research, U.S. Department of Education.

REFERENCES

Barker, E. T., Hartley, S. L., Seltzer, M. M., Floyd, F. J., Greenberg, J. S., Orsmond, G. I. (2011). Trajectories of emotional well-being in mothers and adolescents and adults with autism. *Developmental Psychology, 47*(2), 551–561.

Barnhill, G. P. (2007). Outcomes in adults with Asperger syndrome. *Focus on Autism and Other Developmental Disabilities, 22*(2), 116–126.

Bolman, W. M. (2008). Brief report: 25-year follow-up of a high-functioning autistic child. *Journal of Autism and Developmental Disorders, 38,* 181–183.

Camarena, P. M., & Sarigiani, P. A. (2009). Postsecondary educational aspirations of high-functioning adolescents with autism spectrum disorders and their parents. *Focus on Autism and Other Developmental Disabilities, 24*(2), 115–128.

Cameto, R. Marder, C., Wagner, M., & Cardoso, D. (2003). *Youth employment: A report from the National Longitudinal Transition Study–2 (NLTS-2).* Menlo Park, CA: SRI International.

Centers for Disease Control and Prevention. (2012). Prevalence of autism spectrum disorders: Autism and developmental disabilities monitoring network, 14 sites, 2008. *Morbidity and Mortality Weekly Report, 61*(SS3), 1–19.

Cimera, R. E., & Cowan, R. J. (2009). The costs of services and employment outcomes achieved by adults with autism in the US. *Autism, 13*(3), 285–302.

Cimera, R. E., Wehman, P., West, M., & Burgess, S. (2012). Do sheltered workshops enhance employment outcomes for adults with autism spectrum disorder? *Autism, 16*(1), 87–94.

Daston, M., Riehle, J. E., & Rutkowski, S. (2012). *High school transition that works: Lessons learned from Project SEARCH.* Baltimore: Brookes.

Dew, D. W., & Alan, G. M. (Eds.). (2007). *Rehabilitation of individuals with autism spectrum disorders* (Institute on Rehabilitation Issues Monograph No. 32). Washington, DC: George Washington University, Center for Rehabilitation Counseling Research Education.

Dogoe, M. S., Banda, D. R., Lock, R. H., & Feinstein, R. (2011). Teaching generalized reading of product warning labels to young people with autism using the constant time delay procedure. *Education and Training in Autism and Developmental Disabilities, 46*(2), 204–213.

Garcia-Villamisar, D., & Hughes, C. (2007). Supported employment improves cognitive performance in adults with autism. *Journal of Intellectual Disability Research, 51*(2), 142–150.

Garcia-Villamisar, D., Ross, D., & Wehman, P. (2000). Clinical differential analysis of persons with autism: A follow-up study. *Journal of Vocational Rehabilitation, 14*, 183–185.

Garcia-Villamisar, D., Wehman, P., & Navarro, M. D. (2002). Changes in the quality of autistic people's life that work in supported and sheltered employment: A 5-year follow-up study. *Journal of Vocational Rehabilitation, 17*(4), 309.

Gentry, T., Lau, S., Molinelli, A., Fallen, A., Kriner, R. (2012). The Apple iPod Touch as a vocational support aid for adults with autism: Three case studies. *Journal of Vocational Rehabilitation, 37*(2), 75–85.

Gentry, T., Wallace, J., Kvarfordt, C., & Lynch, K. B. (2010). Personal digital assistants as cognitive aids for high school students with autism: Results from a community-based trial. *Journal of Vocational Rehabilitation, 32*(2), 101–107.

Gerhardt, P. F., & Holmes, D. L. (2005). Employment: Options and issues for adolescents and adults with autism spectrum disorders. In F. R. Volkmar, R. Paul, A. Klin, & D. Cohen (Eds.), *Handbook of autism and pervasive developmental disorders: Vol. 2. Assessment, interventions and policy* (3rd ed., pp. 1087–1101). Hoboken, NJ: Wiley.

Hagner, D., & Cooney, B. F. (2005). "I do that for everybody": Supervising employees with autism. *Focus on Autism and Other Developmental Disabilities, 20*(2), 91–97.

Hendricks, D. (2010). Employment and adults with autism spectrum disorders: Challenges and strategies for success. *Journal of Voctional Rehabilitation, 32*, 125–134.

Hendricks, D., & Wehman, P. (2009). Transition from school to adulthood for youth with autism spectrum disorders: Review and recommendations. *Focus on Autism and Other Developmental Disabilities, 24*(2), 77–88.

Henninger, N., & Taylor, J. (2012). Outcomes in adults with autism spectrum disorders: A historical perspective. *Autism, 17*(1), 103–116.

Hillier, A., Campbell, H., Mastriana, K., Izzo, M., Kool-Tucker, A., Cherry, L., et al. (2007). Two-year evaluation of a vocational support program for adults on the autism spectrum. *Career Development for Exceptional Individuals, 30*(1), 35–47.

Hillier, A., Fish, T., Cloppert, P., & Beversdorf, D. Q. (2007). Outcomes of a social and vocational skills support group for adolescents and young adults on the autism spectrum. *Focus on Autism and Other Developmental Disabilities, 22*(2), 107–115.

Hillier, A. J., Fish, T., Siegel, J. H., & Beversdorf, D. Q. (2011). Social and vocational skills training reduces self-reported anxiety and depression among young adults on the autism spectrum. *Journal of Developmental and Physical Disabilities, 23*(3), 267–276.

Holwerda, A., van der Klink, J. J., Groothoff, J. W., & Brouwer, S. (2012). Predictors for work participation in individuals with autism spectrum disorders. *Journal of Occupational Rehabilitation, 22*(3), 333–352.

Howlin, P. (2000). Outcome in adult life for more able individuals with autism or asperger syndrome. *Autism, 4*(1), 63–83.

Howlin, P., Alcock, J., & Burkin, C. (2005). An 8-year follow-up of a specialist-supported employment service for high-ability adults with autism or Asperger syndrome. *Autism: International Journal of Research and Practice, 9*(5), 533–549.

Hurlbutt, K., & Chalmers, L. (2002). Adults with autism speak out: Perceptions of their life experiences. *Focus on Autism and Other Developmental Disabilities, 17*(2), 103–111.

Hurlbutt, K., & Chalmers, L. (2004). Employment and adults with Asperger syndrome. *Focus on Autism and Other Developmental Disabilities, 19*(4), 215–222.

Jennes-Coussens, M., Magill-Evans, J., & Koning, C. (2006). The quality of life of young men with Asperger syndrome: A brief report. *Autism, 10*, 403–414.

Kandalaft, M. R., Dibehbani, N., Krawczyk, D. C., Allen, T. T., & Chapman, S. B. (2013). Virtual reality social cognition training for young adults with high functioning autism. *Journal of Autism and Developmental Disorders, 43*(1), 34–44.

Katz, E., & Luecking, R. (2009). Collaborating and coordinating with employers (Issue Brief No. 3). New Brunswick, NJ: Rutgers University, National Technical Assistance and Research Leadership Center.

Kessler Foundation/National Organization on Disability. (2010). *2010 survey of employment of Americans with disabilities*. New York: Harris Interactive.

Lattimore, L. P., Parsons, M. B., & Reid, D. H. (2006). Enhancing job site training of supported workers with autism: A reemphasis on simulation. *Journal of Applied Behavior Analysis, 39*, 91–102.

Lawer, L., Brusilovskiy, E., Salzer, M. S., & Mandell, D. S. (2009). Use of vocational rehabilitative services among adults with autism. *Journal of Autism and Developmental Disorders, 39*, 487–494.

Luecking, R. (2004). *Essential tools: In their own words: Employer perspectives on youth with disabilities in the workplace*. Minneapolis: University of Minnesota, Institute on Community Integration, National Center on Secondary Education and Transition.

Luecking, R. (2008). Emerging employer views of people with disabilities and the future of job development. *Journal of Vocational Rehabilitation, 29*, 3–13.

Luecking, R., Cuozzo, L., & Buchanan, L. (2006). Demand-side workforce needs and the potential for job customization. *Journal of Applied Rehabilitation Counseling, 37*, 5–13.

Luecking, R. G., Fabian, E. S., & Tilson, G. P. (2004). *Working relationships: Creating career opportunities for job seekers with disabilities through employer partnerships.* Baltimore: Brookes.

Mawhood, L., & Howlin, P. (1999). The outcome of a supported employment scheme for high functioning adults with autism or Asperger syndrome. *Autism, 3,* 229–254.

Mechling, L. C., Gast, D. L., & Seid, N. H. (2009). Using a personal digital assistant to increase independent task completion by students with autism spectrum disorder. *Journal of Autism and Developmental Disorders, 39*(10), 1420–1434.

Mechling, L. C., & Seid, N. H. (2011). Use of a hand-held personal digital assistant (PDA) to self-prompt pedestrian travel by young adults with moderate intellectual disabilities. *Education and Training in Autism and Developmental Disorders, 46*(2), 220–237.

Migliore, A., & Zalewska, A. (2012a). *Prevalence of youth with autism who received vocational rehabilitation services. DataNote Series* (Data Note 42). Boston: University of Massachusetts, Institute for Community Inclusion.

Migliore, A., & Zalewska, A. (2012b). *What are the employment experiences of youth with autism after high school?* (Data Note 40). Boston: University of Massachusetts, Institute for Community Inclusion.

Morgan, R., & Alexander, M. (2005). The employer's perception: Employment of individuals with developmental disabilities. *Journal of Vocational Rehabilitation, 23,* 39–49.

Müller, E., Schuler, A., Burton, B. A., & Yates, G. B. (2003). Meeting the vocational support needs of individuals with Asperger syndrome and other autism spectrum disabilities. *Journal of Vocational Rehabilitation, 18,* 163–175.

Newman, L., Wagner, M., Cameto, R., & Knokey, A. M. (2009). *The post-high school outcomes of youth with disabilities up to 4 years afer high school. A report from the National Longitudinal Transition Study–2* (NCSER 2009–3017). Menlo Park, CA: SRI International.

Nicholas, R., Krepcio, K., & Kauder, R. (2011). *Ready and able: Addressing labor market needs and building productive careers for people with disabilities through collaborative approaches.* New Brunswick, NJ: Rutgers University, National Technical Assistance and Research Leadership Center.

Nuehring, M. L., & Sitlington, P. L. (2003). Transition as a vehicle: Moving from high school to an adult vocational service provider. *Journal of Disability Policy Studies, 14*(1), 23–35.

O'Brien, M., & Daggett, J. A. (2006). Beyond the autism diagnosis: A professional's guide to helping families. Baltimore: Brookes.

Office of Autism Research Coordination, National Institute of Mental Health & Thomson Reuters, Inc., on Behalf of the Interagency Autism Coordinating Committee. (2012, July). IACC/OARC autism spectrum disorder research publications analysis report: The global landscape of autism research. Retrieved from *https://iacc.hhs.gov/publications-analysis/july2012/index.shtml.*

Rogan, P., & Rinne, S. (2011). National call for organizational change from sheltered to integrated employment. *Intellectual and Developmental Disabilities, 49*(4), 248–260.

Ruef, M. B., & Turnbull, A. P. (2002). The perspectives of individuals with cognitive disabilities and/or autism on their lives and their problem behavior. *Journal of the Association for Persons with Severe Handicaps, 27*(2), 125–140.

Schall, C. (2010). Positive behavior support: Supporting adults with autism spectrum disorders in the workplace. *Journal of Vocational Rehabilitation, 32*(2), 109–115.

Schall, C., Targett, P., & Wehman, P. (2013). Applications for youth with autism disorders. In P. Wehman (Ed.), *Life beyond the classroom: Transition strategies for young people with disabilities* (5th ed.). Baltimore: Brookes.

Schall, C., Wehman, P., & McDonough, J. (2012). Transition from school to work for students with autism spectrum disorders: Understanding the process and achieving better outcomes. *Pediatric Clinics of North America, 59*(1), 189–202.

Schaller, J., & Yang, N. K. (2005). Competitive employment for people with autism: Correlates of successful closure in competitive and supported employment. *Rehabilitation Counseling Bulletin, 49*(1), 4–16.

Shattuck, P. T., Narendorf, S. C., Cooper, B., Sterzing, P. R., Wagner, M., & Taylor, J. L. (2012). Postsecondary education and employment among youth with an autism spectrum disorder. *Pediatrics, 129*(6), 1042–1049.

Shattuck, P. T., Wagner, M., Narendorf, S., Sterzing, P., & Hensley, M. (2011). Post-high school service use among young adults with an autism spectrum disorder. *Archives of Pediatric and Adolescent Medicine, 165*(2), 141–146.

Smith, M. D., & Philippen, L. R. (1999). Community integration and supported employment. In D. E. Berkell Zager (Ed.), *Autism: Identification, education, and treatment* (pp. 493–514). Mahwah, NJ: Erlbaum.

Southall, C., & Gast, D. L. (2011). Self-management procedures: A comparison across the autism spectrum. *Education and Training in Autism and Developmental Disorders, 46*(2), 155–171.

Sperry, L. A., & Mesibov, G. B. (2005). Perceptions of social challenges of adults with autism spectrum disorder. *Autism, 9*(4), 362–376.

Targett, P., & Griffin, C. (2013). Developing jobs for young people with disabilities. In P. Wehman (Ed.), *Life beyond the classroom: Transition strategies for young people with disabilities* (5th ed.). Baltimore: Brookes.

Taylor, J. L., & Seltzer, M. M. (2011). Employment and postsecondary education activities for young adults with autism spectrum disorders during the transition to adulthood. *Journal of Autism and Developmental Disorders, 41*, 566–574.

U.S. Department of Labor, Office of Disability Employment Policy. (n.d.). Employment First. Retrieved June 6, 2013, from *www.dol.gov/odep/topics/EmploymentFirst.htm*.

Wehman, P., Datlow Smith, M., & Schall, C. (2009). *Autism and the transition to adulthood: Success beyond the classroom.* Baltimore: Brookes.

Wehman, P., Lau, S., Molinelli, A., Brooke, V., Thompson, K., Moore, C., et al. (2012). Supported employment for young adults with autism spectrum disorder: Preliminary data. *Research and Practice for Persons with Severe Disabilities, 37*, 160–169.

Wehman, P., Schall, C., Brooke, V., & McDonough, J. (2012, April 26). *The effect of Project SEARCH and supported employment on employment outcomes for adults with ASD.* Lecture presented at the NARRTC annual conference, Alexandria, VA.

Wehman, P., Schall, C., Carr, S., Targett, P., West, M., & Cifu, G. (in press). Transition from school to adulthood for youth with autism spectrum disorder: What we know and what we need to know. *Journal of Disability Policy Studies.*

Wehman, P., Schall, C., McDonough, J., Molinelli, A., Riehle, E., Ham, W., et al. (2013). Project SEARCH for youth with autism spectrum disorders: Increasing competitive employment on transition from high school. *Journal of Positive Behavior Interventions, 15*(3), 144–155.

Westbrook, J., Nye, C., Fong, C., Wan, J., Cortopassi, T, & Martin, F. (2012). Adult employment assistance services for persons with autism spectrum disorders: Effects on employment outcomes. Available at *http://ideas.repec.org/mpr/mprres/7398.html.*

CHAPTER 12

• • • • • •

Facilitating Successful Independent Living Skills for Adults with High-Functioning Autism Spectrum Disorders

• **Brenda Smith Myles, Daniel Steere, Cathy Pratt, Ruth Aspy, Barry G. Grossman, and Shawn A. Henry**

Transitioning to college was difficult for Steve, a 21-year-old young adult with high-functioning autism. Even though he was older than the typical entry-level college-age student, Steve and his family decided that dorm living was a good option for him, both financially and socially. Steve declined to disclose his autism to the university's department of disability services. Steve was assigned a roommate. He rarely left his room except to go to class. Steve did not socialize with others and did not know the names of anyone on his hall. He had a difficult time getting along with his roommate, Mark. Steve demanded complete silence when he studied—even the sound of music coming from Mark's headphones upset him. He was also disturbed by the sound of the beds and asked Mark not to turn over during the night. One day he told Mark that his alarm was too loud. He asked Mark to turn it down or muffle it under his pillow. When Mark explained that there was no volume setting and that he could not sleep with a clock under his pillow, Steve said, "I don't see why you won't compromise with me!" Small changes, such as Mark's having company over or occasionally putting his backpack in a place where he did not normally put it, caused Steve to be upset and demand that it be moved. He commented, "It upsets my homeostasis!" Steve was disorganized and frequently lost books, keys, and even freshly washed clothing. One day, he "lost" his sweater. He systematically knocked on every door on his floor until he found Mark. Steve yelled, "Where did you put my sweater?" Mark was surprised but told Steve that it was hanging to dry by the window. Instead of thanking Mark for his help, Steve blamed Mark for "stealing" his sweater. Steve became increasingly anxious over the course of the semester and had difficulty concentrating when studying. Instead of focusing on academics, he often spent extended periods of time playing chess online or reading *Star Trek* novels. He felt uncomfortable attending large classes and would not ask for help from the professor or teaching assistants. Despite the fact that Steve was very intelligent, his grades were poor. When he talked to his parents, Steve reported that his classes were going well, but that Mark was unreasonable. His parents visited twice and felt that Steve was making progress. Steve received C's in all of his classes that semester, and during the semester break he told his parents that he had no friends and was overwhelmed and depressed. Steve and his parents met with a therapist whom he had seen in the past to discuss how to make the following semester a success, with a focus on developing a social network around recreation and leisure activities.

Henninger and Taylor (2013), in a historical review, reported that outcomes for adults with autism from the 1960s to the present were generally consistent in terms of independent living, developing and maintaining meaningful relationships, and employment. That is, the majority did not experience a high quality of life and were specifically identified as having poor to very poor outcomes. This finding has been validated by self-reports of individuals with high-functioning autism spectrum disorders (HFASD) (Muller, Schuler, & Yates, 2008), as well as by the National Longitudinal Transition Study (NLTS2; Shattuck et al., 2012).

Two studies, however, have shown more encouraging results. The first, conducted by Farley and colleagues (2009), revealed a relatively high level of employment and participation in social activities, along with optimistic self-perceptions among the adults with HFASD. The authors ascribed these results to participants' membership in the Church of Jesus Christ of Latter Day Saints, which places a strong emphasis on community inclusion. In another study, Billstedt, Gillberg, and Gillberg (2005) found average to good outcomes in adults that they attributed to an "autism-friendly environment." This was defined as (1) individualized training with specific skill development, (2) structured environments that meet adult needs, (3) meaningful occupation, and (4) autism knowledge among those who supported the adults on the spectrum.

How can these outcomes be replicated for adults with HFASD? For adults with HFASD who have limitless potential, the process begins with identifying the environmental demands and instructional needs, followed by developing and implementing supports and instruction that are based on individual interests, strengths, and needs, and finally embedding evidence-based practices into a comprehensive plan.

Environmental Demands and Instruction

In order to live as independently as possible in environments of their own choice, individuals with HFASD need to develop skills in a number of different areas. The following skills are deemed important for home living: planning and preparing meals; self-care, bathing, and hygiene; cleaning and care of the home; cleaning and care of clothing; handheld technologies, including telephone and personal digital assistants (PDAs); texting and social media use; leisure activities; safety procedures; time management and scheduling; and self-advocacy, negotiation, and compromising (Agran, 2012; Armstrong, Gentry, & Wehman, 2013; Mechling, 2011; Steere, Burcroff, & DiPipi-Hoy; 2012; Targett & Smith, 2009). Others have identified essential skills that include financial management (e.g., planning bank services, budgeting, managing credit card account information); accessing transportation; exercising; engaging in hobbies and recreation; self-advocacy, negotiating, and compromising; and developing and maintaining relationships with others, including sexual relationships (cf. Agran, 2012; Organization for Autism Research, 2006; Wehmeyer & Webb, 2012). Relationship skills include the ability to get along with others in a home or neighborhood. This can include negotiating chores and duties among people who live together or agreeing upon solutions to challenges that arise among neighbors (e.g., music that is played too loudly at night). Relationship skills is an area in which instruction in appropriate social interaction, including the hidden curriculum or unwritten rules (Myles, Endow, & Mayfield, 2013), is essential.

It is clear that a wide range of skills is necessary for independent living success. These skills include the completion of activities within the home (e.g., cooking a meal, showering, cleaning the living areas, and socializing with others), as well as planning for activities that will take place outside of the home and in the community (e.g., reviewing a bus route in preparation for a trip or writing future events on a calendar) (DiPipi-Hoy, Jitendra, & Kern, 2009; Test, Richter, & Walker, 2012).

In addition, all of the activities listed here increase in functionality when they can be completed in different ways, so it is essential that the generalization of skills be addressed in teaching them. For example, simple meals call for different preparation directions, so the *generalized* ability to follow meal preparation directions leads to increased choices in what to eat. Likewise, the ability to manage time using different approaches (following a "to-do" list; using a paper calendar, a written agenda, or a smartphone) increases the functionality of time-management skills. For this reason, the use of general case programming guidelines to select representative examples of activities is a valuable evidence-based practice (EBP), as described next.

Evidence-Based Practices

Limited research has been conducted on evidence-based strategies and techniques that can be used to teach and support use of the aforementioned skills. However, research has identified evidence-based practices (EBPs) for children, adolescents, and young adults that can easily be translated into work, home, and community for adults with HFASD (Centers for Medicare and Medicaid Services, 2010; National Autism Center, 2009; National Professional Development Center on Autism Spectrum Disorders, 2009). EBPs that translate well into adult environments are described in Table 12.1.

In addition to identifying practices supported by research that promote independent living skills, it is also critical to identify and implement strategies that adults themselves see as essential. Muller and colleagues (2008) summarized the supports that adults on the spectrum identified as helpful. The authors grouped these interventions into four categories: (1) external supports, (2) communication supports, (3) self-initiated supports, and (4) attitudinal supports. These are described further in Table 12.2.

Comprehensive Planning

To maximize positive outcomes, EBPs must be carefully selected to meet individual strengths, needs, and interests, and they must be implemented well in all settings (Fixsen, Blasé, Horner, & Sugai, 2009). This type of comprehensive implementation usually requires changes in the daily activities of staff, related service providers, and family members. Thus it takes cohesive planning, clearly defined objectives, and professional development of those who interact with and support the adult with HFASD to ensure that the chosen strategies are implemented with fidelity and across all settings.

To date, no system has been able to accomplish these lofty goals. This chapter introduces two linked comprehensive planning models—the Ziggurat Model (Aspy & Grossman, 2011) and the Comprehensive Autism Planning System (CAPS; Henry & Myles, 2013; Myles, Grossman, Aspy, Henry, & Coffin, 2007)—that meet these goals.

TABLE 12.1. Evidence-Based Practices

Intervention	CMS	NAC	NPDC
Antecedent interventions			
Interventions put in place before the occurrence of a behavior to prevent it from occurring			
Antecedent package	×	×	×
Structured teaching	×		×
Visual supports			×
Schedules	×	×	
Applied behavior analysis interventions			
Interventions based on the science of applied behavior analysis			
Comprehensive behavioral package	×	×	
Differential reinforcement			×
Discrete trial training			×
Extinction			×
Prompting			×
Time delay			×
Modeling, including video modeling	×	×	×
Reinforcement			×
Response, interruption, redirection			×
Task analysis			×
Functional behavioral assessment			×
Cognitive interventions			
Interventions designed to change negative or unrealistic thought patterns/behaviors to positively influence emotions/life functioning			
Cognitive-behavioral intervention package	×		
Multicomponent interventions			
Interventions involving a combination of multiple treatment procedures that are derived from different fields of interest or different theoretical orientations			
Multicomponent package	×		
Naturalistic teaching strategies			
Instructional strategies used in the individual's natural environments that focus on play, conversation, providing reinforcement, and direct/natural reinforcement.			
Naturalistic teaching strategies	×	×	×
Pivotal response treatment	×	×	×

(continued)

TABLE 12.1. *(continued)*

Intervention	CMS	NAC	NPDC
Non-provider-based interventions			
Interventions provided by parents and peers			
Parent-implemented interventions			×
Peer-training package	×	×	×
Self-management			
Interventions that teach individuals with ASD to regulate their behavior			
Self-management	×	×	×
Social and communication interventions			
Psychosocial interventions that involve targeting some combination of impairments such as pragmatic communication skills and the inability to successfully read social situations			
Joint Attention	×	×	
Picture Exchange Communication System	×		×
Social communication intervention	×		
Social skills groups			×
Social skills package	×		
Story-based intervention package	×	×	
Social narratives			×
Speech-generating devices			×
Technology-based interventions			
The presentation of instructional materials using the medium of computers or related technologies			
Technology-based treatment	×		
Computer-aided instruction			×

Note. NAC, National Autism Center; CMS, Centers for Medicare and Medicaid Services; NPDC, National Professional Development Center on ASD.

The Ziggurat Model

The Ziggurat Model is a comprehensive planning model for individuals with ASD based on the premise that in order for a program to be successful for an individual with ASD, his or her unique needs and strengths must be identified and then directly linked to interventions (Aspy & Grossman, 2011). Therefore, the Ziggurat Model utilizes adults' strengths to address true needs or underlying deficits that result in social, emotional,

TABLE 12.2. Supports Recommended by Adults with HFASD

External supports

- Shared interest activities
- Joint focus activities that require little interaction, such as watching movies or television
- Structured social activities that include a high level of predictability and known social scripts
- One-to-one activities
- Facilitated social interactions, such as having an introduction to an activity by a sibling or friends
- Opportunities to observe and model appropriate behaviors

Communication supports

- Alternative modes of communication, including e-mail, texting, chat groups, and online role-playing games
- Direct and specific communication
- Instruction on how to interpret and use social cues

Self-initiated supports

- Creative and improvisational activities, such as participating in theater groups or bands or playing games (e.g., Dungeons and Dragons)
- Physical and/or outdoor activities that include hiking, running, yoga, and sailing
- Organized religion or spiritual activities
- Time alone
- Objects as bridges to social interactions, such as bringing musical instruments to parties in order to "jam," carrying small objects that can become a conversational topic, or exchanging gifts

Attitudinal supports

- Patient and caring attitudes
- Respect for individual differences and nonjudgmental actions
- Willingness to initiate interactions with greater responsibility on neurotypical individuals for developing and maintaining the relationship

---

and behavioral concerns. In doing so, the Ziggurat approach centers on a hierarchical system consisting of five levels—sensory differences and biological needs, reinforcement, structure and visual/tactile supports, task demands, and skills to teach—that must be addressed for an intervention plan to be comprehensive (see Figure 12.1). The model can be used in two ways: (1) as a planning tool for education, home, workplace, and/or community or (2) as a functional behavior assessment.

When designing a comprehensive program, it is essential to consider the *context of the underlying ASD*. Unfortunately, this is overlooked all too often. Traditional views of program planning that often focus on interventions that address only surface or observable behavior without

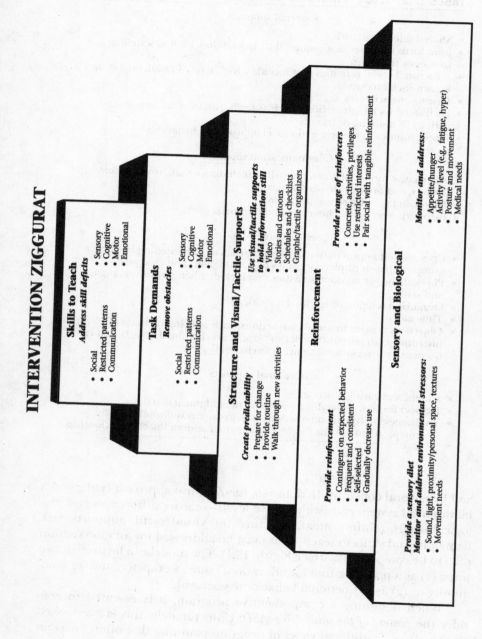

FIGURE 12.1. The Ziggurat Model.

INTERVENTION ZIGGURAT

Skills to Teach
Address skill deficits

- Social
- Restricted patterns
- Communication

- Sensory
- Cognitive
- Motor
- Emotional

Task Demands
Remove obstacles

- Social
- Restricted patterns
- Communication

- Sensory
- Cognitive
- Motor
- Emotional

Structure and Visual/Tactile Supports

Create predictability

- Prepare for change
- Provide routine
- Walk through new activities

Use visual/tactile supports to hold information still

- Video
- Stories and cartoons
- Schedules and checklists
- Graphic/tactile organizers

Reinforcement

Provide reinforcement

- Contingent on expected behavior
- Frequent and consistent
- Self-selected
- Gradually decrease use

Provide range of reinforcers

- Concrete, activities, privileges
- Use restricted interests
- Pair social with tangible reinforcement

Sensory and Biological

Provide a sensory diet
Monitor and address environmental stressors:

- Sound, light, proximity/personal space, textures
- Movement needs

Monitor and address:

- Appetite/hunger
- Activity level (e.g., fatigue, hyper)
- Posture and movement
- Medical needs

consideration of underlying ASD characteristics are potentially less effective and, therefore, less likely to result in sustained behavior change. The Ziggurat Model's approach is different. It targets an individual's specific needs, defined by ASD characteristics. This leads to interventions that are proactive and effective.

The process of intervention design should begin with an assessment of the presenting characteristics of ASD. A thorough assessment of underlying characteristics helps parents and professionals to plan a program that takes into account the individual's strengths and needs. Furthermore, assessment of underlying characteristics provides insight into which skills should be taught and how to design instruction to facilitate learning and bring about meaningful and long-lasting change. The Underlying Characteristics Checklist offers a comprehensive perspective as a basis for program planning.

The Underlying Characteristics Checklist[1] and Individual Strengths and Skills Inventory

The Underlying Characteristics Checklist (UCC; Aspy & Grossman, 2007) is an informal assessment designed to identify ASD characteristics for the purpose of intervention. There are three versions of the UCC, one intended for use with individuals who have high-functioning autism (UCC-HF); one for use with those with a more classic presentation (UCC-CL) in cognition and speech-language skills; and one for young children at the early invention stage (UCC-EI).

Designed to be completed by parents, teachers, individuals on the spectrum, and other service providers, individually or as a team, each of the UCCs comprises the following areas: social; restricted patterns of behaviors, interests, and activities; communication; sensory differences; cognitive differences; motor differences; emotional vulnerability; and medical and other biological factors. Based on the results of completing the UCC, a comprehensive intervention plan is developed that targets the characteristics of the individual's ASD by incorporating each of the five levels of the Ziggurat.

The Individual Strengths and Skills Inventory (ISSI) is built into the UCC and is designed to ensure that an individual's underlying strengths and skills are incorporated in the intervention design process. For example, one adult may have a strength in graphic design, whereas another has an intense interest in and knowledge of animals. These assets can easily become keys to addressing underlying skill deficits. The ISSI parallels

---

[1]UCC items, the ISSI, the Global Intervention Plan, the Ziggurat worksheet, and the CAPS form are presented in the case studies.

the areas of the UCC—social; restricted patterns of behavior, interests, and activities; communication; sensory differences; cognitive differences; motor differences; and emotional vulnerability.

Steve, his parents, and the therapist completed the UCC and ISSI for Steve. During a 20-minute meeting, they candidly discussed Steve's strengths and interests, as well as how his autism affected him. This was the first time that Steve had had the opportunity to have an in-depth discussion about his ASD, and when the UCC and ISSI were completed, Steve said that he had a better understanding of his autism. He agreed with his therapist that his newfound knowledge was empowering.

The Emotional Vulnerability section from Steve's UCC-HF and ISSI are presented in Figure 12.2.

Global Intervention Plan

The Global Intervention Plan helps users complete a person-centered plan by identifying short- and long-term goals and targeting the UCC areas and items that would have the greatest impact on the individual's ability to be independent and experience a sense of well-being across multiple environments. Using this tool, ASD-related areas are selected that will be meaningful in both the short and the long term. Thus the plan will be tied directly to leading a self-determined life as an adult, replete with opportunities, happiness, and other aspects related to a high quality of life (Adreon & Durocher, 2007; Hendricks & Wehman, 2009).

Even though Steve had participated in transition planning in school, this was the first time that Steve felt that he had a role in planning what he wanted to do in school, work, friendships, recreational activities, and daily living skills. This step occurred over a 20-minute period.

Steve's Global Intervention Plan appears in Figure 12.3.

The Intervention Ziggurat

The centerpiece and the framework of the Ziggurat Model is the Intervention Ziggurat (IZ). Designed to avoid overlooking critical areas that affect the effectiveness of any intervention plan, the IZ comprises five critical levels structured into a hierarchy: sensory differences and biological needs, reinforcement, structure and visual/tactile supports, task

UNDERLYING CHARACTERISTICS CHECKLIST—HIGH FUNCTIONING
Ruth Aspy, PhD, and Barry G. Grossman, PhD

Section on Emotional Vulnerability Only

Area	Item		Notes	Follow-Up
EMOTIONAL VULNERABILITY	76. Is easily stressed—worries obsessively	X	Stressed by changes in environment and routine, bus riding, not being able to find things	
	77. Appears to be depressed or sad	X		
	78. Has unusual fear response (e.g., lacks appropriate fears or awareness of danger or is overly fearful)			
	79. Appears anxious	X	Anxious about making friends and school	
	80. Exhibits rage reactions or "meltdowns"	X	Raises voice when upset	
	81. Injures self (e.g., bangs head, picks skin, bites nails until they bleed, bites self)			
	82. Makes suicidal comments or gestures			
	83. Displays inconsistent behaviors			
	84. Has difficulty tolerating mistakes	X	Gets upset when roommate does not follow routine or is messy	
	85. Has low frustration tolerance	X	Easily upset by "small things"—not finding things	
	86. Has low self-esteem, makes negative comments about self			
	87. Has difficulty identifying, quantifying, expressing, and/or controlling emotions (e.g., can only recognize and express emotions in extremes or fails to express emotions—"emotionally flat")			
	88. Has a limited understanding of own and others' emotional responses	X		
	89. Has difficulty managing stress and/or anxiety	X	Easily overwhelmed	

INDIVIDUAL STRENGTHS AND SKILLS INVENTORY: EMOTIONAL	Enthusiastic about interests, takes a walk or leaves the room to cool down, meltdowns are only verbal, recognizes that he does many things well, is getting better about dealing with anxiety

FIGURE 12.2. Steve's UCC and ISSI. From Aspy and Grossman (2007). © 2007 AAPC. Reprinted by permission. All rights reserved, including translation. No part of this form may be photocopied or otherwise reproduced.

GLOBAL INTERVENTION PLAN: GUIDE TO ESTABLISHING PRIORITIES
Ruth Aspy, PhD, and Barry G. Grossman, PhD

Directions: Following completion of the UCC and ISSI, the next step is to identify UCC **areas** and **items** that will result in a *meaningful* Global Intervention Plan. Consideration of priorities and strengths for an individual facilitates selection of UCC areas and items. The following questions are provided as a guide.

Selecting UCC Areas	**Vision** "Begin with the end in mind."—Stephen R. Covey

	• What is the short- and long-term vision of/for the individual? *Note that "short-term" and "long-term" may be defined differently in order to be meaningful.*

<u>Long-term</u>: *Graduate from college, get a good job, participate in chess tournament.*

<u>Short-term</u>: *Make one good friend; get along with roommate; play Dungeons and Dragons and chess; get good grades; find things when needed.*

⊙ Which UCC **areas** would have the greatest impact on achieving this vision?
Social, Restricted Patterns of Behavior, Sensory Differences, Cognitive Differences, Emotional Vulnerability

Settings

• In what settings does the individual participate?
Class, dormitory, campus, home, Dungeons and Dragons, and chess clubs

⊙ Which UCC **areas** have the greatest impact on the individual's ability to function in multiple settings?
Social, Sensory Differences, Cognitive Differences, Emotional Vulnerability

Quality of Life

• What is most important to the individual? What provides a sense of well-being?
Consider independence, relationships, play/leisure activities, safety, health, etc.

My interests (sci-fi, Dungeons and Dragons, chess), learning, having a friend

⊙ Which UCC **areas** have the greatest impact on the individual's quality of life?
Social, Restricted Patterns of Behavior, Cognitive Differences, Emotional Vulnerability

(continued)

FIGURE 12.3. Steve's Global Intervention Plan. From Aspy, R., & Grossman, B. G. (2011). *Designing comprehensive interventions for high-functioning individuals with autism spectrum disorders: The Ziggurat Model.* Shawnee Mission, KS: AAPC (*www.aapcpublishing.net*). Available at no charge from *www.texasautism.com*. Reprinted by permission.

Key UCC Areas

Based on your answers to the questions above, place a check **X** next to the key UCC **areas**. *Transfer to the **Areas of Concern** section of the Ziggurat worksheet.*

- ☒ Social
- ☒ Restricted Patterns of Behavior Interests, and Activities
- ☐ Communication
- ☒ Sensory Differences

- ☒ Cognitive Differences
- ☐ Motor Differences
- ☒ Emotional Vulnerability
- ☐ Known Medical or Other Biological Factors

Key UCC Items

Select key UCC **items** for *each* of the UCC **areas** listed above. Choose items that are essential (necessary for progress) and developmentally appropriate. Emphasize items that are more pivotal (building blocks for additional skills). Avoid selecting redundant items.

Write key item numbers and descriptions below. These items will be used to develop interventions keeping strengths and skills (identified on the ISSI) in mind.

*Transfer items to the **Selected UCC Item** section of the Ziggurat worksheet. Develop interventions.*

#1 Mindblindness
#4 Lacks tact
#5 Difficulty making or keeping friends
#8 Tends to be less involved in group activities
#12 Expresses strong need for routine or sameness
#18 Problems with transition and change

#41 Responds in unusual manner to sounds
#52 Displays poor problem-solving skills
#53 Has poor organizational skills
#60 Has attention problems
#76 Is easily stressed
#89 Has difficulty managing stress and/or anxiety

Selecting UCC Items

FIGURE 12.3. *(continued)*

demands, and skills to teach. The first level, sensory differences and biological needs, addresses basic internal factors that affect functioning. The second level addresses motivational needs prerequisite to skill development. The third level draws on individuals' strength of visual processing and addresses their fundamental need for order and routine. The final two levels of the IZ emphasize the importance of expectations and skill development relative to the characteristics of individuals with ASD.

Each of the levels is essential and contributes to the effectiveness of the others. Thus, if needs on all levels are not addressed, the intervention will not be as effective, and skills will not develop. The following is a brief discussion of the five levels of the IZ.

Sensory Differences and Biological Needs

The first level of the IZ represents what may be considered the foundation of behavior, biology. Consideration of biological factors is important due to the strong genetic and neurological underpinnings of ASD. Sensory differences and biological needs often present some of the greatest challenges for individuals on the spectrum. The existence of one of these areas, sensory, is formalized by its inclusion in the fifth edition of the American Psychiatric Association's (APA) *Diagnostic and Statistical Manual of Mental Disorders* (2013). Many sensory interventions fit into the EBP category of antecedent-based interventions and have a base of research that is considered emerging (cf. Case-Smith, Weaver, & Fristad, in press). Much of the research on biological interventions has centered on the use of medications, both conventional (McPheeters et al., 2011) and complementary and alternative (Hanson et al., 2007).

Reinforcement

All intervention plans ultimately target the development or increase of a behavior or skill. This goal can be accomplished only by incorporating reinforcement into a comprehensive plan given that its purpose is to increase the likelihood that a behavior will occur again. Without reinforcement, there is no intervention. Therefore, reinforcement with an emphasis on interests is included as the second level of the Intervention Ziggurat (see Figure 12.5). The principles of effective reinforcement are well established in the research literature. In fact, the most effective intervention programs deliver reinforcement for positive behaviors and limit access to reinforcement of problem behaviors (cf. Horner, Carr, Strain, Todd, & Reed, 2002).

Structure and Visual/Tactile Supports

Individuals with ASD function best when predictability is established across the day, including schedules, routines, environments, behavioral and occupational expectations, and interpersonal interactions. In order to be successful in home, school, and community, those on the spectrum require preparation. Because verbal communication deficits are evident in HFASD, supports that are visual are critical. For adults with HFASD and a vision impairment, tactile supports should be considered. Visual strategies, such as pictures, written schedules, and video modeling, have been shown to be effective for increasing on-task behavior and enhancing independence (cf. Wang & Spillane, 2009).

Task Demands

The term *task demand* is synonymous with obstacle removal (E. Blackwell, personal communication, July 12, 2007). In designing quality interventions, obstacles that could prevent an individual from succeeding either independently or with assistance should be taken away. For example, for an adult with HFASD who lacks the skills to negotiate peer conflict, a trained mentor during group activities can be provided until he or she is able to master strategies for compromise (Chan et al., 2009). The obstacle is a lack of the skills to negotiate conflict; it is removed through the aid of a trained mentor who can help in situations that require compromise. Task demands in the IZ include work, school, social, communication, organizational, sensory, and other areas of functioning.

Skills to Teach

The first four levels of the Ziggurat set the stage for skill acquisition. It is possible to resolve many issues or concerns using strategies on the first four levels without ever teaching skills. Indeed, many improvements may be seen as a direct result of attending to an individual's biological needs, providing meaningful reinforcers, addressing the need for structure and predictability, and carefully matching demands to ability.

Those who plan programs for adults with ASD may overlook the crucial last level—skills to teach—when success occurs as the result of sensory and biological supports, reinforcement, structure, and matching skills to tasks. However, such a "partial" approach to intervention will have negative long-term outcomes because it does not allow for independence, nor does it promote generalization or growth. It is for this reason that we view skills to teach as the ultimate goal of any intervention plan. Several approaches to teach skills to individuals with ASD have been supported in the literature, including instruction in the natural setting (see Table 12.1).

Using the aforementioned information, the team uses the Ziggurat worksheet to guide them through the development of a comprehensive intervention plan. With a new understanding of the individual's needs and strengths based on (1) completion of the UCC and ISSI and (2) the development of long- and short-term goals and prioritized UCC areas and items using the Global Intervention Plan, the team is prepared to design an intervention plan that is targeted to the individual adult.

Ziggurat Worksheet

All interventions incorporated into the plan must address underlying needs from the UCC. This provides a safeguard against developing a plan that addresses only surface concerns or against recycling interventions that have been used with other adults with ASD without careful consideration of the specific adult. Furthermore, the Ziggurat worksheet promotes collaboration by helping the adult with HFASD, his or her family, and professionals to understand their respective parts in the larger intervention picture. After completion of the Ziggurat worksheet, the team is ready to discuss how these interventions will be embedded throughout the day.

> Steve and his team—therapist and parents—completed the Ziggurat worksheet, matching interventions to Steve's characteristics of autism. This helped everyone better understand the interventions that were needed in (1) sensory and biological areas, (2) reinforcement, (3) structure and visual/tactile supports, (4) task demands, and (5) skills to teach. This step required 30 minutes to complete.

Figure 12.4 shows the task demands section of the Ziggurat worksheet that Steve, his parents, and his therapist created.

The Comprehensive Autism Planning System

Whereas the Ziggurat worksheet allows a team to know that the intervention plan is thorough and targeted, the CAPS provides a structure for implementation, as detailed further below. The CAPS provides an overview of an adult's daily schedule by time and activity and specifies supports needed during each period. Thus the CAPS answers the fundamental question: *What supports does the individual need for each activity?*

The process from Ziggurat to CAPS includes:

- Identifying the individual's needs through completion of the UCC-HF and ISSI.
- Establishing goals for the adult and prioritized UCC items that lead to these goals.
- Developing interventions across the six areas of the Ziggurat that match the UCC- and ISSI-identified strengths and concerns.
- Completing the CAPS.

That is, based on information developed using the Ziggurat Model, the CAPS provides a framework for listing tasks and activities and the times they occur, along with a delineation of the supports needed for success. In addition, the CAPS includes a place for recording the results of ongoing data collection and consideration of how skills are to be generalized to other settings, as needed.

ZIGGURAT WORKSHEET (task demands only)
Ruth Aspy, PhD, and Barry G. Grossman, PhD

Behavior/Areas of Concern Social, Restricted Patterns of Behavior, Sensory Differences, Cognitive Differences, Emotional Vulnerability	For FBA Operationalized Behaviors	Selected UCC Items	Check all that apply		
			A	B	C
Task Demands		#1 Mindblindness #4 Lacks tact #5 Difficulty making or keeping friends #8 Tends to be less involved in group activities #12 Expresses strong need for routine or sameness #18 Problems with transition and change			
		#41 Responds in unusual manner to sounds #52 Displays poor problem-solving skills #53 Has poor organizational skills #60 Has attention problems #76 Is easily stressed #89 Has difficulty managing stress and/or anxiety	X	X	
	Task Demand Intervention:	• Hire personal organizer to organize and label dorm room (mother). Also, have personal organizer make a schedule of activities. • Engage a laundry service to do laundry for next semester. • Use directions (written by therapist) for riding bus to Dungeons and Dragons. • Enroll in classes that have study sessions and teaching assistants. • Arrange through Student Support Center to have professors provide copies of class notes or have a peer take notes. • Use ToDo app on iPad to record assignments, tests, study time, D&D time, and chess time. • Use script (written by therapist and Steve) on how to address issues with roommate. • Disclose autism to Mark. • List of kind versus rude words (therapist and Steve). • Educate the resident assistant (RA) about autism. Notify him when a conflict occurs between Mark and you. When possible, have the RA mediate by helping you understand how your roommate feels or how your behavior may affect Mark, and vice versa. • Post on computer and iPad stickies with phrases that can be used to help when Mark and you disagree. • Talk with Mark about using an Incredible 5-Point Scale to help each of you understand the other. Use for yourself, even if Mark does not want to.			
	Underlying Characteristics Addressed:	#1 Difficulty recognizing the feelings and thoughts of others (mindblindness) #53 Has poor organizational skills #60 Has attention problems #76 Is easily stressed			

FIGURE 12.4. Steve's Ziggurat worksheet (partial). From Aspy, R., & Grossman, B. G. (2011). *Designing comprehensive interventions for high-functioning individuals with autism spectrum disorders: The Ziggurat Model.* Shawnee Mission, KS: AAPC (*www.asperger.net*). Reprinted by permission. A, antecedent; B, behavior; C, consequence.

The CAPS contains the following components:

1. *Time and Activity.* This section indicates the clock time of each activity that the adult engages in throughout the day. This includes *all* tasks and activities throughout the day in which the adult requires support. Academic periods (e.g., reading), nonacademic times (e.g., recess, lunch), and transitions between classes are all considered activities.

2. *Targeted Skills to Teach.* This includes skills that lead to success for a given adult.

3. *Structure/Modifications.* Structures/modifications can consist of a wide variety of supports, including placement in the classroom, visual supports, peer networks, and instructional strategies (e.g., priming, self-monitoring).

4. *Reinforcement.* Adult access to specific types of reinforcement, as well as reinforcement schedules, are listed here.

5. *Sensory Supports.* Sensory supports and strategies identified by an occupational therapist or others are listed in this CAPS area.

6. *Social Skills/Communication.* Specific communication goals or activities, as well as supports, are delineated in this section. Goals or activities may include (a) requesting help, (b) taking turns in conversation, or (c) protesting appropriately. Supports may encompass scripts, enlisting the help of a mentor, or social narratives.

7. *Data Collection.* This space is for recording the type of data, as well as the behavior to be documented during a specific activity. Typically, this section relates directly to individualized education program (IEP) goals and objectives.

8. *Generalization.* Because individuals with HFASD often have problems generalizing information across settings, this section of the CAPS was developed to ensure that the adult with HFASD has written ideas about when supports can be used in other situations.

The next step for Steve and his team was to create the CAPS. Steve's therapist suggested that Mark join the team. Mark consented. They created a CAPS that addressed the important activities in life, focusing on college work, leisure activities, and daily living skills. This meeting was also used to introduce Mark to Steve's autism using some video clips from the television show *The Big Bang Theory*.

The CAPS appears in Figure 12.5 (pp. 284–285).

Summary

In order to assist adults in meeting their potential, comprehensive planning is necessary. The comprehensive planning process begins with an understanding of the adult's autism—both strengths and concerns—and continues with establishing long- and short-term goals and developing an implementation plan. This process can aid adults, such as Steve, learn and apply the myriad skills, including independent living skills, that can allow them to be successful.

ACKNOWLEDGMENT

The case study of Steve in this chapter was adapted from Aspy and Grossman (2011).

REFERENCES

Adreon, D., & Durocher, J. (2007). Evaluating the college transition needs of individuals with high-functioning autism spectrum disorders. *Intervention in School and Clinic, 42,* 271–279.

Agran, M. (2012). Health and safety skills. In P. Wehman & J. Kregel (Eds.), *Functional curriculum for elementary and secondary students with special needs* (3rd ed., pp. 471–495). Austin, TX: Pro-Ed.

American Psychiatric Association. (2013). *Diagnostic and statistical manual of mental disorders* (5th ed.). Arlington, VA: Author.

Armstrong, A., Gentry, T., & Wehman, P. (2013). Using technology from school to adulthood: Unleashing the power. In P. Wehman (Ed.), *Life beyond the classroom: Transition strategies for young people with disabilities* (5th ed., pp. 285–308). Baltimore: Brookes.

Aspy, R., & Grossman, B. (2007). *Underlying characteristics checklist: High-functioning autism (UCC-HF), classic autism (CL), early intervention (EI).* Shawnee Mission, KS: AAPC.

Aspy, R., & Grossman, B. (2011). *Designing comprehensive interventions for high-functioning individuals with autism spectrum disorders: The Ziggurat Model.* Shawnee Mission, KS: AAPC.

Billstedt, E., Gillberg, I. C., & Gillberg, C. (2005). Autism after adolescence: Population-based 13– to 22–year follow-up study of 120 individuals with autism diagnosed in childhood. *Journal of Autism and Developmental Disorders, 35,* 351–360.

Case-Smith, J., Weaver, L. L., & Fristad, M. A. (in press). A systematic review of sensory processing interventions for children with autism spectrum disorders. *Autism.*

Centers for Medicare and Medicaid Services. (2010). *Autism spectrum disorders: Final report on environmental scan.* Washington, DC: Author.

COMPREHENSIVE AUTISM PLANNING SYSTEM

Name _Steve_

Activity	Targeted Skills to Teach	Structure/ Modifications	Reinforcement	Sensory Supports	Social Skills/ Communication	Data Collection	Generalization
Dorm Room	Cooperation with roommate. Maintain room neatness.	Book or video on autism for RA. Use RA as mediator. Put everything away before going to bed (following professional organizer structure). Drop laundry off at laundry service each Saturday; pick up Monday afternoon.	Star Trek or Halo (with roommate or headphones).	Noise-canceling headphones, as needed.	Conversation starters with roommates. List of kind versus rude words posted on board. Script on addressing issues with roommate. Social autopsy with RA when challenges occur with Mark.	Cooperative (Y/N) rated by Steve and Mark.	Use kind words throughout the day.
Classes	Class attendance. Relaxation. Organization.	Early-morning or late-evening classes (low enrollment). Ensure that each class has a teaching assistant (TA). Attend all study sessions. Get class notes from help center. Arrive early and sit in first row (midway from door). Laptop.	30 minutes to 1 hour of leisure time before beginning homework after classes.	Deep breathing before class. Walk before and after class.	Prepare written questions for professor or RA. Meet with professor or TA 1 week before test.	Class notes (Y/N). Assignments in phone (Y/N). Supplies needed (Y/N). Relaxed (Y/N).	Laptop and phone (ToDo app) as organizing tools.

284 •

Homework (studying)	Phone with ToDo for schedule. Use library or help center for study when possible. Use ToDo for study schedule: at least 4 hours per day.	Assignment completion. Being prepared for tests.	Star Trek or Halo after studying 15 minutes or preferred activity after every hour of study.	Noise-canceling headphones. Deep breathing every 30 minutes. Walk before and after studying.	List of polite ways to say "be quiet."	Grades on tests and assignments.	Deep breathing and brief walks throughout the day, as needed.
Dungeons and Dragons	Instructions for bus riding. List of supplies needed for D&D.	Cooperation with others. Enjoy games with others.	Game is reinforcing.	Noise-canceling headphones on bus.	Conversation starter cards.	Outing at least once per week (Y/N). Enjoyed D&D (Y/N).	Think about asking a D&D player to go to a movie or play Halo after about 1 month.
Other extra-curricular	Join chess club or science fiction club. Attend class on organization and study skills. Meet with therapist in the fall to identify other important classes to take. Attend local high-functioning autism adult group.	Cooperation with others. Enjoy games with others.	None other than activities.	Learn relaxation and self-understanding in counseling sessions.	Conversation starter cards.	Communicate with others (Y/N). Go out at least one time per week (Y/N).	Enjoy activities and remain calm throughout the day.

FIGURE 12.5. Steve's CAPS.

Chan, J. M., Lang, R., Rispoli, M., O'Reilly, M., Sigafoos, J., & Cole, H. (2009). Use of peer-mediated interventions in the treatment of autism spectrum disorders: A systematic review. *Research in Autism Spectrum Disorders, 3,* 876–889.

DiPipi-Hoy, C., Jitendra, A., & Kern, L. (2009). Effects of time management instruction on adolescents' ability to self-manage time in a vocational setting. *Journal of Special Education, 43,* 145–159.

Farley, M. A., McMahon, W. M., Fombonne, E., Jenson, W. R., Miller, J., Gardner, M., et al. (2009). Twenty-year outcome for individuals with autism and average or near-average cognitive abilities. *Autism Research, 2,* 109–118.

Fixsen, D., Blasé, K., Horner, R., & Sugai, C. (2009). *Concept paper: Develop the capacity for scaling up the effective use of evidence-based programs in state departments of education.* Unpublished manuscript, University of North Carolina, Chapel Hill.

Hanson, E., Kalish, L. A., Bunce, E., Curtis, C., McDaniel, S., Ware, J., et al. (2007). Use of complementary and alternative medicine among children diagnosed with autism spectrum disorder. *Journal of Autism and Developmental Disorders, 37,* 628–636.

Hendricks, D., & Wehman, P. (2009). Transition form school to adulthood for youth with autism spectrum disorders. *Focus on Autism and Other Developmental Disabilities, 24,* 77–88.

Henninger, N. A., & Taylor, J. L. (2013). Outcomes in adults with autism spectrum disorders: A historical perspective. *Autism, 17,* 103–116.

Henry, S. A., & Myles, B. S. (2013). *The Comprehensive Autism Planning System (CAPS) for individuals with autism spectrum disorders and related disabilities: Integrating evidence-based practices throughout the student's day* (2nd ed.). Shawnee Mission, KS: AAPC.

Horner, R. H., Carr, E. G., Strain, P. S., Todd, A. W., & Reed, H. K. (2002). Problem behavior interventions for young children with autism: A research synthesis. *Journal of Autism and Developmental Disorders, 32,* 423–446.

McPheeters, M. L., Warren, Z., Sathe, N., Bruzek, J. L., Krishnaswami, S., Jerome, R. N., et al. (2011). A systematic review of medical treatments for children with autism spectrum disorders. *Pediatrics, 127,* 1312–1321.

Mechling, L. C. (2011). Review of twenty-first century portable electronic devices for persons with moderate intellectual disabilities and autism spectrum disorders. *Education and Training in Autism and Developmental Disabilities, 46,* 479–498.

Muller, E., Schuler, A., & Yates, G. B. (2008). Social challenges and supports from the perspectives of individuals with Asperger syndrome and other autism spectrum disabilities. *Autism, 12,* 173–190.

Myles, B. S., Endow, J., & Mayfield, M. (2013). *The hidden curriculum of getting and keeping a job: Navigating the social landscape of employment: A guide for individuals with autism spectrum disorders and other social-cognitive challenges.* Shawnee Mission, KS: AAPC.

Myles, B. S., Grossman, B. G., Aspy, R., Henry, S. A., & Coffin, A. B. (2007). Planning a comprehensive program for students with autism spectrum disorders using evidence-based practices. *Education and Training in Developmental Disabilities, 42,* 398–409.

National Autism Center. (2009). *National standards report: Addressing the need for evidence-based practice guidelines for autism spectrum disorders.* Randolph, MA: Author.

National Professional Development Center on Autism Spectrum Disorders. (n.d.). Evidence-based practice briefs. Retrieved April 10, 2010, from *http:// autismpdc.fpg.unc.edu/content/briefs.*

Organization for Autism Research. (2006). *Life journey through autism: A guide for transition to adulthood.* Arlington, VA: Author.

Shattuck, P. T., Narendorf, S. C., Cooper, B., Sterzing, P. R., Wagner, M., & Taylor, J. L. (2012). Postsecondary education and employment among youth with an autism spectrum disorder. *Pediatrics, 129,* 1–8.

Steere, D., Burcroff, T., & DiPipi-Hoy, C. (2012). Living at home: Skills for independence. In P. Wehman & J. Kregel (Eds.), *Functional curriculum for elementary and secondary students with special needs* (3rd ed., pp. 389–417). Austin, TX: Pro-Ed.

Targett, P. S., & Smith, M. D. (2009). Living in the community. In P. Wehman, M. D. Smith, & C. Schall (Eds.), *Autism and the transition to adulthood: Success beyond the classroom* (pp. 233–250). Baltimore: Brookes.

Test, E. W., Richter, S., & Walker, A. R. (2012). Life skills and community-based instruction. In M. L. Wehmeyer & K. W. Webb (Eds.), *Handbook of adolescent transition education for youth with disabilities* (pp. 121–139). New York: Routledge.

Wang, P., & Spillane, A. (2009). Evidence-based social skills interventions for children with autism: A meta-analysis. *Education and Training in Developmental Disabilities, 44,* 318–342.

Wehmeyer, M. L., & Webb, K. W. (2012). *Handbook of adolescent transition education for youth with disabilities.* New York: Routledge.

CHAPTER 13

● ● ● ● ● ●

Aging, Estate Planning, and Funding Services for Adults with Autism Spectrum Disorders

● **Carol Markowitz**

Aging successfully has been defined as maintaining good health, physically as well as mentally. It requires appropriate environments for living and recreation, social relationships, and the opportunity for active engagement in life (Perkins & Berkman, 2011). For people both with and without disabilities, successful aging includes access to good health care and to preferred recreation and leisure pursuits, a comfortable place to live, a social network consisting of family and friends, and an appropriate level of care or support (Reichstadt, Sengupta, Depp, Palinkas, & Jeste, 2010). Arranging for these services and supports can be costly. For people with autism spectrum disorders (ASD), obtaining the funds to ensure that supports are present is central to the challenge of aging successfully. Early, thoughtful planning by family members or guardians and by the individual him- or herself is essential for an older adult with ASD to enjoy a good quality of life.

A summary of prevalence statistics was included in the report of the Centers for Disease Control and Prevention (CDC) (Baio, 2012). The CDC reported a dramatic increase in the population of individuals with ASD. In 2004 the estimated prevalence was 8 per 1,000 children, or 1 in 125. In 2006, the prevalence increased to 1 in 110. By 2008, the CDC counted 11.3 per 1,000, or 1 in 88. A recent CDC report cites a rate of 1 in 50

(Blumberg et al., 2013). The CDC did not speculate as to a specific cause for the increase but stated that "ASDs continue to be an important public health concern in the United States, underscoring the need for continued resources to identify potential risk factors, and to provide essential supports for persons with ASDs and their families" (Baio, 2012, p. 2).

In their book *The Autism Matrix*, Eyal, Hart, Onculer, Oren, and Rossi (2010) contend that the increase in autism prevalence is due in part to the deinstitutionalization movement. In the 1950s it was common for children with ASD to be placed in state institutions. The development of meaningful educational opportunities reversed this trend. Children with ASD could now be diagnosed and identified. Increased availability of community-based educational placements coupled with the advent of family support has led to a growing adult population living in the community with family members or in community placements such as group homes and supported apartments (Eyal et al., 2010).

In the 1980s an increased awareness of the differing needs of adults with ASD led to an emerging emphasis on employment and residential options to assist individuals and their families across the lifespan (Gerhardt & Holmes, 2005). However, employment outcomes for adults with ASD continue to be poor, with higher rates of unemployment than among their nondisabled peers (deFur, 2003). Parents of adults with ASD are often poorly informed about work and residential options and about funding for these options (deFur, Todd-Allen, & Getzel, 2001). As they and their children age, a common theme emerges: "What will happen to him when we're no longer here to support him?" (Seventh Voice, 2012). Current outcome studies suggest that many adults with ASD rely heavily on their families for support, for living arrangements, and for transportation (Howlin, Goode, Hutton, & Rutter, 2004). More than 25% of adults with intellectual disabilities (ID) live with parents who are 60 years old or older (President's Committee for People with Intellectual Disabilities, 2004). Parental anxiety about their children's future is justified. Many adults with disabilities are unemployed, with estimates as high as 75% (Gerhardt & Holmes, 2005, p. 1088). Barriers to employment include communication and skill deficits and lack of access to transportation and job coaching (Gerhardt & Holmes, 2005).

As the number of children with ASD increases, the number of older adults is increasing as well (Bruder, Kerins, Mazzarella, Sims, & Stein, 2012). Heller and Factor (2004) estimated that there were more than 641,000 adults with ASD over the age of 60 living in the United States in the year 2000. By 2030, they estimate that the number will increase to 1.2 million. Fisher and Kettl (2005) report similar numbers, estimating that the number of people with ID over 60 years of age will be in the millions by the year 2030. There is a shift in the population in disability services to a greater number of people over 50 (Janicki, 2009). The current life expectancy is 66 years (Fisher & Kettl, 2005). As life expectancy continues to increase, the population of older adults with ASD will increase further.

Although there have been numerous studies of older individuals with ID, there is less information about older adults with ASD (Stuart-Hamilton & Morgan, 2011). Until recently many of these individuals lived out their lives in state institutions. "Empirical studies including samples aged 50+ are practically absent in the literature" (Perkins & Berkman, 2011, p. 9). This chapter discusses issues in successful aging and enhanced quality of life for older individuals with ASD. These issues include obtaining appropriate medical care, the role of parents and guardians as planners and advocates, the transition from employment to retirement, residential alternatives, and access to funding needed to support these activities.

Access to Appropriate Medical Care

The life expectancy of people with disabilities has improved over the past 30 years. Mortality rates are now similar to those of the general population. The adult population with ASD may experience fewer risk factors, such as smoking, drinking alcohol, occupational accidents, and suicide. However, adults with ASD may have increased risk of other factors. Shavelle, Strauss, and Pickett (2001) report seizures, drowning, and other accidents as the most common causes of death for adults with ASD. As individuals with ASD live longer, they encounter the same health issues as the typical aging population (Drum, Krahn, Peterson, Horner-Johnson, & Newton, 2009). This highlights the importance of access to quality medical care, attention to wellness, preventive practices, and dental care, and access to the same screening procedures and diagnostic tests that exist for the typical aging population (Bruder et al., 2012).

However, there is a disparity in the provision of health care for adults with disabilities. For example, the U.S. Department of Health and Human Services reported in 2005 that fewer women over the age of 40 with disabilities received annual mammograms than women in the general population and that only 37% of children and adults with disabilities had annual dental visits, compared with 46% without disabilities (Drum et al., 2009). There are "disparities in health outcomes, access, and health promotion and health behaviors" (Bruder et al., 2012, p. 2498). In 2002, the surgeon general issued a call to action to improve the health and wellness of persons with disabilities (U.S. Public Health Service, 2002). The surgeon general's report outlined the disparities that exist in health care for people with disabilities and identified goals for improving the health care of people with ID. These included integration of health promotion into community environments for people with ID and improving the quality of health care. Also included were recommendations for specialized training for health care providers and ensuring that health care financing produces good health outcomes (U.S. Public Health Service, 2002). In 2005, the surgeon general addressed the issues again, highlighting the fact that "health care providers have the knowledge and tools to screen, diagnose and the treat the whole person with a disability with dignity" and that "persons with disabilities can promote their own good health by developing and maintaining healthy life styles" (U.S. Department of Health and Human Services, 2005, p. 21). He also stated that "accessible health care and support services promote independence for people with disabilities" (U.S. Department of Health and Human Services, 2005, p. 21).

Barriers to appropriate medical care include health insurance limitations, restricted access to community-based care, lack of training of some physicians in characteristics of ASD, and lack of implementation of a medical model that reflects best practices. Most adults with ASD have Medicaid as their primary insurance coverage. This coverage is frequently a requirement made by states' departments of human services to ensure that the state is reimbursed for services provided under the Medicaid waiver (Division of Developmental Disabilities, 2013). This process limits the selection of physicians and other specialists. It also limits medications that can be prescribed, resulting at times in changes of medications and changes in treating physicians due to insurance coverage.

A study published in 2012 by Bruder and colleagues surveyed physicians in the state of Connecticut related to provision of health care services to persons with ASD. Responses to the survey revealed that the physicians who treated adults with ASD felt that they could benefit from more training and that there was a lack of adequate training available. Many of the physicians surveyed did not treat patients with ASD at all. Only 36% of respondents reported that they had received any training in caring for patients with ASDs (Bruder et al., 2012). Understanding the needs of people with ASD and providing them with high-quality medical care is a specialized area requiring ongoing training and increased attention by medical schools.

As adults with ASD age in their own homes and in community placements, age-related health issues will appear. "As life expectancy of individuals with ID increases, experts are learning more about the aging process, and about the emergence of secondary conditions later in life" (Nehring & Betz, 2007). Osteoporosis, arthritis, high blood pressure, decreased vision or hearing, type II diabetes, and cardiac issues can all occur in individuals with or without disabilities. Seizure disorders diagnosed in childhood or adolescence often persist into adulthood. Long-term use of psychotropic medications can result in side effects such as the early onset of osteoporosis. Behavioral difficulties have been shown to persist into adulthood for many individuals with ASD. In a review of the literature, Shea and Mesibov (2005) found that "adults with autism are reported by their parents to exhibit significant behavior problems, including resistance to change, compulsions, unacceptable sexual behavior, tantrums, aggression, and self-injurious behavior" (p. 290). Davidson and colleagues (2003) found that "behavioral disorders, which are often coincident with functional decline in older persons with intellectual and developmental disabilities, may be more related to medical morbidity than previously reported" (p. 424). Health problems may be the cause of the behavioral disturbance and may be "sentinels for medical morbidity" (Davidson et al., 2003, p. 424). This problem highlights the importance of good communication between caregivers and medical professionals and careful attention to diagnosis of difficult-to-detect underlying medical problems.

Decades of self-injurious head hitting can lead to retinal detachment. Postconcussive syndrome can also occur after prolonged years of head hitting (Erlanger, Kutner, Barth, & Barnes, 1999). The symptoms that have been reported in football players, such as early-onset dementia, depression, and sleep disturbances (Pilon & Belson, 2013), may be appearing in adults with ASD and may go undetected. Years of pica and rumination can lead to gastrointestinal disorders such as chronic gastroesophageal reflux disease (GERD). Access to quality medical care is therefore critical to maintaining and improving the health status of the aging population with ASD.

High-quality health care is characterized by accessibility, a focus on wellness and preventative care, continuity, health promotion, evidence-based practice, and care coordination. The medical home model may provide an answer to these needs. "A medical home is not a house, office or hospital but rather an approach in providing comprehensive primary care. In a medical home a clinician works in partnership with the family or patient to assure that the medical and non-medical needs of the patient are met" ("What Is a Medical Home?," n.d.). This model is characterized by access to routine care, a personal doctor or nurse to provide continuity of care, referrals to specialists when needed, and person-centered care (Larson & Reid, 2010). The medical home model emphasizes putting the patient first and provides coordination of care, an important aspect for people with ASD who may not understand medical needs or act on their own behalf. Working in partnership with family or guardians is emphasized in this model. The National Committee for Quality Assurance (NCQA; 2010) has established standards for medical homes. These standards include access, care management, referral tracking, and advanced electronic communications. Older adults with ASD will benefit substantially from these services, especially as their parents age and have difficulty attending to their medical care. This model can provide guardians with needed support when they take on this responsibility.

Parents and Guardians as Advocates
. . . .

"The need for parents to forcefully advocate on behalf of their son or daughter does not, in most instances, diminish with age" (Gerhardt & Holmes, 2005, p. 1093). Parents of adults with ASD express a common fear: "What will happen to him when we're not here to take care of him?" This fear is well founded, as many adults with ASD are highly dependent on parents or family members for their care, living arrangements, and financial needs into older adulthood (Howlin et al., 2004). As parents age and find their own health declining, this problem becomes urgent. Planning for the future requires parents to confront their mortality and acknowledge that they will not live forever, even in the face of great family need.

Launching a child out of the family home is a positive and expected part of parenting. For parents of individuals with ASD it can be a fearful and negative experience, related to an inability to continue to provide care and feelings of mortality "marked by turmoil and disequilibrium in the family" (Lounds & Seltzer, 2007, p. 562; see also Wehmeyer & Zager, Chapter 3, this volume, for a discussion of parenting adult children with ASD). Karl Greenfeld, the brother of Noah (the subject of *A Child Called Noah*), expressed his view of the difficult situation of aging parents: "Noah's condition persists; an immovable psychic object. . . . My father is in his 80s now, my mother in her late 70s. They will go on as long as they can. Then I will try to step in. Will I always be there for Noah, as my parents have been? I wish I could say, Yes, definitely I will be there. But I honestly don't know"(2009, p. 6). He is not alone in this view; siblings can exhibit a lack of emotional closeness and may be pessimistic about the future for their sibling with ASD (Orsmond & Seltzer, 2007).

"Older caregivers of individuals with intellectual and developmental disabilities have significant challenges including the long duration of their care giving roles, experiencing the onset of their own age-related health issues, as well as those of the care recipient" (Haley & Perkins, 2004). Stress as a source of health impairments is well documented in research (Schultz & Beach, 1999). Stress-related medical conditions or problems that can be made worse by stress include coronary heart disease, hypertension, asthma, migraine, depression, and insomnia (Lehrer & Woolfolk, 1993). These conditions can lead to diminished health in caregivers, resulting in lessened ability to provide care.

Lounds and Seltzer (2007) found that mothers are often the primary caregivers of children with ASD. The health and well-being of the mother is improved when she has the support of a spouse or other children in managing the care of the individual with ASD. "Increased feelings of closeness to the child with autism led to mothers feeling more optimistic, and subsequently reporting better psychological well being and fewer depressive symptoms" (Lounds & Seltzer, 2007, p. 561). Mothers who used coping strategies that focused on problem solving were closer to their children with ASD than those who used emotional coping strategies (Lounds & Seltzer, 2007). Coping strategies that result in action or problem resolution appear to be more effective strategies. Barbosa, Figueiredo, Sousa, and Demain (2011) also found that in both primary and secondary caregivers "emotion–cognitive strategies are less efficient. . . . Common problem solving strategies adopted by both types of caregivers rely on their own experience and expertise and addressing and finding a solution to the problem" (p. 490).

Parents typically depend on their nondisabled children to become the secondary caregivers. This reliance is more likely to be successful if the nondisabled siblings have a close relationship with their siblings with ASD. "Nondisabled siblings seem to have the best outcomes, particularly in terms of psychological well-being, when they have close ties to the family of origin and particularly with their siblings with intellectual or developmental disability" (Lounds & Seltzer, 2007, p. 566). Orsmond, Kuo, and Seltzer (2009) also found that coping that focused on problem solving fostered better sibling engagement with the sibling with ASD and that parental support of the sibling resulted in more positive sibling relationships.

Aging caregivers may find it increasingly difficult to participate in support groups or get information in person. Perkins and LaMartin (2012) suggest that information available on the Internet and Internet-based support groups can be beneficial to aging caregivers. This material can take the form of shared strategies or experiences and can have educational content. Sources for accurate information can improve the problem-solving coping strategies referenced by Lounds and Seltzer (2007) and Barbosa and colleagues (2011). "74% of family carers surveyed by the National Alliance of Caregivers (2011) asserted that technology had the potential to increase their effectiveness as a carer and reduce stress" (Perkins & LaMartin, 2012, p. 57).

Heller and Kramer (2009) found that 38% of siblings felt that they would someday assume responsibility for the care of their siblings with developmental disabilities. Many felt that they had not been included in the planning process. These findings suggest that enhanced relationships within families improve the outcomes when the family must address difficult transitional issues in adulthood. Parents who include their adult nondisabled children in the planning process are more likely to find that those children assume the caregiver roles effectively. Supports given to families must promote effective problem solving and not simply offer emotional support. Parents who use information to solve problems are more likely to experience better outcomes and lower stress.

The law presumes that individuals are legally competent at age 18. Some individuals with ASD are competent, but most will need a guardian to make informed decisions about health care, living arrangements, and finances. If guardianship is needed, it should be used as necessary to protect the individual's rights, as well as to provide for his or her needs (Arc for People with Intellectual and Developmental Disabilities, 2009). Full legal guardianship is appropriate if the family decides it is necessary and if the court agrees that the individual is not capable of making any medical or financial decisions on his or her own. For adults with ASD who have the ability to make some decisions, there are other alternatives to full guardianship. For example, a conservator can be appointed who makes only financial decisions, or a limited guardian can be appointed who makes only medical decisions. A joint bank account can be opened with the individual with ASD to help him or her manage money (Rudy, 2011).

If parents are the guardians, it is critical for them to plan for the time when they will no longer fill this role. They should determine a coguardian or designate a new guardian who will take on the responsibilities and is willing to do so. Guardians should be designated in a will. The guardian needs to understand the person and the situation well enough to take the person's preferences into account when making decisions. He or she may need to decide where the person will live and to manage finances, income, or trust funds. The guardian may need to make difficult medical decisions. Anyone assuming guardianship must be cognizant of the requirements and be ready to carry them out. Parents should be very clear about the preferences and needs of their adult child in communicating with the designated guardian (Bala, 2013). Parents can make their wishes and preferences known during the planning process. This plan can include information about religious preferences, preferred living arrangements, educational and medical history, where records are stored, and goals for work placements. The designated guardian should spend time with the family and the individual with ASD to best understand his or her role. Trusted guardians can act more effectively as advocates when they clearly understand the parents' intentions.

The Transition from Employment to Retirement

Although federal law guarantees every child the right to a "free and appropriate education" (U.S. Department of Education, 2012), there are no guarantees for services for adults with disabilities. As a result, the process of obtaining employment or day programs for adults with ASD is a difficult one. Allen, Burke, Howard, Wallace, and Bowen (2012) cited a statistic of 90% unemployment for adults with ID, taken from the President's Committee for People with Intellectual Disabilities (2004). Jefferson and Putnam (2002) identify lack of specific job skills, and the need for better social skills training as obstacles to increasing rates of employment of adults with ASD (Jefferson & Putnam, 2002). Many of the adults who are employed work for only a few hours a week. In her article "Transition to Living," Jeanne Repetto (2003) discusses the skills that adults with disabilities need for "life beyond work." She contends that work occupies a small portion of time for individuals with or without disabilities and that it is therefore important to be prepared for a full range of adult roles and activities: "family member, friend, consumer and community member," among others (p. 79). There is a need to balance work and other pursuits to maintain a good quality of life.

Engagement with life, self-growth, social interactions, and novel pursuits all contribute to quality of life for many retired adults (Reichstadt et al., 2010). Lloyd and Auld (2002) also found that a "person-centered leisure attribute, leisure satisfaction, was the best predictor of quality of life" (p. 43). What does this mean for those adults with ASD who may have been employed full or part time and are now reaching typical retirement age? These adults often have limited choice-making skills, have few friends, and rely on a daily routine that involves a job or day program. In many cases family or guardians continue to provide practical support, transportation, living arrangements, meals, and assistance with medical care, as well as emotional support. These individuals may need other sources of support as well, such as access to the community or quality daytime activities (Bureau of Facility Standards, 2012).

For some adults with ASD full-time work may not be appropriate, and choice-making skills about daily activities are desirable. As one example, the Carolina Living and Learning Centers provide alternate activities that may continue to be appropriate into retirement age. These centers offer activities such as gardening, facility maintenance, community recreation, cooking, and crafts (Shea & Mesibov, 2005). The Creative Living Program of North Carolina provides day services with opportunities to participate in music, art, community trips, and volunteer activities at places such as animal shelters and libraries (Shea & Mesibov, 2005). (For more information on recreation and leisure skills for adults with ASD, see Coyne & Fullerton, Chapter 10, this volume).

Wilson, Stancliffe, Bigby, Balandin, and Craig (2010) described a "person-centered support model" for older adults with intellectual disabilities (ID). This model includes active treatment to assist the older adults in maintaining physical well-being and fitness, social engagement, and teaching or practice to maintain adaptive skills. The individual is assessed so that a plan can be designed that is appropriate for his or her chronological age and level of independence and that meets his or her needs and interests. "A disconnect prevails between what disability services can offer and what older people with ID want from their retirement years" (Wilson et al., 2010). They also offered "active mentoring" as a strategy to reduce this disconnect and facilitate the transition to retirement. Instead of going to his or her job or day program, the older person with ID spends one day a week engaged in activities that reflect typical retirement activities. This pattern is analogous to job sampling done during the transition from school to work. In this study 30 older individuals were supported in specific community or volunteer activities according to their interests. Mentors were recruited and trained from groups of typical retirees to assist the people with ID. The study revealed some of the challenges associated with the transition to retirement, including getting families and the individuals with ID to buy into the idea, working around group home schedules, and providing ongoing support. Individuals with no stated interests had more difficulty; at least one of these individuals returned to full-time day placement. Many were successful, however, and continued to participate in their "retirement" groups with support from their mentors.

Wilson and colleagues (2010) also found that case managers who are used to working with people in work placements did not have the orientation or skills to assist in transitions to retirement for the people on their caseloads. As the older population with ASD and ID increases, there will be a need for case managers with the skills and focus to assist individuals with ASD with the transition to retirement.

As they approach retirement years, adults with ASD need the opportunity to make real choices. There is no "one size fits all" age or model for retirement. For example, typical adults in many fields are choosing to work well into their 70s and 80s if their physical health allows them to. Some adults with ASD similarly may benefit from continuing to be engaged in gainful employment. Notwithstanding the age of retirement, older adults with ASD who have planned for retirement can enjoy a positive quality of life well into old age.

Residential Alternatives

For many older adults, aging successfully depends on living in a community that supports their needs and reflects their preferences. Many individuals move into "over-55" communities or supported living facilities where meals, transportation and other supports are available. Some complexes have movie theaters, stores, and hair salons on their sites. Swimming pools, golf courses, tennis courts, and game rooms may be available for onsite recreation. As the generation of baby boomers ages, the availability and variety of these communities has proliferated.

Similarly, older adults with ASD may find that circumstances dictate a need for a change in living arrangements. These adults may have lived with parents or family members until later in life. A change in health status of the parents may be one reason that the older adult with ASD needs a new place to live, or the adult her- or himself may have declining health and require more medical supports.

Placing a family member in a residential setting is often a difficult decision for a family. Some families put off this decision because of fears about the quality of life in residential services (Lounds & Seltzer, 2007). Finding the right placement with sufficient staff support and a philosophy of service provision in line with the family's ideas is important to a family seeking a residential placement for their family member with ASD.

"The characteristics of peoples' homes and the nature of their home life are likely to have a significant influence on their overall quality of life" (Felce & Perry, 2007, p. 410). The deinstitutionalization movement led researchers to identify quality indicators for residential settings. There are certain variables that seem to consistently contribute to quality in residential settings. Although the size of the program or facility in itself is not an indicator, staff ratio as related to the needs of the residents is an important variable. Personalization of the space or "home-likeness," level of staff–resident interaction, social climate, and individualization are other indicators of program quality (Felce, Jones, Lowe, & Perry, 2003). Choice, privacy, and relationships with parents and staff were also identified as important to quality of life for group home residents (Moss, 1994).

Older individuals with ASD can experience a variety of medical problems associated with aging, such as decreased vision or hearing and decreased mobility. An optimal living situation will include supports that enable these individuals to age in place. When selecting a group home or other living arrangement, families need to look well into the future and consider the ability of the agency or facility to adapt to the needs of aging individuals with ASD. With proper planning, group homes and apartments can incorporate these supports and accommodations, allowing the individual to age in place.

There is a need to support people through changes in their physical abilities as they age (Moss, 1994). The physical structure of the home or apartment is important. Location on one floor or a ground floor, an uncluttered environment without tripping hazards, adequate lighting, and comfortable furniture make the environment optimal for the older adult.

A well-planned environment will promote independence and autonomy as appropriate to the person. Aging individuals with ASD will need access to their own doctors and to specialists, as well. "They should have the potential to make choices, have close personal relationships for support, and the pursuit of leisure" (Moss, 1994, p. 231). Proximity to family members will promote continued closeness and frequent visits.

One example of a community that promotes aging in place is the Creative Living Community of Connecticut, which provides housing for adults with and without disabilities. It is an integrated farming community of 80 people, 20 of whom have ID. Residents run an agricultural business, and there is horticultural therapy available for senior citizens with or without developmental disabilities (visit *www.creativelivingofct.org* for details).

For individuals aging in their group homes or apartments, residential staff need training in sensitivity to issues of aging. Staff must monitor nutritional needs and weight gain or loss and must be sensitive to changes in behavior or habits that may indicate the onset of a medical problem. With appropriate supports in place and knowledge of the needs of older individuals with ASD, aging in place is an achievable goal.

Medical needs sometimes arise that may make it necessary to consider a nursing home placement for the aging individual with ASD. A family or guardian looking for a nursing home should consider quality indicators such as person-centered care and consistent assignment. In person-centered care, residents are given choices about their daily schedules, what time they get up, shower, or have meals. Consistent assignment is accomplished by assigning aides, nurses, and doctors to the same patients each shift. This arrangement promotes consistency and decreases errors in providing treatment or dispensing medication. Consistent assignment also allows closer relationships to develop between patients and staff (Konrad, 2010). An appropriate nursing home will be ready to meet the needs of the individual with ASD and will modify its system of service delivery to meet that person's unique needs. Information about nursing homes, including ratings of specific nursing homes and checklists for family members, is available at *www.medicare.gov*.

Before making a nursing home placement, it is important to explore supports that might allow the individual to remain in his or her own home. The state of Maryland, for example, has a Medicaid waiver that specifically addresses the needs of adults over age 50 who have low monthly income and assets below $2,000 and who qualify for nursing home level of care (Hilltop Institute, 2010). Services can be provided in the individual's home or in an assisted living facility. Included are services such as personal care, home-delivered meals, respite care, nutritionist services, assistive devices, environmental modifications, and case management.

Maryland's older-adult waiver does not specifically target individuals with ASD. However, it does offer an opportunity to address the changing needs of older adults with ASD, allowing them to remain in their homes or supervised apartments. Services such as medical day care provided in a group home setting also make it possible for some individuals to age in place.

Funding and Estate Planning

Historically, Medicaid was the funding source for institutional placements in the United States. When public policy shifted from institutions to community services, Medicaid permitted states to request waivers to use those funds to support community-based services instead. As a result, most services available today to adults with developmental disabilities are Medicaid-funded services. Because states are permitted some latitude in developing these waiver services, the rules and regulations vary from state to state. It is, therefore, essential to become familiar with the rules and regulations in the state in which the individual is seeking services (Arc for People with Intellectual and Developmental Disabilities, 2012). Specifically, families may need to understand the eligibility criteria, the application process, and any documents that may be required in order to receive services under the waiver. For example, in the state of New Jersey, in order to be eligible an individual must be a U.S. citizen and a New Jersey resident with limited income and resources. The individual must meet the functional criteria for the Division of Developmental Disabilities and the clinical criteria for level of care in an intermediate care facility for individuals with intellectul disabilities (ICF/ID), and must have been determined to be blind or disabled by the Social Security Administration or the Division of Medical Assistance and Health Services. Finally, the individual must be determined to be in need of, and use, a monthly waiver service. It is important to keep in mind that adult services are not an entitlement program. Eligibility, by itself, does not guarantee service. "Enrollment into the program is based on availability of a funded slot" (Division of Developmental Disabilities, 2013).

Medicaid eligibility requires that the individual with disabilities have limited income and resources. "The 2013 monthly income limit is $2,130 and resource limit is $2,000" (Division of Developmental Disabilities, 2013). Therefore, careful estate planning will be an essential element of proper planning for adults with ASD. For example, if an individual with ASD is named as a beneficiary in a will, it may jeopardize his or her eligibility for services. As an alternative, many legal and financial advisors recommend establishing a trust in the individual's name.

"A Trust is a legal document containing instructions directing the management and distribution of the resources placed in the Trust" (National Alliance on Mental Illness, 2013). The person who establishes the trust will appoint a person to manage it. A supplemental, or special needs, trust protects the individual's ability to qualify for government funding. This type of trust can provide supplemental funds to support a better quality of life for the individual with disabilities (Hannibal, 2013). Trusts can be used to supplement what is provided through government funding. Trusts can fund access to social events, vacations, or trips. If an advocate is needed to attend meetings or to visit the individual with ASD and monitor his or her care, a trust can provide an appropriate source of funds. It can also fund travel for family members' visits (Minde, 2011). These trusts can become particularly important when the parents or primary guardians are no longer alive or otherwise cannot participate actively.

Instead of setting up an individual trust, the parent or guardian may prefer to use a group trust to manage these assets. A group or pooled special needs trust is managed by a nonprofit organization set up specifically for this purpose. These nonprofits hire professionals to manage the trusts who are knowledgeable about the regulations and about individuals with disabilities. These pooled trusts may be useful if the family does not have a trustee to designate. Pooled trusts, however, have some limitations; for example, the assets cannot be moved after the trust is established. This potential limitation makes it important to fully investigate the organization before signing on. Comparing the rates and services of several pooled trusts is important before signing up to ensure that the organization meets the needs of the family and the individual with ASD (Hannibal, 2013).

The laws governing funding and estate planning vary from state to state. This chapter offers only a brief overview of these issues. It is strongly recommended that family members contact an attorney and a financial advisor with expertise in disability law for advice on these issues. Qualified attorneys and financial planners can be found through national, state, or local disability advocacy agencies. For example, Autismspeaks has listings, by state, of attorneys and financial planners on their website (*www.autismspeaks.org*), which includes contact information and a description of their services.

Case Example: John

John is a 52-year-old man with ASD and ID. He communicates verbally in short phrases and expresses his needs and preferences. He can make meaningful choices, and offering him choices is a positive strategy that helps reduce his frustration. He does have difficulty at times with articulation, which can make it difficult to understand him. Problems in communication can at times frustrate him, leading to aggressive grabbing of others or self-injurious head hitting. Changes in schedule or the inability to have a desired item can also lead to these behaviors. Program staff use preventive strategies with John to address his frustration; most effective are preparing him for changes in routine with verbal prompting and making a change on his written schedule. His receptive understanding of language is good, and he can indicate when he is not feeling well. He completes most daily living activities with minimal supervision; he dresses and feeds himself and prepares simple meals. He requires supervision for safety when cooking and cannot travel without supervision. He reads and uses a written schedule to help organize his day.

John began attending a day program for adults with ASD after he graduated from school. He has a part-time job doing building maintenance at a local office. He works with the supervision of a job coach, who provides transportation to his job. When he is not at his job, he goes to the day program, where he participates in subcontract mailing work, collating, labeling, and affixing stamps. John enjoys watching television, especially football, and looking at books or magazines. He likes to do puzzles, play Scrabble, and jet ski. He enjoys community outings, bowling, shopping, and trips to the library.

At age 34, John moved into a group home, where he lives with five other men with ASD with full-time staff supervision. His sister described the move to the group home as difficult for her mother. She had concerns that he would not be taken care of properly or would be unhappy there. The family convinced her of the need for the move; the parents were getting older and could no longer care for John's needs or deal with his behavioral challenges. Since that time both his parents have passed away, leaving his care and guardianship to his two siblings.

Because of their concerns about John's future, his parents planned carefully, and the results have been positive. They chose a group home operated by the same agency that provides his day services. This selection has provided continuity of programming for him and coordination of his goals in both settings. The quality of life in his home has been good, with his preferred leisure activities available. The home is not far from his siblings, who visit frequently and participate in house social events. His housemates have been the same for many years, providing a stable environment. When new staff members are hired, they receive extensive agency training to ensure that all staff fully understand his needs.

In addition to planning for an appropriate day program and a good place to live, his parents also made sure that his needs would continue to be met after they were gone. His brother is his legal guardian, and his sister provides emotional support to him as well. A special needs trust was set up for John. The funds from the trust have made it possible for him to vacation in places like Disney World. His siblings have also used the trust's funds to employ an outside consultant to attend meetings when needed and provide them with advice. As John ages, his family has plans to use the trust to fund modifications to the home to allow him to age in place.

His sister reported that her family always discussed these issues openly. She and her brother knew that they would someday become the caretakers for John. They are both older than John, so there is a plan in place for the next generation in the family to take over as guardians. The family supports each other and relies on information and support from the agency. When John was hospitalized, his sister reported that group home staff stayed with John at the hospital and made sure that his care was appropriate.

His sister does worry about the future, about John's health and "what will happen when I'm gone," just as so many other family members do. Will her nieces be ready for the responsibility, and will they visit as often as she does? These concerns are echoed by many other family members with ASD and are noted repeatedly in the literature. Because of the loving concern and detailed plans that his family have for him, it is probable that John's future outcomes will be good and that, as he grows older, his quality of life will continue.

Conclusions

There has been a good deal of attention in recent years to planning for children as they move from early intervention to school and also to transition services from school to adulthood. As adults with ASD age in the community, it is time for professionals, planners, policymakers, and service providers to place greater focus on the needs of this growing population. There is limited research on older adults with ASD. Existing research, however, does point to factors that contribute to their quality of life. Research on the typical aging population, as well as adults with ID, can also offer direction.

A study of 819 older adults with ID, with or without ASD, was conducted by Totsika, Felce, Kerr, and Hastings in 2010. They found that "older adults with ASD did not differ from those with ID in terms of behavior problems, psychiatric disorder, and quality of life." They went on to say that "differences in skills of adults with ASD were associated with decreased adaptive skills and not ASD per se" (Totsika et al., 2010, p. 1171). Adaptive skills and the ability to take care of oneself may be the best indicators of an enhanced quality of life for older adults with ASD.

Teaching adaptive skills in childhood and ensuring that they are maintained will pay a lifetime of dividends. Decisions made in the individual's childhood will have a great influence on the life of an aging adult.

Quality of life is promoted by living arrangements that reflect personalization and positive attention from support staff. Access to preferred leisure and recreation, proximity to family and friends, and engagement in daily activities in the community are also important components. Quality health care is essential to aging successfully. Challenges identified in 2002 in the surgeon general's report have yet to be addressed. Disparities in health care in the 2005 "call to action" still exist. Access to person-centered health care and a "medical home" remain out of reach for many adults with ASD. Strategies that promote aging in place should be considered in any public policy forum addressing the needs of those individuals aging with ASD.

For individuals with ASD and ID, aging successfully requires careful planning by parents and guardians. Parents who use coping mechanisms related to problem solving, who have access to accurate information, and who create a next generation of caregivers through family closeness and honest discussion are more likely to achieve desired outcomes. This type of success is borne out in interviews with family members of older adults with ASD. Family support services that go beyond "emotional support," that put an emphasis on improving the knowledge and coping skills of family members, and that encourage siblings to be part of the educational and therapeutic process will also improve outcomes. Family members who were interviewed emphasized the need for guardians who "can handle it"; who are up to the challenges and will remain actively involved with the individual with ASD. "Bring the next generation to visit the adult with ASD and encourage them to visit often"; "be realistic and have a plan"; and stay abreast of changes in laws and regulation that will affect the individual with ASD. One mother acknowledged that services have improved greatly over her son's lifetime but said "I keep moving forward." There are still many improvements that are needed and can be made.

REFERENCES

Allen, K. D., Burke, R. V., Howard, M. R., Wallace, D. P., & Bowen, S. L. (2012). Use of audio cuing to expand employment opportunities for adolescents with autism spectrum disorders and intellectual disabilities. *Journal of Autism and Developmental Disorders, 42*(11), 2410–2419.

Arc for People with Intellectual and Developmental Disabilities. (2009). Guardianship. Retrieved April 8, 2013, from *http://thearc.org/page.aspx?pid=2351.*

Arc for People with Intellectual and Developmental Disabilities. (2012). Medicaid reference desk. Retrieved April 8, 2013, from *www.thedesk.info.*

Baio, J. (2012). Prevalence of autism spectrum disorders: Autism and Developmental Disabilities Monitoring Network, 14 sites, United States, 2008. *MMWR Surveillance Summaries, 61*(5503), 1–19.

Bala, S. (2013, January 11). Autism transition handbook: Guardianship and financial planning. Retrieved April 8, 2013, from *www.autismhandbook.org*.

Barbosa, A., Figueiredo, D., Sousa, L., & Demain, S. (2011). Coping with the caregiving role: Differences between primary and secondary caregivers of dependent elderly people. *Aging and Mental Health, 15*(4), 490–499.

Blumberg, S. J., Bramlett, M. D., Kogen, M. D., Schieve, L. A., Jones, J. R., & Lu, M. C. (2013). *Changes in prevalence of parent-reported autism spectrum disorder in school-aged U.S. children. 2007 to 2011–2012* (National Health Statistics Reports No. 65). Hyattsville, MD: U.S. Department of Health and Human Service, Centers for Disease Control and Prevention, National Center for Health Statistics.

Bruder, M., Kerins, G., Mazzarella, C., Sims, J., & Stein, N. (2012). Brief report: The medical care of adults with autism spectrum disorders: Identifying the needs. *Journal of Autism and Developmental Disorders, 11*, 2498–2504.

Bureau of Facility Standards. (2012, July 13). Retirement for people with intellectual disabilities. Retrieved March 19, 2013, from *www.healthandwelfare.idaho.gov/portals/0/medical/licensingcertification/icfidretirement.pdf*.

Davidson, P. W., Janicki, M. P., Ladrigan, P., Houser, K., Henderson, C. M., & Cain, N. N. (2003). Associations between behavior disorders and health status among older adults with intellectual disability. *Aging and Mental Health, 7*(6), 424–431.

deFur, S. H. (2003). IEP transition planning: From compliance to quality. *Exceptionality, 11*, 115–129.

deFur, S. H., Todd-Allen, M., & Getzel, E. E. (2001). Parent participation in the transition planning process. *Career Development for Exceptional Individuals, 24*, 37–50.

Division of Developmental Disabilities. (2013, February). Medicaid eligibility for the CCW. Retrieved April 8, 2013, from *http://ccwmedicaidfactsheetgraphicfinal2.11.12(green).pdf*.

Drum, C. E., Krahn, G. L. Peterson, J. J., Horner-Johnson, W., & Newton, K. (2009). Health of people with disabilities: Determinants and disparities. In C. E. Drum, G. L. Krahn, & H. Bersani, Jr. (Eds.), *Disability and public health* (pp. 125–144). Washington, DC: American Association on Intellectual and Developmental Disabilities.

Erlanger, D. M., Kutner, K. C., Barth, J. T., & Barnes, R. (1999). Neuropsychology of sports-related head injury: Dementia pugilisticato post concussive syndrome. *Clinical Neuropsychologist, 13*(2), 193–210.

Eyal, G., Hart, B., Onculer, E., Oren, N., & Rossi, N. (2010). *The autism matrix: The social origins of the autism epidemic.* Cambridge, UK: Polity.

Felce, D., Jones, E., Lowe, K., & Perry, J. (2003). Rational resourcing and productivity: Relationships among staff input, resident characteristics, and group home quality. *American Journal on Mental Retardation, 108*, 161–172.

Felce, D., & Perry, J. (2007). Living with support in the community: Factors associated with quality of life outcome. In S. L. Odom, R. H. Horner, M. E. Snell,

& J. B. Blacher (Eds.), *Handbook of developmental disabilities* (pp. 410–428). New York: Guilford Press.

Fisher, K., & Kettl, P. (2005). Aging with mental retardation: Increasing population of older adults with mental retardation require health interventions and prevention strategies. *Geriatrics, 60*(4), 26–29.

Gerhardt, P., & Holmes, D. (2005). Employment: Options and issues for adolescents and adults with autism spectrum disorders. In F. R. Volkmar, R. Paul, A. Klin, & D. Cohen (Eds.), *Handbook of autism and pervasive developmental disorders* (3rd ed., pp. 1087–1101). Hoboken, NJ: Wiley.

Greenfeld, J. (1972). *A child called Noah: A family journey*. New York: Holt, Rinehart & Winston.

Greenfeld, K. T. (2009, May 25). Growing old with autism. *Time*. Retrieved April 8, 2013, from *www.time.com/time/magazine/article/0,9171,1898322,00/html*.

Haley, W. E., & Perkins, E. A. (2004). Current status and future directions in family caregiving and aging people with intellectual disabilities. *Journal of Policy and Practice in Intellectual Disabilities, 1*, 24–30.

Hannibal, B. S. (n.d.). Pooled special needs trusts. Retrieved April 8, 2013, from *www.nolo.com/legal-encyclopedia/pooled-special-needs-trusts.html.*.

Heller, T., & Factor, A. (2004). *Older adults with mental retardation and their aging family caregivers*. Chicago: University of Illinois, Rehabilitation Research and Training Center on Aging with Developmental Disabilities.

Heller, T., & Kramer, J. (2009). Involvement in adult siblings of persons with developmental disabilities. *Intellectual and Developmental Disabilities, 47*, 208–219.

Hilltop Institute. (2010, December 3). Medicaid long-term supports and services in Maryland: The older adults waiver. Retrieved April 18, 2013, from *www.hilltopinstitute.org/publications/dhmhltsschartbook-olderadultswaiver-December2010.pdf*

Howlin, P., Goode, S., Hutton, J., & Rutter, M. (2004). Adult outcome for children with autism. *Journal of Child Psychology and Psychiatry, 45*(2), 212–229.

Janicki, M. P. (2009). The aging dilemma: Is increasing longevity among people with intellectual disabilities creating a new population challenge in the Asia-Pacific region? *Journal of Policy and Practice in Intellectual Disabilities, 6*(2), 73–76.

Jefferson, G. L., & Putnam, R. F. (2002). Understanding transition services: A parent's guide to legal standards and effective practices. *Exceptional Parent, 32*, 70–77.

Konrad, W. (2010, March 18). Stressful but vital: Picking a nursing home. *New York Times*, p. B1.

Larson, E. B., & Reid, R. (2010). The patient-centered medical home movement. *Journal of the American Medical Association, 303*(16), 1644–1645.

Lehrer, P. M., & Woolfolk, R. L. (1993). *Principles and practice of stress management* (2nd ed.). New York: Guilford Press.

Lloyd, K. M., & Auld, C. J. (2002). The role of leisure in determining quality of life: Issues of content and measurement. *Social Indicators Research, 57*(1), 43–71.

Lounds, J. J., & Seltzer, M. M. (2007). Family impact in adulthood. In S. L.

Odom, R. H. Horner, M. E. Snell, & J. P. Blacher (Eds.), *Handbook of developmental disabilities* (pp. 552–569). New York: Guilford Press.

Minde, J. H. (2011). Supplemental needs trusts: Some frequently asked questions. Retrieved April 8, 2013, from *www.nsnn.com/frequently.htm*.

Moss, S. (1994). Quality of life and aging. In D. Goode (Ed.), *Quality of life for persons with disabilities: International perspectives and issues* (pp. 218–234). Cambridge, MA: Brookline Books.

National Alliance on Mental Illness. (2013). Special needs estate planning. Retrieved April 8, 2013, from *www.nami.org/template.cfm?section=special_needs_estate_planning&template=/contentmanagement/contentdisplay.cfm&contentid=8936*.

National Committee for Quality Assurance. (2010, June 2). Leveraging health IT to achieve ambulatory quality: The patient-centered medical home. Retrieved March 20, 2013, from *www.ncqa.org/portals/0/publicpolicy/himss_ncqa_pcmh_factsheet.pdf*.

Nehring, W. M. & Betz, C. L. (2007). General health. In S. L. Odom, R. H. Horner, M. E. Snell, & J. B. Blacher (Eds.), *Handbook of developmental disabilities* (pp. 79–97). New York: Guilford Press.

Orsmond, G., Kuo, H., & Seltzer, M. M. (2009). Siblings of individuals with an autism spectrum disorder: Sibling relationships and well-being in autism and adulthood. *Autism, 13*(1), 59–80.

Orsmond, G. I., & Seltzer, M. M. (2007). Siblings of individuals with autism or Down syndrome: Effect on adult lives. *Journal of Intellectual Disability Research, 51*(9), 682–696.

Perkins, E. A., & Berkman, K. (2011, June 7). Aging adults with autism spectrum disorders. Retrieved January 12, 2013, from *www.aaidd.org/docs/default-source/annual-meeting/aaidd_gerontology_division_symposium_aging_with_autism_submittedtoaaidd.pdf?sfvrsn=2..*

Perkins, E., & LaMartin, K. (2012). The Internet as social support for older carers of adults with intellectual disabilities. *Journal of Policy and Practice in Intellectual Disabilities, 9*(1), 53–62.

Pilon, M., & Belson, K. (2013, January 10). Seau suffered from brain disease. *New York Times*, p. B13.

President's Committee for People with Intellectual Disabilities. (2004). A charge we have to keep. Available at *www.acf.hhs.gov/programs/pcpid/2004_rpt_pres/2004_rpt_pg7.html*.

Reichstadt, J., Sengupta, G., Depp, C. A., Palinkas, L. A., & Jeste, D. V. (2010). Older adults' perspectives on successful aging: Qualitative interviews. *American Journal of Geriatric Psychiatry, 18*(7), 567–575.

Repetto, J. B. (2003). Transition to living. *Exceptionality, 11*, 77–87.

Rudy, L. J. (2011, September 6). Guardianship for ASD adults. Retrieved April 8, 2013, from *www.autismafter16.com/print/18*.

Schultz, R., & Beach, S. R. (1999). Caregiving as a risk factor for mortality: The caregiver health effects study. *Journal of the American Medical Association, 15*, 2215–2219.

Seltzer, M. M., Krauss, M. W., & Hong, J. (1996). Midlife and later-life parenting of adult children with mental retardation. In C. D. Ryff & M. M. Seltzer (Eds.), *The parental experience in midlife* (pp. 459–489). Chicago: University of Chicago Press.

Seventh Voice. (2012, May 6). Aging and autism: Insights from the perspectives of adults with high-functioning autism. Retrieved March 12, 2013, from *http://seventhvoice.wordpress.com/2012/05/06/aging-and-autism-insights-from-the-perspectives-of-adults-with-high-functioning-autism*.

Shavelle, R. M., Strauss, D. J., & Pickett, J. (2001). Causes of death in autism. *Journal of Autism and Developmental Disorders, 31*, 569–576.

Shea, V., & Mesibov, G. (2005). Adolescents and adults with autism. In F. R. Volkmar, R. Paul, A. Klin, & D. Cohen (Eds.), *Handbook of autism and pervasive developmental disorders* (3rd ed., pp. 288–311). Hoboken, NJ: Wiley.

Stuart-Hamilton, I., & Morgan, H. (2011). What happens to people with autism spectrum disorders in middle age and beyond?: Report of a preliminary online study. *Advances in Mental Health and Intellectual Disabilities, 5*(2), 22–28.

Totsika, V., Felce, D., Kerr, M., & Hastings, R. P. (2010). Behavior problems, psychiatric symptoms, and quality of life for older adults with intellectual disability with and without autism. *Journal of Autism and Developmental Disorders, 40*(10), 1171–1178.

U.S. Department of Education. (2012, May). Building the legacy: IDEA. Retrieved April 11, 2013, from *http://idea.ed.gov/explore/home*.

U.S. Department of Health and Human Services. (2005). The Surgeon General's call to action to improve the health and wellness of persons with disabilities. Retrieved from *www.ncbi.nlm.nih.gov/books/nbk44667*.

U.S. Public Health Service. (2002). Closing the gap: A national blueprint for improving the health of individuals with mental retardation: Report of the Surgeon General's conference on health disparities and mental retardation. Retrieved from *www.ncbi.nlm.nih.gov/books/nbk44346*.

What is a medical home? (n.d.). Retrieved February 5, 2014, from *www.medical-homeportal.org*.

Wilson, N. J., Stancliffe, R. J., Bigby, C., Balandin, S., & Craig, D. (2010). The potential for active mentoring to support the transition into retirement for older adults with a lifelong disability. *Journal of Intellectual and Developmental Disabilities, 35*(3), 211–214.

CHAPTER 14

● ● ● ● ● ● ●

Legal Issues
and Autism Spectrum Disorders

● **Beverly L. Frantz and David W. Zellis**

This chapter examines the challenges faced by individuals with autism spectrum disorders (ASD) and their involvement with the criminal justice system. The existence of misconceptions surrounding people with ASD and violence is skewed and perpetuated by popular media. The fifth edition of the *Diagnostic and Statistical Manual of Mental Disorders* (DSM-5; American Psychiatric Association, 2013) states that symptoms associated with ASD include a range of social and communication problems and restrictive and repetitive behaviors. The communication deficiencies frequently possessed by persons with ASD, such as responding inappropriately in conversations, misreading nonverbal interactions, or having difficulty building age-appropriate relationships, are not indicators of criminal pathology. Nor is repetitive motor behavior, such as hand flapping when others are not engaged in such action.

The Sandy Hook Elementary School shooting is an example of how popular media exploited a perceived relationship between ASD and violence, reigniting the debate on whether individuals with high-functioning autism spectrum disorders (HFASD) are at an increased risk for committing criminal behavior. Friends and people interviewed by the FBI described Adam Lanza, the identified shooter, as having HFASD. He was described as a "shut-in," "avid [video] gamer," "deeply uncomfortable in social situations," "never seen with anyone, either socializing or as a friend," and obtaining "good grades" (Kleinfield, Rivera, & Kovaleski, 2013). By attempting to draw a causal correlation between ASD and criminal behavior, the media unintentionally reinforce fallacies and perpetuate stereotypes that create discomfort, and even fear, about people with ASD.

Haskin and Silva (2006) found that people with Asperger syndrome are overrepresented among the delinquent or criminal offending population compared with the general population. For clarification, this chapter uses the term *Asperger syndrome* when citing research that was conducted prior to the publication of DSM-5.

Weiss (2011) suggests that in a cultural milieu in which citizens are asked to report "suspicious behavior," it is not difficult to see how oddly behaving individuals can become the focus of concern. Individuals exhibiting "suspicious behavior" are not exclusively people with autism or other disabilities. The 2012 shooting death of Trayvon Martin by a neighborhood watch captain is such an example. According to police reports, the neighborhood watch captain called 9-1-1 to report that he was following "a suspicious person [Trayvon Martin]."

Howlin (2004) argues that any connection between Asperger syndrome and crime is "the result of a small number of cases which have given rise to much publicity and to (speculative) causal attributions in the media" (p. 302). A diagnosis of Asperger syndrome is not an inevitable risk factor for committing a criminal act, nor does everyone with Asperger syndrome commit a crime. Similarly, Murrie, Warren, Kristiansson, and Dietz (2002) state that the majority of people with Asperger syndrome are law abiding. Ghaziuddin (1991) concurs, reporting that, in a review of 132 published case studie of people with Asperger syndrome between 1944 and 1990, only three (2.27%) had a clear history of violence. Hippler, Viding, Klicpera, and Happé (2010) reported that the average proportion of convictions in their sample (1.3%) is comparable to that in the general male population (1.25%). Woodbury-Smith, Clare, Holland, and Kearns's (2006) community study indicated "that the rate of law-breaking, including offending, was very low" (p. 108). Studies that report higher prevalence rates of people with HFASD committing violent acts compared with people in the general population were primarily of two kinds. These are retrospective studies that explored whether people convicted of serious crimes showed any autistic characteristics and studies that were conducted in forensic psychiatric hospital and custodial settings.

Wing (1981) identified six core clinical characteristics typical of individuals with Asperger syndrome: (1) minimal empathy; (2) naive, inappropriate, one-sided social interactions and limited capacity to form relationships; (3) pedantic and repetitive speech; (4) poor nonverbal communications; (5) intense preoccupation with circumscribed topics; and (6) clumsy movements, poor coordination, and odd posture.

Several of these characteristics, such as lack of empathy, naive, inappropriate one-sided interactions, inability to develop and sustain friendships, and poor communication skills, increase the probability of a person's contact with the criminal justice system. What the disability community sees as an individual's unique attributes or idiosyncratic behavior, the criminal justice system sees as a person's unwillingness to cooperate, lack of remorse, defiance, unwillingness to follow directions, and disrespect for authority.

The following case example illustrates the collision between ASD and the criminal justice system.

Case Example: AB

AB was a 20-year-old man who lived with his parents in an apartment complex. One evening AB was home alone. A neighbor called 9-1-1 to report loud music coming from AB's apartment. A police officer responded, knocked on AB's apartment door, and identified himself as a police officer. There was no response. The police officer knocked again with a bit more force and loudly announced, "Police, open the door."

Again, there was no response. Inside the apartment AB heard the knocks on the door and the police officer's command to open the door. AB was frightened and panicked. He did not understand why a police officer was at his front door, but he thought that if he hid in his closet, the police officer would go away.

However, the police officer did not go away. He continued to knock and then bang on the door while continuing to ask that the apartment door be opened. When that failed, the police officer located the apartment's maintenance supervisor, who unlocked the apartment door. Upon entering the apartment, the police officer, using a very authoritative and loud voice, identified himself. There was no response. The officer lowered the volume of the music and was about to search the apartment when he heard a noise coming from a back room. The officer proceeded toward the noise, identifying himself and ordering whoever was in the room to come out with his hands on top of his head.

AB was screaming from inside his bedroom closet. The police officer proceeded cautiously toward the noise while continuing to identify himself and asking the person to come out with his hands on his head. AB became increasingly fearful and grabbed a baseball bat from inside the closet. When his bedroom door was opened and the police officer entered, AB charged out of the closet swinging the bat. In an instant, the police officer, fearing for his own life, fired a single shot at AB. AB died.

Tragic situations such as this can be prevented. Similar to the African proverb "It takes a village to raise a child," it takes multiple systems and individuals to keep people with ASD safe. Personal safety skills need to be first taught at a young age, with repeated trainings at regular intervals through adulthood. The frequency, depth of information, and safety strategies need to be appropriate for the person's chronological and development ages.

Similar to person-centered planning, making a safety plan involves a group of people from various systems working together to create guidelines and build alliances that make sense to the individual with ASD in order to create and maintain safety at home, at work, and in the community. The development of a safety plan should involve a series of meetings that include the individual with ASD so as to identify the best way to approach that person. Such factors include the name the individual likes to be called, his or her interests, and other information that may be helpful in calming the individual. The types of sensory stimulation, if any, that are disturbing to the individual and how the person responds to being touched should be identified.

In AB's case, the safety plan should have been shared with several neighbors and the maintenance supervisor and registered with the local 9-1-1 emergency system Premise Alert program. Safety plans should be brief and bulleted. Police officers have just a few seconds to assess a situation and determine an appropriate response in order to maintain a safe environment and ensure their own safety. A prominently displayed autism ribbon, puzzle logo, or similar symbol can alert a police officer that a person with autism lives at the address and may have difficulty responding to police commands.

If a police officer has probable cause to believe that a suspect poses a significant threat or serious bodily injury to the officer or others, then the use of deadly force is justified. Law enforcement officers follow a six-level force continuum in determining the required force needed for any situation. The levels are designed to be flexible as the need for force changes as a situation develops.

The six levels of the force continuum are: (1) officer presence; (2) verbal commands; (3) empty-hand control; (4) pepper spray, baton, taser; (5) less lethal techniques; and (6) deadly force. In AB's case the combination of the presence of a police officer and shouted verbal commands had the reverse effect. Rather than deescalating the situation, the shouting of commands by the police officer only served to make it worse. The outcome of this situation may have been different if the police officer had known that an individual with ASD lived in the apartment and responded negatively to people "yelling" and if AB had been taught the importance of following police commands.

Police need to receive training in the unique attributes of juveniles and adults with autism; in the best practices for identifying and deescalating situations involving people with ASD; and in understanding that an officer's badge or other reflective insignia on their uniforms may cause a person with ASD to impulsively reach out in an attempt to touch the officer's badge. This "reaching out" action can be misunderstood and perceived by the police officer as an aggressive act. Conversely, educating people with ASD and their families about the role and responsibilities of law enforcement and the importance of following a police officer's verbal command is essential in deescalating dangerous situations. Common verbal commands are "stop," "don't move," "be quiet," "show me your hands," or "let me see your ID."

There is considerable research supporting the theory that people who are exposed to particular risk factors are more likely to become involved in offending behaviors. The Office of Juvenile Justice and Delinquency Prevention in the U.S. Department of Justice (Shader, 2003) recognizes the Mrazek and Haggerty (1994) definition of risk factors as "those characteristics, variables, or hazards that, if present for a given individual, make it more likely that this individual, rather than someone selected from the general population, will develop a disorder" (p. 495). Conversely, Allen, Evans, Hider, and Peckett (2008) state that individuals on the spectrum "may be particularly vulnerable to exploitation as stooges in criminal activities as a result of their failure to understand social relationships" (p. 758).

Although risk factors are used by researchers to detect the likelihood of offending behaviors, there are many individuals who possess those risk factors who never commit a delinquent or violent act (Browning & Caulfield, 2011). The prevalence of offending behaviors among people with HFASD/Asperger syndrome is difficult to determine because the majority of research is drawn from individuals who are already in forensic settings (Allen et al., 2008; Hippler et al., 2009; Scragg & Shah, 1994).

The term *forensic setting* generally refers to behavioral/mental health units in state and federal prisons or units within a psychiatric facility designated for offenders. What is missing from the research are studies that investigate the prevalence of offending behaviors among people with ASD in county jails. The terms *jail* and *prison* are frequently used interchangeably; however, they are entirely different entities.

Jails are run by county governments. They are a place to hold a person who is not able to make bail in custody prior to trial; they are a place for people convicted of relatively minor crimes with sentences that rarely exceed 2 years. Psychological testing is not considered a necessity in county jails. Prisons are run by state governments. Inmates entering a state prison system are required to undergo a rigorous comprehensive intake process, which may include medical and psychological examinations.

The importance of understanding the distinction between county jails and state prisons is that judges are more inclined to sentence a person with a disability, especially intellectual and developmental disabilities, to a county jail rather than a state prison. The advantage of a sentence to a county jail is that the individual will be closer to his or her family. The disadvantage of county jails is that they are not designed to, nor do they have the resources to, provide the types of supports a person with an intellectual disability or ASD requires.

A 2006 community-based study conducted by Woodbury-Smith and colleagues refutes previous research findings that suggest a causal correlation between Asperger syndrome and offending behaviors. Most studies of people with ASD and the criminal justice system focus on the relationship between ASD and aggression or acts of violence. Palermo's (2004) research suggests that aggression in individuals with ASD can be attributed to comorbid psychiatric disorders.

Studies do exist that document the increased risk of individuals with HFASD and Asperger syndrome to engage in illegal behaviors (Howlin, 1997; Plimley & Bowen, 2007), including inappropriate sexual behaviors (Baron-Cohen, 1988; Haskin & Silva, 2006), and to have increased contact with the criminal justice system at the state level, including forensic correctional facilities. The term *inappropriate sexual behavior* is not a legal term. It is frequently used when attempting to mitigate circumstances surrounding nonconsensual touch between an individual with an intellectual disability (ID) and a person with or without a disability.

The American criminal justice system has been described as the best in the world because it is based on the U.S. Constitution. The legal principles of "innocent until proven guilty," "being judged by a jury of your peers," "the right to remain silent," and "the right to an attorney" are all based on the Constitution. These and other Constitutional protections are intended to protect all citizens from the government and, in particular, law enforcement. The fundamental public policy issue that is beginning to bubble to the surface is whether the American criminal justice system can ensure that the Constitution will continue to protect all citizens, including citizens with ASD.

The following two case examples illustrate the potential traps within the criminal justice system that may ensnare individuals with ASD.

Case Example: TL

TL was a 26-year-old man diagnosed with Asperger syndrome at age 15. He is a high school graduate with average intelligence and good verbal skills. He has difficulty carrying on a conversation, walks away from confrontational and stressful situations, and has no history of violent behavior. His family reports he has never had any friends, struggles to maintain employment, and flirted with drug and alcohol use when he was a minor. From age 19 he had been arrested six times and charged with various counts of burglary, use/possession of drug paraphernalia, receiving stolen property, recklessly endangering another, simple assault, corruption of minors, supplying liquor and other illegal substances to minors, possession of a small amount of marijuana for personal use, and criminal trespassing. His first several encounters with the criminal justice system resulted in the court's placing him on probation. He violated his probation several times and is currently incarcerated in a county jail.

TL has a supportive family who retained a criminal attorney to represent him when he was arrested. He is currently represented by a public defender for probation violations. TL received court-ordered inpatient drug and alcohol treatment. According to court documents, TL successfully completed the drug and alcohol inpatient treatment program. However, approximately 18 months after his "successful completion of the program," TL was arrested for probation violations, including drug and alcohol use. The drug and alcohol program that he had previously successfully completed would not consider his application for readmission, nor would the program suggest other appropriate programs.

TL's case is not unusual and illustrates the dilemma individuals with ASD face when they encounter the criminal justice system. His impaired social reciprocal skills—his history of not having friends, inability to pick up social cues, communication deficiencies, and repetitive behavior—made him a prime candidate to be a repeat offender. A review of the circumstances and charges against TL exemplifies how individuals with ASD become ensnarled in the criminal justice system.

TL wants a life like his siblings. He wants friends, a girlfriend, a job, and independence. Although he "hung out" with some students in high school, he did not have any friends. When he graduated, he did not have anyone to "hang out" with. He obtained a part-time job in the food service industry. He learned that if he bought alcohol for underage youth, they would invite him to their parties. By supplying underage students with alcohol, he thought he would fit in and have friends—a one-sided approach to social interactions.

Law enforcement officials are frustrated with him due to their perception of his indifference and repetitive criminal activities. The courts view his probation violations and continued offending behaviors as acts of defiance and as demonstrating no remorse for his actions. But, in fact, his repetitive criminal offenses are traceable in part to a desire to fit in, coupled with a poor understanding of social cues and social consequences, as is common in persons with HFASD.

Legal Perspective

In an effort to protect TL, educators, family members, and possibly even law enforcement may have rationalized and excused TL's questionable actions as a combination of juvenile behavior and an HFASD diagnosis. However, at 26 years of age, TL is not a teenager, and his HFASD diagnosis is no longer an excuse for his behavior, especially his criminal behavior.

A diagnosis of ASD is not a legal defense. Law enforcement officers, prosecutors, judges, probation/parole officers, and correctional officers may not understand how an ASD diagnosis may affect the respective roles and responsibilities of their positions. This is not to suggest that they are not empathetic to TL or other individuals with disabilities. However, the current criminal justice system exists to efficiently and effectively move thousands of individuals charged with minor to serious crimes through the system, which is overburdened and underfunded.

As a result, when faced with a repeat offender such as TL, the typical response by police officers, prosecutors, and judges is to assume that the offender "does not get it." In other words, as long as TL continues to "act out" or "engage in criminal behavior," he leaves "us," the judicial system, no choice but to "lock him up" in order to "protect the community." Without an understanding of the idiosyncratic behaviors of persons with ASD, the judicial system interprets the person's behavior as noncompliant, defiant, and lacking remorse. Unless a defense attorney introduces ASD into evidence as a mitigating factor, it may never be considered during the court process. TL and other persons with ASD involved in the criminal justice system may find themselves trapped in the system's continuously revolving door.

Discussion

Regardless of the support provided by his family, TL requires intense and ongoing support from a trained professional, ideally someone with knowledge of applied behavior analysis. Without such intervention, it is unlikely that TL's behavior will change. He will continue to have contact with police and may eventually be charged as a repeat offender and sentenced to a state prison or a psychiatric forensic facility.

Haskin and Silva (2006) discuss the frequency of HFASD being misdiagnosed as schizoid and schizotypal disorders. This suggests that HFASD can be misdiagnosed and that diagnosis can be substantially complicated when other, co-occurring conditions are present.

Case Example: XY

U.S. Immigration and Customs Enforcement (ICE) agents arrived at XY's home while he was attending classes at the community college. They identified themselves to his mother as ICE agents assigned to the child pornography unit. They informed her that they had a warrant to search XY's bedroom and to remove his computer and other electronic devices, including discs and flash drives. Upon leaving, the lead agent strongly suggested to XY's mother that the family consider retaining legal counsel for their son. In similar situations, some parents have argued that their adolescent or adult child accidentally opened a child pornography website. According to the FBI, when searches are authorized, they are based on numerous and repeated visits to child pornography sites from a specific computer over a period of time.

XY had installed peer-to-peer software, also known as P2P, on his computer. P2P is a software file transfer service that allows users to share computer files through the Internet. P2P services are designed to allow users to search for and download files of others to their computers and to enable other users to download from their computers (*www.nsf.gov/oig/peer.pdf*).

XY's parents retained a criminal defense attorney for him. He began seeing a sex addiction therapist and participating in outpatient group therapy. It has been over a year, and criminal charges have still not been filed. Through his attorney, XY was informed that it may be an additional 6 months or more before a determination is made as to whether charges will be filed, and, if filed, what the charges would be.

Diagnosed at an early age, XY exhibits classic attributes of Asperger syndrome, such as the inability to pick up social cues, a history of not being able to make friends, communication deficiencies, and a preoccupation with specific areas of interest, computers in XY's case.

Legal Perspective

XY finds himself in serious trouble even though criminal charges have yet to be filed. There is little doubt that, once the forensic computer examinations are completed, criminal charges will be filed against XY for possession and distribution of child pornography. Ultimately, if XY is convicted or pleads guilty, he could face a significant amount of time in a state or federal prison.

In XY's situation, his only protector against being treated inappropriately and unfairly by the criminal justice system is his lawyer. A critical decision made by XY and his family was which attorney should represent him. Clearly, XY's case is too serious for a family attorney to handle. Family law attorneys generally handle issues concerning estate planning and administration (e.g., living will trusts, power of attorney, and guardianship), divorce, adoptions, contract matters, and other noncriminal issues. XY requires an attorney who specializes in criminal defense.

XY's family took the necessary steps of hiring an attorney by interviewing a number of criminal defense attorneys and asking important relevant questions. The purpose of the interview process was to gather information about the attorney's experience and knowledge in handling similar cases. The family asked each attorney the following questions: (1) Have you ever handled cases with clients who were on the autism spectrum, especially individuals with Asperger syndrome? (2) If so, how many cases, how long ago, and what were the criminal charges? and (3) Would you be receptive to speaking to experts in the field of autism in order to gain additional knowledge concerning the behaviors of XY?

Although XY's attorney took the proactive approach of recommending therapy with an addiction professional, it is unclear what knowledge and experiences the attorney and addiction professional have with Asperger syndrome. Therein lies another trap within the criminal justice system: defense attorneys who lack the knowledge and skill set required to work with people with Asperger syndrome. A criminal defense attorney is not just responsible for protecting XY's rights but is also responsible for zealously advocating on behalf of XY.

Zealous advocacy includes educating law enforcement and prosecutors about XY's diagnosis and explaining the impact it has on his ability to function and adhere to the law. In order to fulfill such a function and perhaps minimize the charges before they are filed, the defense attorney must take the time to obtain a comprehensive understanding of XY and be able to convey such information to law enforcement and prosecutors. The problem for XY and others like him is that most public defenders and private criminal defense attorneys do not have the time or patience to become knowledgeable about an ASD diagnosis.

It is incumbent upon XY's family to carefully choose a defense attorney who has the willingness, time, patience, and knowledge to represent XY's unique circumstances. Furthermore, XY's family can help and has an obligation to educate the defense attorney about XY, but in a manner which is sensitive to the attorney's time constraints. One way the family can assist is by collecting XY's medical, psychological, and school records for the attorney to review and by making a list with contact information of the professionals with knowledge of XY's ASD.

If XY's attorney presents his case to the prosecutor and the judge as though this is a sex addiction issue without giving consideration to his Asperger syndrome diagnosis, the prosecutor and the judge will ignore XY's special needs as a mitigating circumstance.

Discussion

The sexual development of individuals with HFASD and Asperger syndrome is comparable to that in the general population (Henault, 2006). (See Travers & Whitby, Chapter 9, this volume, for additional discussion of sexuality and people with ASD.) Yet parents frequently have a difficult time speaking to their children about sexuality. Many parents fear that if they talk about sexuality, their children will want to explore it.

A comprehensive social sexual history of XY would identify at what age he first became curious about and explored sexuality. Did his parents ever notice any interest in sexually explicit materials, sexualized gestures, or talk that would be considered inappropriate for his age? Sexual interest and arousal are normal developmental stages for adolescent males. Whether XY attended sex education classes in high school, discussed sexuality with his parents, and/or exhibited any interest in sexuality is unknown. Rather than restricting healthy sexual curiosity, urges, and desires, these urges should be directed toward appropriate socially accepted expressions.

It is unclear whether the addiction professional has experience working with individuals with Asperger syndrome and what type of assessment, if any, was used to ascertain whether XY actually has a sexual addiction. Or is XY's behavior, albeit illegal, a characteristic of his Asperger syndrome? That is, is his behavior not an addiction but rather severe and sustained impairment in social interactions and the development of restricted, repetitive patterns of behaviors, interests, and activities (American Psychiatric Association, 2013).

Suggestions for Selecting a Criminal Defense Attorney

Advertisements for lawyers bombard us on billboards, television, and radio and in newspapers, direct mail, and social media. Attorneys spend a lot of money on advertising and marketing. But will lawyer advertising assist you in selecting the best attorney for your legal situation? It may, but it may not.

When choosing an attorney, think of the attorney–client relationship like the doctor–patient relationship. Just like a patient meeting a prospective doctor, a client searching for an attorney is also facing serious and personal circumstances. Although, when searching for a doctor, you may consider advertisements, it should not be a substitute for engaging in your own research before making a final decision. There are many guiding principles when choosing a lawyer, but perhaps the five most important points to consider are the following:

1. Identify the type of attorney necessary to deal with the problem that needs to be resolved. Lawyers have become very specialized, and one lawyer today may not be capable of handling all of your different legal needs. This principle is even truer when it comes to attorneys who handle issues involving adults with disabilities who happen to be in trouble with the law. There are many criminal defense attorneys, but there may only be a few who can appreciate and effectively represent an adult with a disability. Therefore, it is important to use the next four principles to select the right attorney for the legal situation.

2. Although it may sound too simple, you should trust and rely on your instincts when selecting any attorney. To do this, it helps to ask the following questions:

    a. Does the lawyer seem as if he or she wants to be there meeting with you?

    b. Do you feel like just another client?

    c. Does the attorney take the time to *listen* to you and answer your questions?

If you feel that the attorney is not engaged with you or taking you or your problem seriously, a lack of trust will probably exist. A lack of trust will make your job and your attorney's job harder and will take the focus away from the best handling and resolution of the case.

3. Your responsibility to yourself and the accused is to ask questions and get answers from the lawyer. An attorney's job is not only to go to court on behalf of the client but also to educate the client so that the client can make an informed decision. To select the right attorney, you should prepare questions to ask the attorney. In addition, you have to know what you are looking for and determine whether the attorney is knowledgeable enough to represent your interests. This is not to say that the attorney is "bad" if he or she cannot answer every question off the top of his or her head. The law is voluminous, always changing, and very complex. Many times the attorney needs to do research to determine the correct answers. Ultimately, when asking questions of an attorney, you need

to determine whether he or she seems knowledgeable, as well as upfront, about your circumstances.

4. A cardinal principle governing the search for an attorney is that guarantees are only worth as much as the paper they are written on. There are cases in which an attorney can anticipate possible outcomes, and there are "standard" cases that may make predictions more likely to come true. However, no matter how many years of practice an attorney has, the outcome cannot be guaranteed. Guarantees are worthless because each case has its own judge, prosecutor, law enforcement officer, and set of facts, which can change the outcome of the case. An attorney who you can trust should be upfront about this, and you need to be skeptical of anyone who guarantees an outcome.

A skilled attorney can do a lot to put the case in the best position to benefit the accused, but the attorney cannot predict the future. It may make you feel better when you go home with a guarantee, but this is an illusion, as there is no guaranteed result for any case.

5. A final consideration is that attorneys cost money, and oftentimes you get what you pay for, just as with many other things in life. Many people engage in "attorney shopping" and call around to see who can do the work at the lowest price. But you would not choose a doctor simply because he or she could do the procedure at the lowest price. You would not choose a doctor by the lowest price because it involves your life and it is serious. Although attorney fees are certainly a significant factor in determining which attorney to retain, you are taking a huge risk if price is your sole or most important consideration.

Discussion

The aim of this chapter is to dispel the misconception that persons with ASD are at a higher risk than persons in the general population for committing crimes. Characteristics associated with ASD, such as social and communication deficits—including responding inappropriately in conversations, misreading nonverbal interactions, and having difficulty building age-appropriate relationships—are not indicators of criminal pathology. Nor are restrictive and repetitive behaviors, such as hand flapping, an indicator for criminal behavior. Conversely, these same behaviors may contribute to the vulnerability of a person with ASD to becoming a crime victim or an alleged offender. Irrespective of how a person with ASD comes into contact with the criminal justice system, his or her idiosyncratic behavior may be misunderstood. Professionals working within law enforcement, the courts, and correctional facilities may attribute these unique behaviors of a person with ASD as an unwillingness to cooper-ate, lack of remorse, disrespect for authority, and unwillingness to follow directions.

A cross-system, cross-discipline, systemic approach, including edu-cation, intervention, and risk reduction strategies, is essential to reduc-ing the risk of people with ASD encountering the criminal justice system as victims, witnesses, or offenders. For example, parents need to begin "safety" discussions with their child with ASD at an early age and con-tinue those discussions through adulthood. These "safety" discussions need to be chronologically and developmentally age appropriate.

Once the child enters an educational setting, the "safety" discussion should continue, but it should also become a safety plan and be included in the student's individualized educational plan (IEP). The safety plan is a mechanism for sharing with a wider audience typical emergency informa-tion (name, address, telephone number of emergency contact), and also information such as whether the student has any sensory issues; his or her favorite toys, subjects, or other topics the student enjoys; best approaches and deescalation techniques; and the most effective method of commu-nication (verbal, nonverbal, written, drawings, etc.). This information should also be provided to the local 9-1-1 Premise Alert system.

A training paradigm shift is slowly developing within the criminal justice and disability communities. The new paradigm shifts attention away from diagnostic labels, such as intellectual disability, autism, mental health, and others, to recognizing and understanding a person's func-tional ability. Law enforcement officers should not be expected to do an "on the street/on an incident" diagnosis with training. The specialized training should be skill-based, providing law enforcement officers with the tools to access, communicate in, and deescalate a confrontation with anyone, not just a person with ASD.

Parents, persons with ASD, educators, and criminal justice profes-sionals need to embrace a commitment to building strong public aware-ness and education campaigns to keep people with ASD safe at home, school, work, and in the community. We are not suggesting that people with ASD should not be held accountable for their actions. Rather, the criminal justice and disability systems should work together to develop specialized courts and diversion programs. An example might be a hybrid program that offers both appropriate punishment (criminal justice per-spective) and rehabilitation (disability system).

Although a number of studies have been conducted that examine autism and offending behaviors, with the exception of Woodbury-Smith and colleagues' (2006) community survey, the other studies drew their samples from forensic hospitals and other secure correctional facilities. Many of these studies suggest that people with ASD are overrepresented in the correctional facilities. However, these studies relied on small sample sizes and many individuals with comorbidity. Larger research studies are needed to investigate what is often referred to as the "swinging door" of the local criminal justice system; that is, county jails. County jails can process hundreds of inmates a day, and these inmates can be incarcerated for a day, a week, a month, a year, or more. How many inmates are persons with ASD, what were their charges, were they habitual offenders, at what age did they commit their first offense, and what were their dispositions are all questions that research needs to ask.

Collateral consequences, the penalties or disadvantages imposed on a person as a result of a criminal conviction, are another important area of study. Common collateral consequences may include denial of access to government benefits, voting rights, housing, and educational student loans, as well as a registration requirement for sex offenders. To our knowledge there have been no studies exploring the impact of collateral consequences on persons with ASD. Without larger and more in-depth research studies, it is difficult to rationalize the development of disability courts, diversion programs, and specialized training for criminal justice professionals.

REFERENCES

Allen, D., Evans, C., Hider, A., & Peckett, H. M. (2008). Offending behaviours in adults with Asperger syndrome. *Journal of Autism and Developmental Disorders, 38*(4), 748–758.

American Psychiatric Association. (2013). *Diagnostic and statistical manual of mental disorders* (5th ed.). Arlington, VA: Author.

Baron-Cohen, S. (1988). An assessment of violence in a young man with Asperger's syndrome. *Journal of Child Psychology and Psychiatry, 29*(3), 351–360.

Browning, A., & Caulfield, L. (2011, April). The prevalence and treatment of people with Asperger's syndrome in the criminal justice system. *Criminology and Criminal Justice, 11*(2), 165–180.

Ghaziuddin, M. (1991). Violence in Asperger syndrome: A critique. *Journal of Autism and Developmental Disorders, 21*(3), 349–354.

Haskin, B. G., & Silva, J. A. (2006). Asperger's disorder and criminal justice behavior: Forensic-psychiatric considerations. *Journal of the American Academy of Psychiatry and the Law, 34*, 374–384.

Howlin, P. (1997). *Autism: Preparing for adulthood.* London: Routledge.

Howlin, P. (2004). *Autism and Asperger syndrome: Preparing for adulthood.* London: Routledge.

Henault, I. (2006). *Asperger's syndrome and sexuality.* London: Jessica Kingsley.

Hippler, K., Viding, E., Klicpera, C., & Happé, F. (2010). Brief report: No increase in criminal convictions in Hans Asperger's original cohort. *Journal of Autism and Developmental Disorders, 40*(6), 774–780.

Kleinfield, N. R., Rivera, R., & Kovaleski, S. F. (2013, March 28). Newtown killer's obsessions, in chilling detail. *New York Times.*

Mrazek, P. B., & Haggerty, R. J. (1994). *Reducing risks for mental disorders: Frontiers for preventive intervention research.* Washington, DC: National Academy Press.

Murrie, D. C., Warren, J. I., Kristiansson, M., & Dietz, P. E. (2002). Asperger's syndrome in forenic settings. *International Journal of Forensic Mental Health, 1*(1), 59–70.

Palermo, M. T. (2004). Pervasive developmental disorders, psychiatric comorbidities, and the law. *International Journal of Offender Therapy and Comparative Criminology, 48*(1), 40–48.

Plimley, L., & Bowen, M. (207). *Social skills and autism spectrum disorders.* London: Chapman.

Scragg, P., & Shah, A. (1994). Prevalence of Asperger's syndrome in a secure hospital. *British Journal of Psychiatry, 165*(5), 679–682.

Shader, M. (2003). *Risk factors for delinquency: An overview.* Washington, DC: U.S. Department of Justice Office of Juvenile Justice and Delinquency Prevention. Retrieved from *www.ncjrs.gov/html/ojjdp/jjjournal_2003_2.*

Weiss, K. J. (2011). Autism spectrum disorder and criminal justice: Sqare peg in a round hole? *American Journal of Forensic Psychiatry, 32*(3), 3–19.

Wing, L. (1981). Asperger's syndrome: A clinical account. *Psychological Medicine, 11*(1), 115–129.

Woodbury-Smith, M., Clare, I., Holland, A., & Kearns, A. (2006). High-functioning autistic apectrum disorders, offending and other law-breaking: Findings from a community sample. *Journal of Forensic Psychiatry and Psychology, 17*(1), 108–120.

Index

Page numbers in *italic* indicate a figure or a table